THE HEART

STRUCTURE IN HEALTH AND DISEASE

Robert H Anderson BSc, MD, FRCPath

Joseph Levy Professor of Paediatric Cardiac Morphology

National Heart and Lung Institute

Royal Brompton National Heart and Lung Hospital

London, UK

Anton E Becker MD

Professor of Pathology

Head, Department of Cardiovascular Pathology

Academic Medical Centre

University of Amsterdam

The Netherlands

Gower Medical Publishing · London · New York

Distributed in the USA and Canada by:
Raven Press Ltd
1185 Avenue of the Americas
New York
New York 10036
USA

Distributed in the rest of the world by:
Gower Medical Publishing
Middlesex House
34–42 Cleveland Street
London W1P 5FB
UK

Project Editor:	Claire Burdett
	Zak Knowles
Design:	Balvir Koura
Illustration:	Lynda Payne
	Sue Tyler
	Lee Smith
Layout:	Tim Friers
	Mark Willey
Paste-up:	Olgun Hassan
	Ruth Miles
Index:	Ann McCarthy
Production:	Susan Bishop
Publisher:	Fiona Foley

British Library Cataloguing in Publication Data:
Anderson, R.H.
 The heart: structure in health and disease.
 — New ed.
 I. Title   II. Becker, A.E.
 616.1

Library of Congress Cataloging-in-Publication Data:
Available upon request.

ISBN 0-397-44719-1

Originated by Mandarin Offset (HK) Ltd, Hong Kong
Produced by Imago Productions, Singapore
Printed and bound in Singapore
Typesetting by M to N Typesetters, London
Text set in Baskerville and Gill.

A Slide Atlas of Cardiac Structure in Health and Disease, based on the contents of this book, is available. In the slide atlas format, the material is split into volumes, each of which is presented in a binder together with numbered 35mm slides of each illustration. Further information can be obtained from:

Gower Medical Publishing	Gower Medical Publishing
101 Fifth Avenue	Middlesex House
New York	34–42 Cleveland Street
NY 10003	London W1P 5FB
USA	UK

Preface

The Heart – Structure in Health and Disease is a consolidation and expansion of our two previous enterprises with Gower Medical Publishing, namely *Cardiac Anatomy* and *Cardiac Pathology*. These earlier volumes succeeded beyond our wildest dreams in presenting the somewhat dry aspects of morbid material in vivid fashion, and bought, as judged from reviews and personal contacts, the crucial morphological details of the normal and diseased heart to the fingertips of clinicians in many and varied disciplines. But even morphology is not a purely static subject. Our perceptions of the structure and interpretation of the normal and abnormal hearts have undergone marked evolution since we wrote these earlier volumes, and saw them published in 1980 and 1983, respectively. You now hold in your hands the product of an additional decade of experience of the authors in research, diagnosis and teaching. The format of the new book is unchanged, since the Text and Colour Atlases as pioneered by Gower Medical have shown their worth in many fields subsequent to the appearance of *Cardiac Anatomy*. In *The Heart – Structure in Health and Disease*, we have tried to take the best of our previous volumes and combine them in to a single book that will satisfy the morphological needs of the clinician into the twenty-first century.

Much of the material from our first attempts have been retained, particularly in the sections concerned with acquired diseases of the heart. The sections concerned with congenital diseases of the heart have been somewhat curtailed, but have been supplemented by many new illustrations and by a total revision of the text, this representing the major improvements in understanding which have occurred over the past decade, improvements of a magnitude sufficient to relegate arguments concerning nomenclature to a minor role. The wealth of material concerning normal anatomy has also been greatly curtailed to produce a single section, yet not, we believe, to the detriment of the topic itself. Finally, recognizing the importance of strides taken in transplantation, a section has been devoted to the pathological aspects of this important new therapy.

As always, the book could not have been completed without the untiring help of our many colleagues. It is often invidious to single out some at the expense of others, and we apologize in advance to any who think they should have been mentioned by name, but the contributions of a few do stand out. First in this group must be Dr. Jessica Mann, Lecturer in Pathology at St. George's Hospital, who completed the chapter concerned with transplantation in double-quick time. Then there are our many colleagues who helped in the acquisition of photographs and material, notably Dr. James R. Zuberbuhler, University of Pittsburgh; Dr. Benson R. Wilcox, University of North Carolina; and Dr. Siew Yen Ho, Royal Brompton National Heart and Lung Institute. The excellent photographs of the hearts exhibiting acquired pathology were largely produced by Wilfred Means, and to him we offer special thanks. The book could also not have been completed without the secretarial assistance of Marsha Schenker and Christine Anderson. The team from Gower Medical Publishing, led by Zak Knowles and ably guided, as always, by Fiona Foley, ensured the production of a splendid book. As with the previous editions, if not more so, the finished product is as much a work of art as an account of cardiac morphology.

RHA, AEB
London & Amsterdam
November 1991

Contents

14   PERICARDIAL HEART DISEASE

15   THE AGEING HEART

16   TUMOURS OF THE HEART AND PERICARDIUM

17   TRANSPLANTATION

INDEX

Anatomy

ANATOMY OF THE HEART

1

▌ CARDIAC ANATOMY

RELATIONSHIPS OF THE HEART

The heart lies in the mediastinum with its long axis orientated from the hypogastrium towards the right shoulder (Fig. 1.1). Apart from a small bare area, its anterior surface is covered by the overlapping lungs contained in their pleural sacs (Fig. 1.2), the whole being contained within the thoracic cavity. Although the heart is usually described in terms of a triangle, considered in this way to have a base and an apex, in reality its silhouette is trapezoidal. The so-called base, formed by the junction of the atriums, ventricles, and great arteries, is the diagonal of this trapezoid, whilst the apex extends out towards the left hypogastrium (Fig. 1.3). The overall mass of the heart is tethered to adjacent structures by the arteries and veins which leave and enter its chambers. It is tightly enclosed in a fibrous bag, the pericardium, which is itself firmly attached to the diaphragm, providing still further anchorage. When considered in cross-section the ventricular mass is pyramidal in shape. Its surfaces are the anterior sternocostal surface, the inferior diaphragmatic surface, and the more rounded superior surface which abuts against the lingula of the left lung. The edge between sterno-costal and diaphragmatic surfaces is sharp and is termed the acute margin, whilst the edge between sternocostal and pulmonary surfaces is much more rounded, and is known as the obtuse margin (Fig. 1.4).

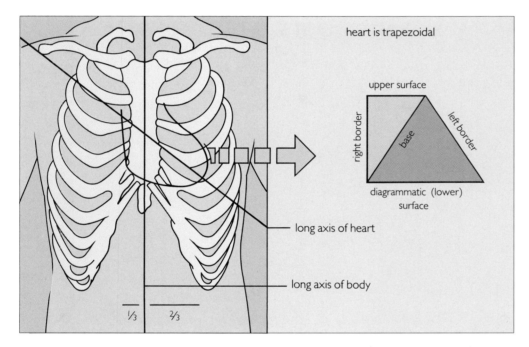

Fig. 1.1 This diagram illustrates the basic arrangement of the heart within the chest.

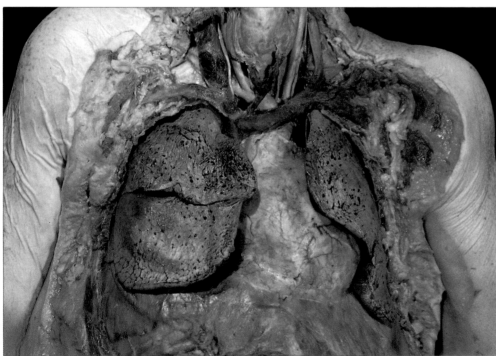

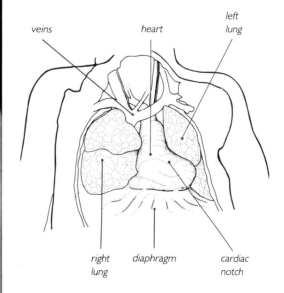

Fig. 1.2 This dissection shows the position of the heart relative to the other organs of the thorax. The anterior wall has been removed.

Two great veins descend and ascend anteriorly, joining the right atrium to form the right border of the cardiac silhouette. The intrathoracic segment of the inferior caval vein is a short channel, ascending from the substance of the liver to pierce the diaphragm and enter the floor of the right atrium. The superior caval vein is much longer, being formed by the union of right and left brachiocephalic veins before descending, receiving the azygos vein *en route*, to reach the upper margin of the right atrium (Fig. 1.5).

The great arteries leave the left side of the cardiac base, the pulmonary trunk running anterior and to the left of the aorta (Fig. 1.5). Having emerged from the ventricular mass, the trunk passes posteriorly, dividing into right and left pulmonary arteries which pass into the hilums of the lungs. The aorta swings up from the midportion of the cardiac base and, as it ascends, it curves first to the right, then upwards, leftwards and backwards to cross over the right side of the pulmonary bifurcation and descend to the left of the vertebral column, finally passing down

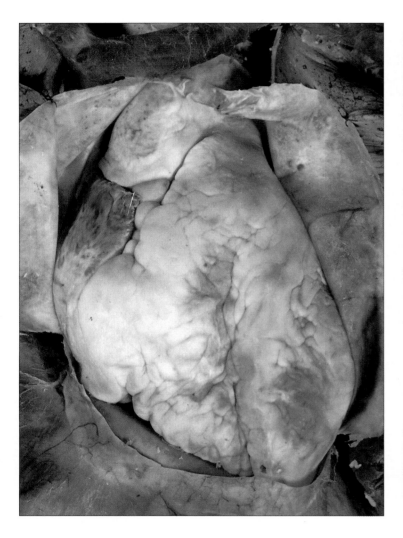

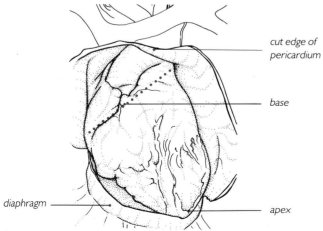

Fig. 1.3 A further step of the dissection of the heart shown in Fig. 1.2. The pericardium has been incised.

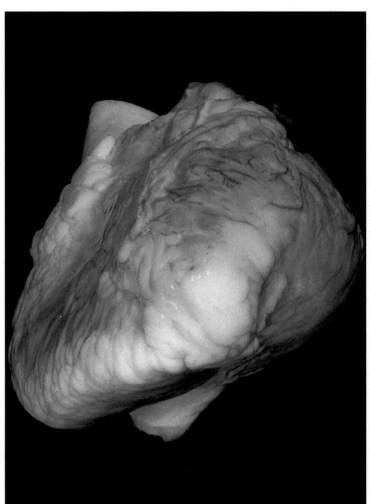

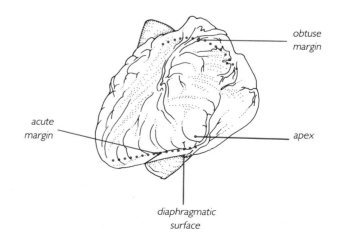

Fig. 1.4 This isolated heart is viewed from the apex of the ventricular mass, showing its surfaces.

to exit through the diaphragm. As the arch of the aorta swings backwards, it gives off the arterial branches to the head and arms, namely the brachiocephalic trunk (which soon divides into right subclavian and common carotid arteries), the left common carotid, and the left subclavian arteries.

Extending down into the thorax behind these arteries is the trachea, which bifurcates into the right and left bronchi at the level of the aortic arch. These then run on towards the hila of the lungs, curling beneath the branches of the pulmonary trunk as they do so. There is an important difference in the branching pattern of right and left pulmonary arteries (Fig. 1.6). The right

main bronchus gives off its first branch before it is crossed by the right pulmonary artery, and this then runs on towards the upper lobe, therefore arising above and posterior to the pulmonary artery. It is termed an eparterial (above the artery) bronchus. In contrast, the left pulmonary artery crosses over the left main bronchus before the latter divides into branches supplying the upper and lower lobes. The bronchus therefore said to be hyparterial (below the artery). This asymmetric pattern of branching means that the morphologically left bronchus is approximately twice the length of the morphologically right bronchus.

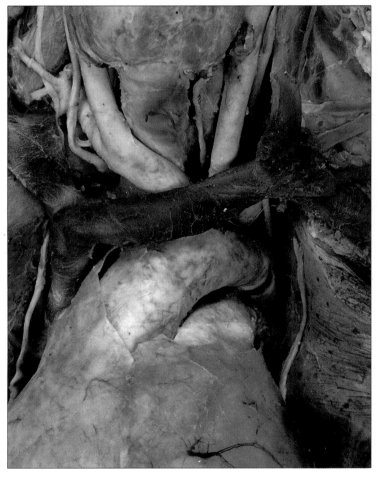

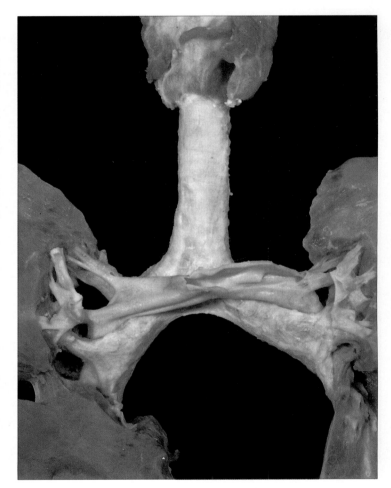

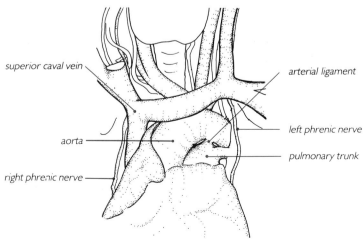

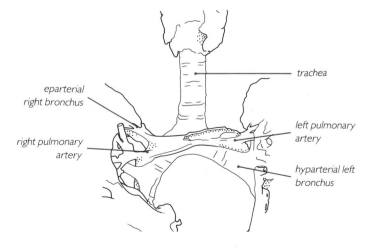

Fig. 1.5 This dissection shows the relationships of the vagus and phrenic nerves at the thoracic inlets.

Fig. 1.6 The bronchial tree has been isolated and is viewed from the front.

The pulmonary veins run inward from the hila of the lungs to enter the posterior aspect of the cardiac base. Branches from the upper and lower lobes of both lungs pass centripetally to enter the four corners of the posterior aspect of the left atrium. Also running through the thorax, posterior to the trachea and to the right of the aortic arch and descending aorta, is the oesphagus. Immediately below the tracheal bifurcation, the oesophagus is related to the posterior wall of the left atrium, running behind this chamber to enter the abdomen through the right crus of the diaphragm (Fig. 1.7).

Two pairs of important nerves, the phrenic and vagus nerves, extend throughout the mediastinum. The phrenic nerves, branches of the cervical plexus, originate in the neck and enter the thoracic inlet on the surface of the anterior scalene muscle (Figs 1.8 & 1.9). The right phrenic nerve then runs along the right brachiocephalic and the superior caval veins, and extends across the right margin of the pericardium to the diaphragm (Fig. 1.5). The left phrenic nerve passes behind the left sub-clavian vein as it enters the thorax, crossing behind the internal mammary artery to run over the aortic arch and left pulmonary

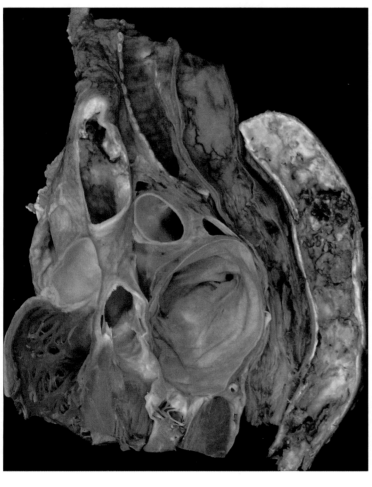

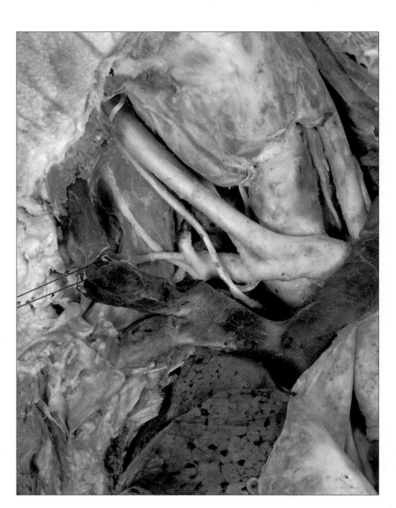

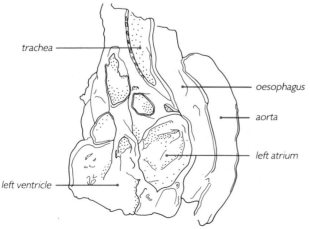

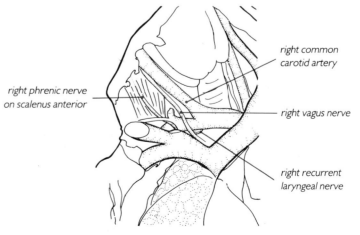

Fig. 1.7 This long axis section shows the relationship of the oesophagus to the left atrium.

Fig. 1.8 This dissection shows the origin of the right recurrent laryngeal nerve from the vagus nerve.

artery, before passing over the left margin of the pericardial bag to reach the left dome of the diaphragm (Fig. 1.5). The vagus nerves, the tenth cranial nerves, are more intimately related to the arteries of the head and neck. The right vagus nerve enters the thoracic cavity on the anterior surface of the right common carotid artery, immediately giving off the right recurrent laryngeal nerve, which passes beneath the right subclavian artery and

ascends into the neck (Fig. 1.8). Also recurring around the right subclavian artery is the subclavian loop (ansa subclavia), an important branch from the stellate ganglion which conveys sympathetic fibres to the head, particularly the iris. The right vagus nerve, having given off the recurrent laryngeal nerve, passes along the brachiocephalic trunk and behind the union of the right and left brachiocephalic veins (Fig. 1.10). It then angles

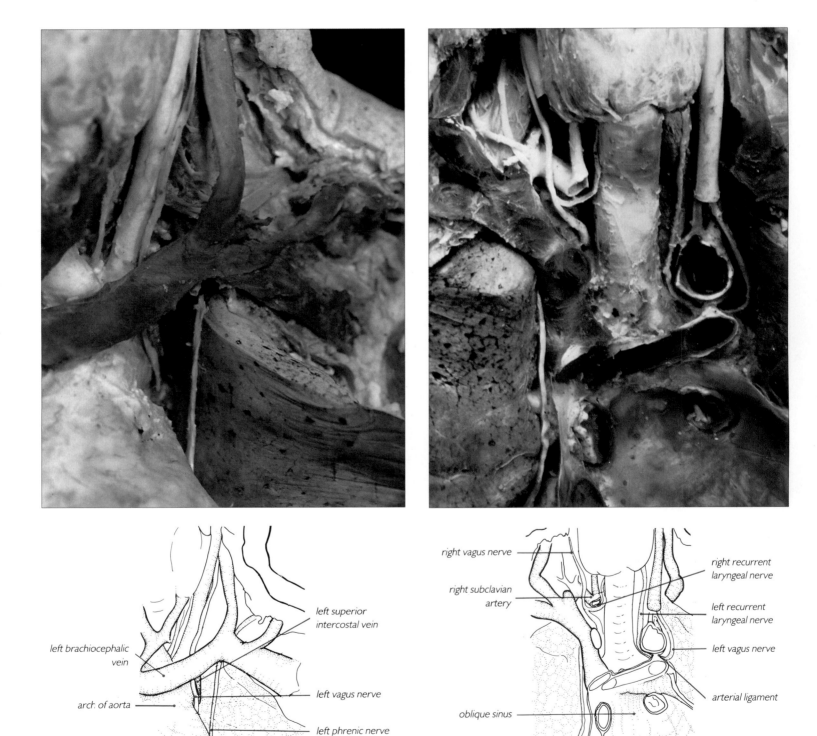

Fig. 1.9   This dissection shows the relationship of the left vagus and phrenic nerves at the thoracic inlet.

Fig. 1.10   The heart has been removed from its pericardial cradle, showing the site of the oblique sinus.

backwards across the trachea and runs onto the oesphagus behind the pulmonary hilum, intermingling with the left vagus to form the pulmonary plexus. From there it extends backwards over the hilum, running along the pericardium and continuing down to pass through the diaphragm with the oesphagus. The left vagus nerve enters the thoracic cavity between the left common carotid and subclavian arteries, close to the phrenic nerve (Fig. 1.9). As the phrenic nerve runs down towards the pulmonary trunk, the left vagus angles back towards the pulmonary hilum, the left superior intercostal vein passing between the nerves as the vein crosses the aortic arch. The vagus then continues backwards to pass behind the pulmonary hilum and joins the oesophagus. As it passes the lower edge of the aortic arch, it gives off the left recurrent laryngeal nerve, which recurs round the arterial ligament and the aorta before ascending towards the thoracic inlet (Fig. 1.10).

The heart itself is enclosed in a firm fibrous sack, the pericardium, which covers the apex of the heart like a bag and encloses it up to the base, where it clothes the arterial vessels entering and leaving the heart for about 1–2cm before merging with their walls. The layer which clothes the diaphragmatic surface of the heart is firmly attached to the diaphragm in the area of the central tendon. Loose fibroareolar tissue is the only other connection between diaphragm and pericardium. The bag is also attached to the posterior surface of the sternum by superior and inferior sternopericardial ligaments. Elsewhere, the pericardium is covered by the pleural cavities, apart from the bare area where it abuts directly against the anterior chest wall (Fig. 1.2). The pericardium is lined by a much thinner serous envelope which lines the surfaces of both fibrous pericardium and the heart, the pericardial fluid being present between the two serous surfaces. The layer covering the surface of the cardiac chambers is the epicardium. The outer, parietal layer is an integral part of the fibrous pericardium (Fig. 1.11). The layers of serous pericardium are continuous with each other at the entrances and exits of the vessels but, because of the arrangement of the vessels, two recesses (or sinuses) are present within the cavity. One, the transverse sinus, lines the inner curvature of

the heart, being positioned between the anterior surface of the atriums and the posterior surface of the great arteries. The other recess, the oblique sinus, is behind the left atrium, and is limited by the reflection of the four pulmonary veins and the inferior caval vein (Fig. 1.10).

Position of the heart within the thorax

One of the major impediments in relating cardiac anatomy to clinical settings has been the penchant of morphologists to illustrate and describe the heart as though it sits upright on its apex. If descriptions are to be of value to the clinician, they must account for the heart as it lies in the body. It is important, therefore, to emphasize the position of the heart relative to the surface markings of the thorax, and then to describe the relationships of the cardiac chambers within the cardiac silhouette.

In its normal position, the heart occupies the inferior part of the mediastinum with two-thirds of its bulk to the left of the midline (Fig. 1.1) and, as discussed, the cardiac silhouette is trapezoidal in shape. Its lower border lies on the diaphragm while its upper border lies behind the sternum. Its right margin is more or less vertical but its left margin angles out to the apex. The ribs provide good markers for charting the silhouette, and give some guide as to whether or not cardiac position is normal (Fig. 1.12). The base of the heart is at the level of the second and third costal cartilages, hidden behind the sternum. The second cartilage is easily identified, since it articulates at the angle of the sternum. The body of the heart extending to the apex is behind the fourth and fifth interspaces, the position of the apex usually being taken to be the fifth intercostal space in the midclavicular line. The lower border of the silhouette is directly on the dia-

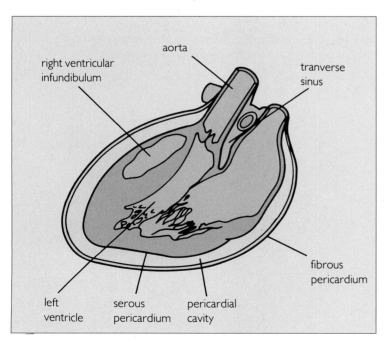

Fig. 1.11 This diagram illustrates the components of the pericardium and their relationship to the heart.

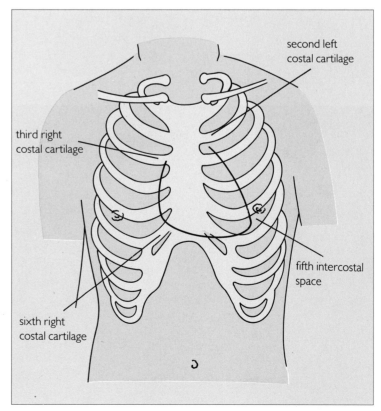

Fig. 1.12 This drawing marks the relationships between the rib cage and the cardiac silhouette.

phragm and is seen as a horizontal line at the level of the sixth rib, extending across to the sixth costal cartilage at the right border of the sternum. The right border of the heart is then a slightly curved line between the sixth and third right cartilages, and can just be seen behind the right border of the sternum.

Cardiac chambers relative to the silhouette

The position of the chambers within the silhouette can be located once the normal position of the heart relative to the frontal view of the chest has been established. As already discussed, the superior caval vein enters the upper border of the right margin of the base while the pulmonary trunk exits from the left upper border (Fig. 1.13). The anterior interventricular groove, marked by the interventricular branch of the left coronary artery, descends to the apex almost parallel to and close to the left

cardiac margin (Fig. 1.14). As the heart lies in the chest, therefore, the so-called right-sided chambers are anterior to their left-sided counterparts, and the anterior projection of the cardiac silhouette is made up, for the most part, by the right atrium and the right ventricle. The right atrium forms the entire right border of the silhouette, with the superior caval vein forming its top and the entrance of the inferior caval vein its bottom. The right lower border of the silhouette marks the inferior point of the atrioventricular junction, where the right atrium joins the right ventricle. The right ventricle forms the horizontal inferior border of the silhouette to the apex, beyond which the left ventricular apex protrudes (Fig. 1.14). The pulmonary trunk helps form the left border, the rest being made up from the only left-sided structures to contribute, namely, the left margin of the left ventricle and the left atrial appendage. Consequently, although the aorta arises from the left ventricle, it is to the right

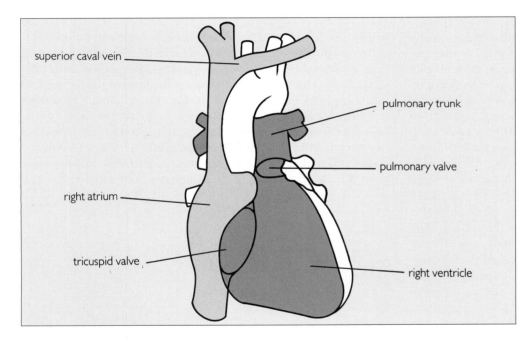

Fig. 1.13 This diagram shows how the structures of the right heart occupy most of the frontal aspect of the cardiac silhouette.

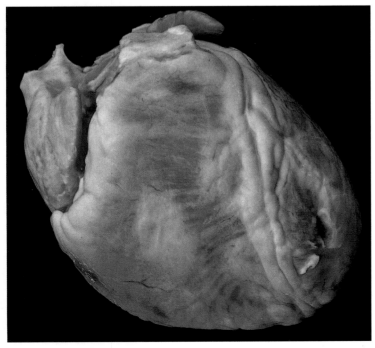

Fig. 1.14 This isolated heart is shown in its anatomic orientation. Most of the frontal surface is occupied by the right atrium and ventricle.

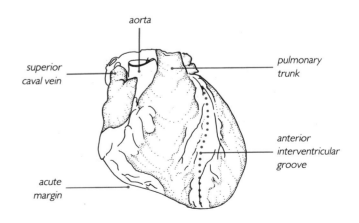

of the pulmonary trunk at their ventricular origins. The left atrium is the most posterior structure of the heart, lying directly adjacent to the oesophagus in the bifurcation of the trachea. It is overlaid anteriorly by part of the right atrium, the ascending aorta and the pulmonary trunk (Fig. 1.7). Only its appendage pokes round the pulmonary trunk to form part of the cardiac silhouette (Fig. 1.13). The left ventricle is behind the outflow tract of the right ventricle but does not reach the left edge of the cardiac silhouette. The aorta is a deep structure, springing from between the right atrium and the pulmonary trunk and only becoming part of the silhouette as its arch extends upwards and backwards.

A further important consideration in clarifying cardiac anatomy is the location of the four cardiac valves within the cardiac silhouette. Since the plane of the atrioventricular and ventriculo–arterial junctions is oblique, with its axis veering towards the vertical, the valves will occupy a similar orientation. The most superior valve is the pulmonary valve, which is a horizontal structure lying behind the third costal cartilage (Fig. 1.15). The aortic valve lies behind and below the pulmonary valve and above the tricuspid valve. This last continues the downward arc from the obtuse to the acute margins of the silhouette. The mitral valve is more posterior and lies behind the aortic valve, overlapping the tricuspid valve.

It is particularly important to understand the precise position of the aortic valve, which lies posterior to the right ventricle, occupying a position more or less in the middle of the heart. This is best appreciated by viewing a section of the base of the heart from the right shoulder (Fig. 1.16). This shows the central position of the aorta, which is the key to full understanding of cardiac anatomy.

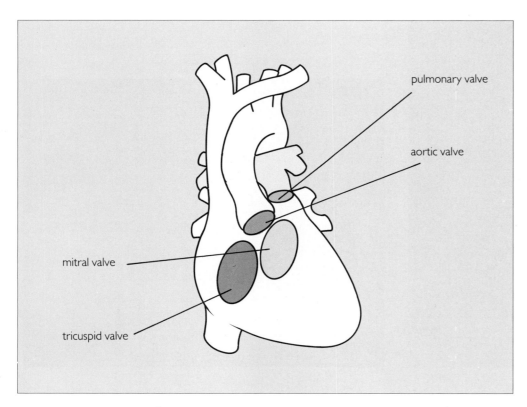

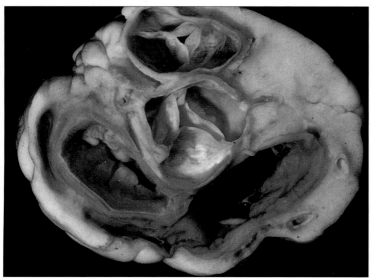

Fig. 1.15 This drawing shows the relationships of the cardiac valves within the cardiac silhouette.

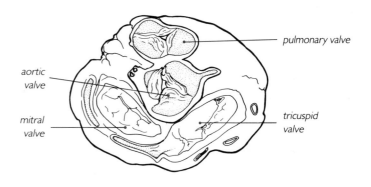

Fig. 1.16 This short axis section through the atrioventricular junction is viewed from above having removed the musculature of the atrial chambers together with the arterial trunks.

Anatomy of individual chambers

Having established the relations of the heart and the locations of its chambers, we are now in a position to discuss the morphology of the individual chambers. This is important because, in some congenitally malformed hearts, these chambers may not occupy their anticipated positions. It is essential, therefore, to emphasize those features which give the atriums and ventricles their morphologically rightness or leftness.

The morphologically right atrium

In the normal heart, the right atrium forms the rightward and anterior part of the cardiac mass. This overlaps the right hand margin of the left atrium and joins the right side of the right ventricle. Externally, the chamber consists of a venous sinus (sinus venarum), which receives the superior and inferior caval veins, and an anterior part, the appendage, which extends forwards to encircle the right border of the aorta (Fig. 1.17). The border between the two is marked by the terminal groove (sulcus terminalis). This varies in development and may be inconspicuous in some hearts. The leftward margin of the right atrium is marked posteriorly by the groove, named for either Waterston or Sondergaard, which lies between the superior caval vein and the right pulmonary veins. The groove is infolded to form the upper rim of the oval fossa (Fig. 1.18).

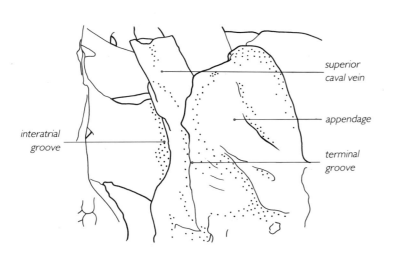

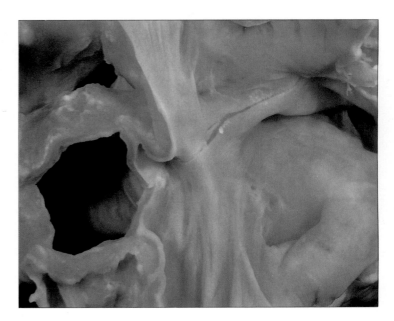

Fig. 1.17 This figure shows the external appearances of the morphologically right atrium.

Fig. 1.18 This heart has been dissected to show the site of the interatrial groove (Waterston's groove).

When the atrium is opened, the distinction between the posterior smooth-walled venous sinus and the anterior appendage lined with its pectinate muscles is much more apparent (Fig. 1.19), with the junction between the two marked by the well-formed terminal crest (crista terminalis). The vestibule of the tricuspid valve orientates obliquely to the right (Fig. 1.19), and forms the third component of the right atrium. The orifice of the superior caval vein is in the roof of the chamber with the septal surface running from a right posterior to left anterior

position. The terminal crest runs from the anterior part of the septal surface and swings in front of the orifice of the superior caval vein, the vein entering the right atrium between the crest and the superior rim of the oval fossa. In fetal life, the margin of the crest is reinforced by sheet-like structures which separate the orifices of the inferior caval vein and coronary sinus from the atrial appendage, directing the richly oxygenated blood coming from the placenta towards the oval fossa. These structures become the valves of the inferior caval vein (Eustachian valve) and coronary sinus (Thebesian valve), and remain visible to some extent even in adult hearts (Fig. 1.20). Remnants of the extensive valves found during fetal life may persist to form so-called Chiari networks, and similar remnants may be seen across the oval fossa.

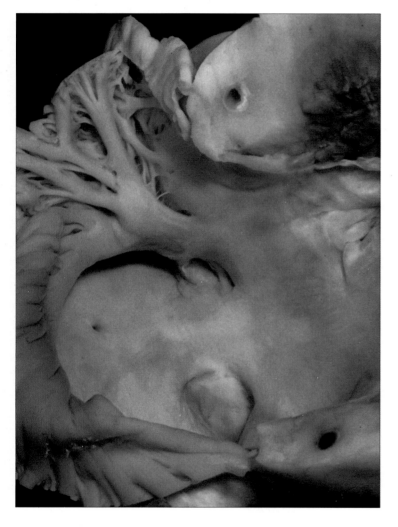

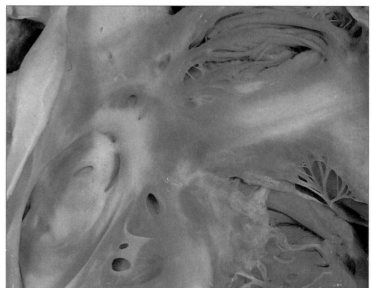

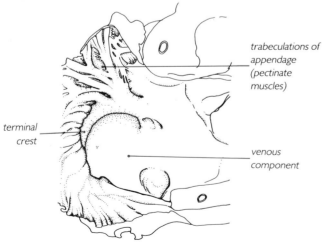

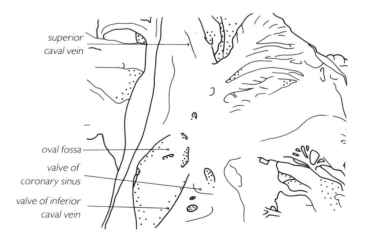

Fig. 1.19 This view of the internal aspect of the right atrium contrasts the arrangement of the pectinate muscles within the appendages with the smooth-walled venous component.

Fig. 1.20 This internal view of the right atrium shows a typical arrangement of the valves guarding the orifices of the inferior caval vein and the coronary sinus (Eustachian and Thebesian valves).

The posteroseptal surface of the chamber is, at first sight, extensive. It is characterized by the oval fossa, and the orifice of the coronary sinus which is the third of the systemic venous channels which drain to the right atrium (Fig. 1.21). The fossa is the depression marking the site of the fetal interatrial communication, the hole which permits the richly oxygenated blood coming from the placenta through the inferior caval vein to reach the left atrium. It has a well-marked rim which, superiorly, is often described as the "septum secundum", although this is no more than infolded atrial walls between the superior caval and the

pulmonary veins (Fig. 1.18). Anteriorly, the rim is the interatrial groove whilst, inferiorly, it overlies the central fibrous body and continues backwards as the structure separating the orifice of the coronary sinus from that of the inferior caval vein. This structure is termed the sinus septum and through it extends a tendinous structure which, in most hearts, is the continuation of the commissure between Eustachian and Thebesian valves. Termed the tendon of Todaro, it runs intramyocardially to insert into the central fibrous body. It is a vital structure in demarcating the position of the atrial component of the axis of atrioventricular conduction tissue (see below) and is easily demonstrated by superficial dissection (Fig. 1.22). The posterior rim of the oval fossa is very variable in its formation – in some hearts, a well-formed posterior lip is seen (Fig. 1.21), whilst in others the posterior wall of the fossa is directly continuous with

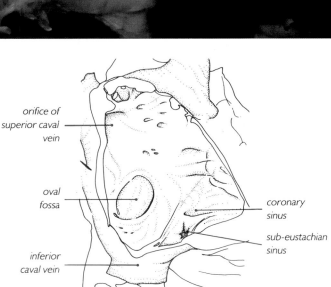

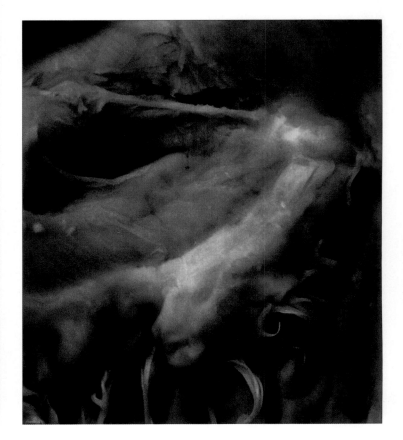

Fig. 1.21   This view of the internal aspect of the right atrium shows the typical arrangement of the oval fossa.

Fig. 1.22   This dissection shows how the commissure of the Eustachian and Thebesian valves (the tendon of Todaro) forms one boundary of the triangle of Koch. The location of the membranous septum is shown by transillumination.

the left wall of the inferior caval vein. The floor of the oval fossa is a thin fibromuscular partition known as the flap valve (Fig. 1.23). In normal hearts this is of sufficiently large size to close the fossa completely, although it is not always adherent at its superior margin. In approximately 30% of normal hearts, a probe can be passed through it from the right to the left atrium, producing a so-called probe-patent oval foramen. Because of the valve-like architecture, such a probe-patent foramen does not permit an interatrial shunt as long as the left atrial pressure is higher than that of the right atrium.

An extensive band of atrial muscle is present inferior to the orifice of the coronary sinus which extends into the leaflets of the tricuspid valve. Although this is the wall of the right atrium, it also overlies the ventricular musculature, since the leaflet of the tricuspid valve is attached more towards the ventricular apex than is that of the mitral valve. The area between these two attachments is the muscular component of the atrioventricular septum (Fig. 1.24). A prominent depression, the sub-Eustachian sinus (Fig. 1.21), is often seen inferior and posterior to the orifice of the coronary sinus.

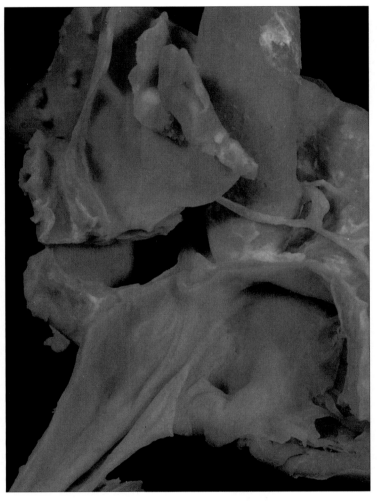

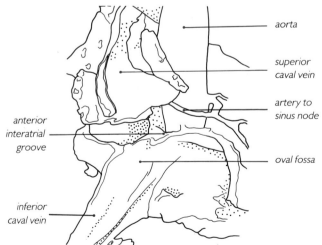

Fig. 1.23 This dissection, viewed from behind, shows the arrangement of the oval fossa and its boundaries.

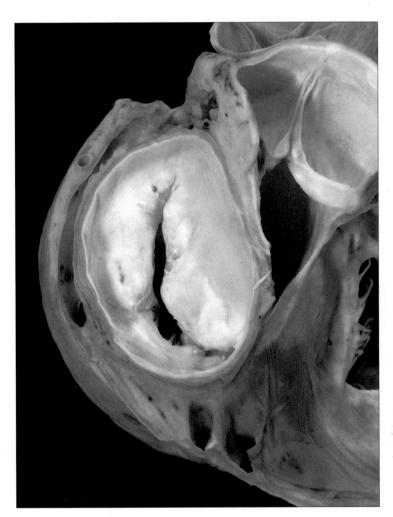

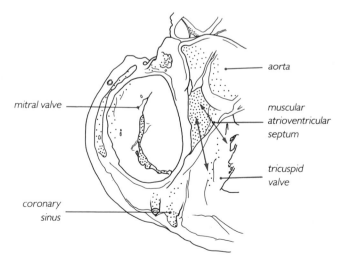

Fig. 1.24 This dissection, made by removing the non-facing sinus of the aortic valve along with its leaflet, shows the location of the muscular component of the atrioventricular septum.

The anterior wall of the right atrium is the appendage which, seen externally, has a characteristically blunt triangular shape (Fig. 1.25). Internally, the appendage is lined by the pectinate muscles which extend at right angles to the terminal crest all along its length, continuing inferiorly into the sub-Eustachian sinus. In the roof of the atrium one of the muscles is frequently prominent and is sometimes called the septum spurium.

The morphologically left atrium

This is the most posterior chamber in the heart (Fig. 1.7) and, like the right atrium, has a smooth-walled venous component, an appendage, and a vestibule surrounding the orifice of the mitral valve (Fig. 1.26). The appendage, which is tubular and hooked, is the only part of the left atrium to project directly on the cardiac silhouette (Fig. 1.27). The junction between the venous component of the atrium and the appendage is much smaller than that of the right atrium and is not marked by any specific crest or groove. The venous component of the atrium receives the four pulmonary veins at its corners (Fig. 1.26) and is considerably larger than the appendage.

Inferiorly, the coronary sinus is found along the posterior wall of the left atrium within the left atrioventricular groove (Fig. 1.24). Sometimes a persistent left superior caval vein drains to the coronary sinus as an extensive channel between the left atrial appendage and the left pulmonary veins, although usually

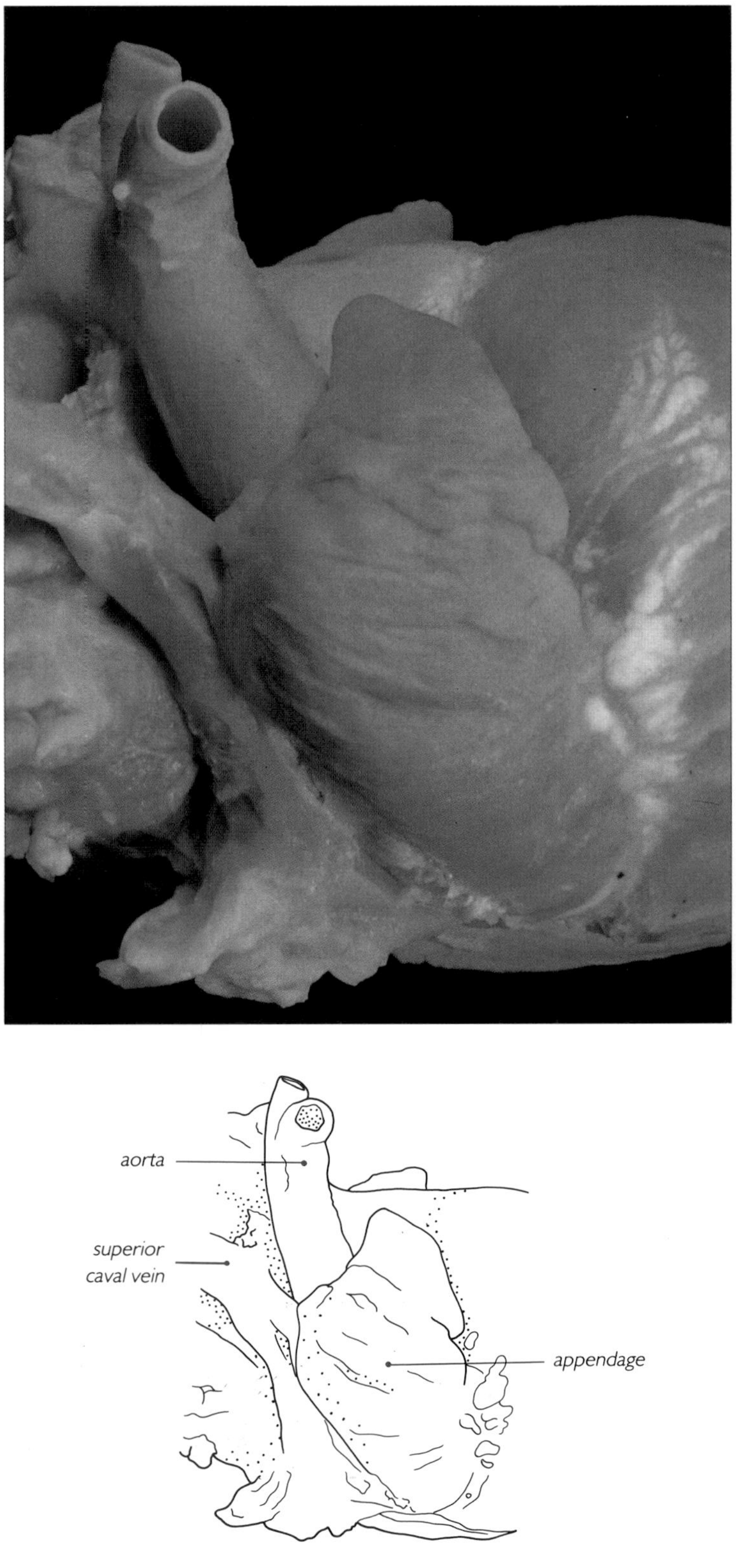

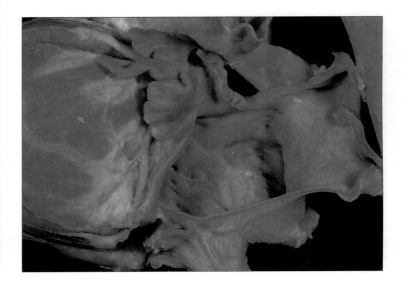

Fig. 1.25 This view of the external aspect shows the typical arrangement of the morphologically right atrial appendage.

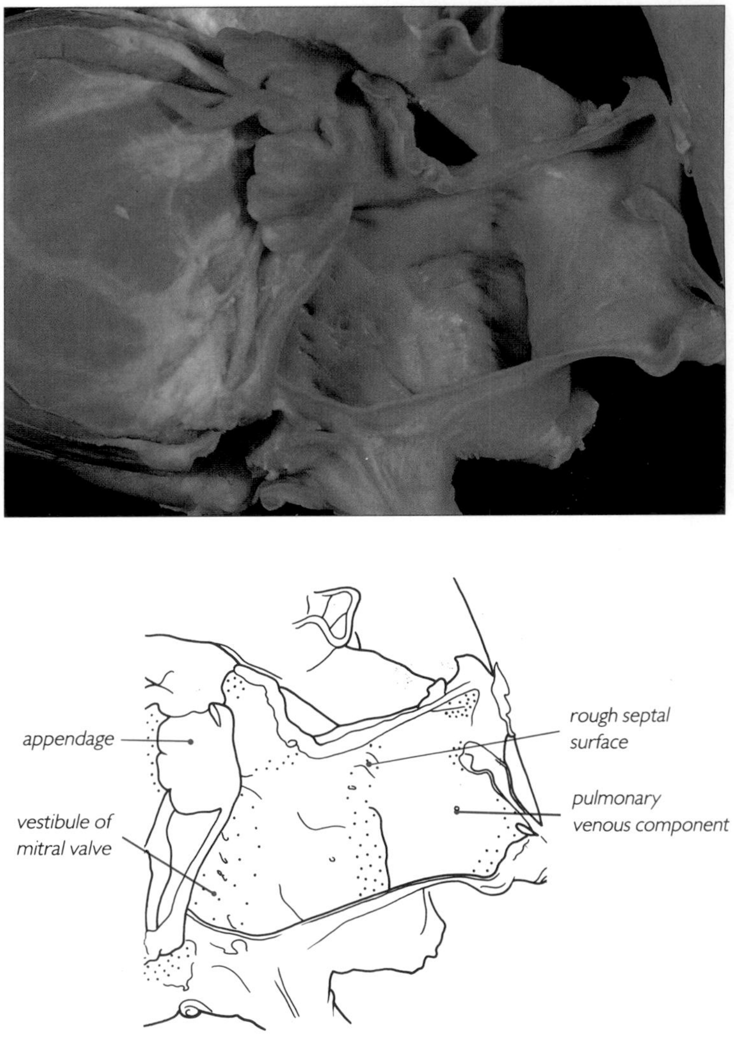

Fig. 1.26 This dissection shows the characteristic features of the morphologically left atrium.

the vein regresses, only persisting as the oblique vein of the left atrium. To the right, the right pulmonary veins are separated from the right atrium by the deep groove (Waterston's groove) which marks the site of the superior rim of the oval fossa. Internally, the appendage of the left atrium is trabeculated, as is the right appendage, although the junction of pectinate muscles and venous atrium on the left is not marked by the presence of any structure comparable to the terminal crest, and the pectinate muscles themselves are less pronounced. The septal surface of the left atrium consists of the flap valve of the oval fossa which is usually plastered down onto the anterior wall, whilst the roof above the septum has a characteristic rough appearance. Transillumination shows that the floor of the oval fossa is posterior to the rugose area of the left atrial wall (Fig. 1.28).

The interatrial septum

The true interatrial septum occupies only a small part of the atrial walls that are often held to represent the "septal surface".

Much of the superior rim is simply the infolded groove between superior caval and the right pulmonary veins (Fig. 1.23). The anterior rim is mostly the anterior atrial wall and, in this position, is in direct relation to the root of the aorta. The inferior rim is, in part, true atrial septum, but, owing to the more distal attachment of the leaflets of the tricuspid valve relative to that of the mitral valve, much of the inferior rim is positioned between the right atrium and the inlet portion of the left ventricle (Fig. 1.24). Similarly, the anterior part of the rim overlying the central fibrous body is continuous with the atrioventricular component of the membranous septum, the latter structure being located between the right atrium and the subaortic outflow tract. The area around the coronary sinus is related directly to the atrioventricular groove and consequently is not strictly part of the septum. The area of the posterior rim is directly continuous with the wall of the inferior caval vein, and only a small part is true atrial septum. This fact will be of major importance when we come to discuss the morphology of interatrial communications (see Chapter 6).

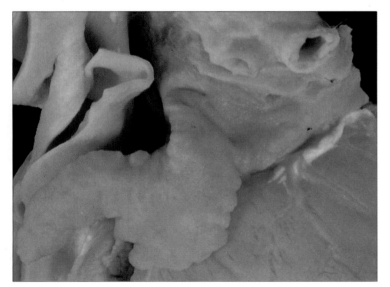

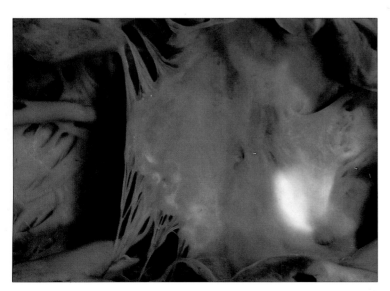

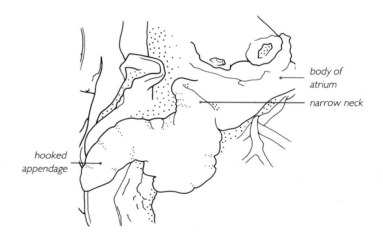

Fig. 1.27 This view of the external aspect shows the typical features of the morphologically left atrial appendage.

Fig. 1.28 This view of the internal aspect of the left atrium with transillumination shows the position of the floor of the oval fossa.

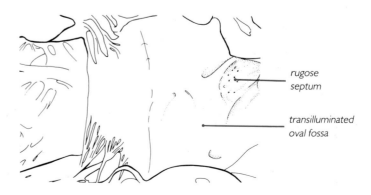

The morphologically right ventricle

The morphologically right ventricle occupies most of the anterior part of the frontal projection of the cardiac silhouette, swinging up from the inferiorly positioned tricuspid valve to the antero-superior pulmonary valve (Fig. 1.29). It passes from beneath to above the left ventricle when seen in lateral projection (Fig. 1.30). In shape, it is like an additional slice of tissue wrapped around the circular left ventricle, particularly when viewed in a section across the short axis of the ventricular mass. Its right-sided inlet component contains the tricuspid valve. The limit of the inlet zone is the attachment of the papillary muscles, although there is no distinct line between inlet and trabecular portions (Fig. 1.31). The apical trabecular zone extends inferiorly and more horizontally beyond the attachments of the papillary muscle towards the ventricular apex, the wall of which is thinner than the remainder of the wall. The trabecular zone extends out from the mainstream of inlet and outlet portions (Fig. 1.32).

The outlet portion of the right ventricle, or the infundibulum, is a free-standing muscular tube which supports the pulmonary valve (Fig. 1.33), the larger part of which can be removed completely from the heart without entering the left ventricle (Fig. 1.34). The postero-inferior component of the tube separates the

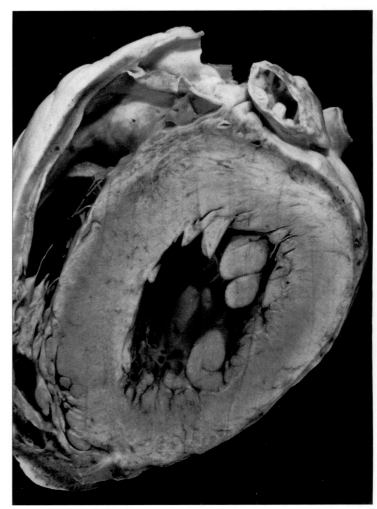

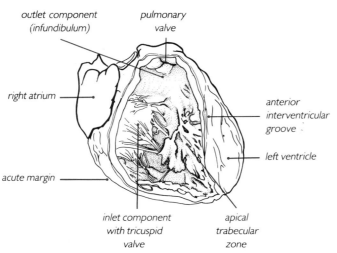

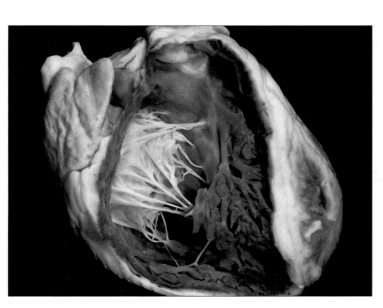

outlet component (infundibulum)   pulmonary valve

right atrium

acute margin

inlet component with tricuspid valve   apical trabecular zone

anterior interventricular groove

left ventricle

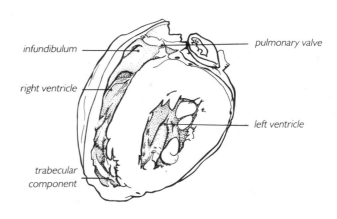

infundibulum

right ventricle

trabecular component

pulmonary valve

left ventricle

Fig. 1.29 This heart, shown in anatomical orientation, has been prepared by removing the anterior wall of the right ventricle.

Fig. 1.30 This section along the long axis of the heart itself shows the relationships of the right and left ventricles.

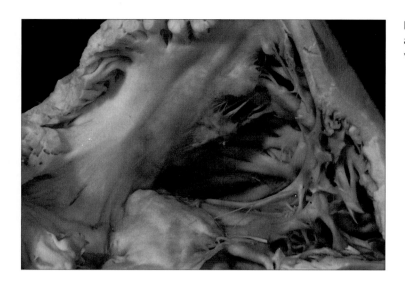

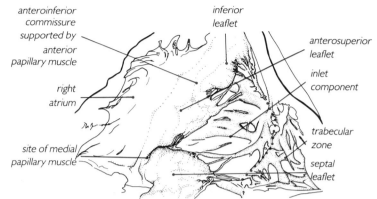

Fig. 1.31 This heart has been opened through the back of the right atrioventricular junction to show the location of the leaflets of the tricuspid valve.

anteroinferior commissure supported by anterior papillary muscle

right atrium

site of medial papillary muscle

inferior leaflet

anterosuperior leaflet

inlet component

trabecular zone

septal leaflet

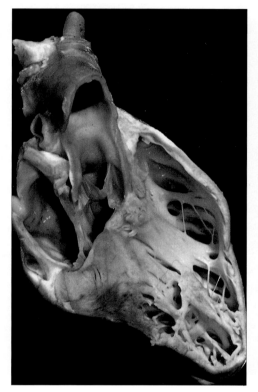

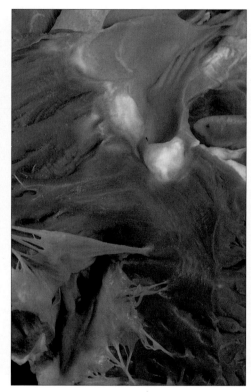

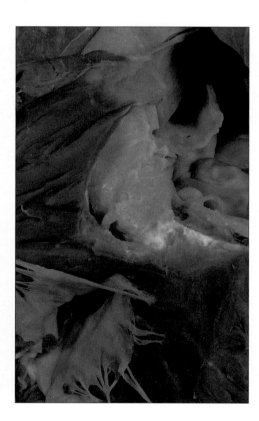

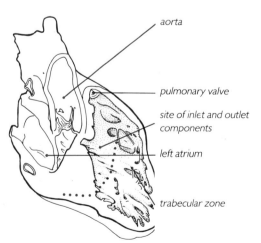

aorta

pulmonary valve

site of inlet and outlet components

left atrium

trabecular zone

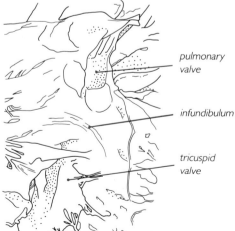

pulmonary valve

infundibulum

tricuspid valve

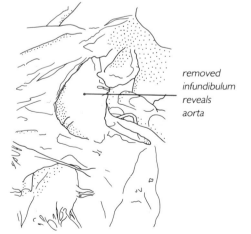

removed infundibulum reveals aorta

Fig. 1.32 This section obliquely across the right ventricle shows how the apical trabecular component "hangs down" from the inlet and outlet components.

Fig. 1.33 This heart is prepared to show the location of the infundibulum of the right ventricle.

Fig. 1.34 Further dissection of the heart shown in Fig. 1.33 reveals that the infundibulum is a free standing structure, since it can be removed without disturbing the structure of the left ventricle.

attachments of the tricuspid and pulmonary valves (Fig. 1.35). This is largely made up of the inner curvature of the heart wall, or the ventriculo–infundibular fold (Fig. 1.36), and is usually described as the supraventricular crest (crista supraventricularis). Only a very small part of the crest, where it merges with the septum, is a true septal structure. This component (Fig. 1.37) inserts to the septum between the limbs of a prominent right ventricular landmark, the septomarginal trabeculation, which is a muscle strap plastered onto the right ventricular aspect of the

septum (Fig. 1.38). A distinct raphe is often visible at the site of its junction with the supraventricular crest (Fig. 1.38), whilst in other hearts the crest merges imperceptibly with the trabeculation (Fig. 1.39). The septomarginal trabeculation itself bifurcates in the outlet component of the ventricle into two limbs which clasp the supraventricular crest. The anterior limb then ascends to support the leaflets of the pulmonary valve whilst the posterior limb runs onto and overlays the ventricular septum, giving rise to the medial papillary muscle complex and other cords supporting

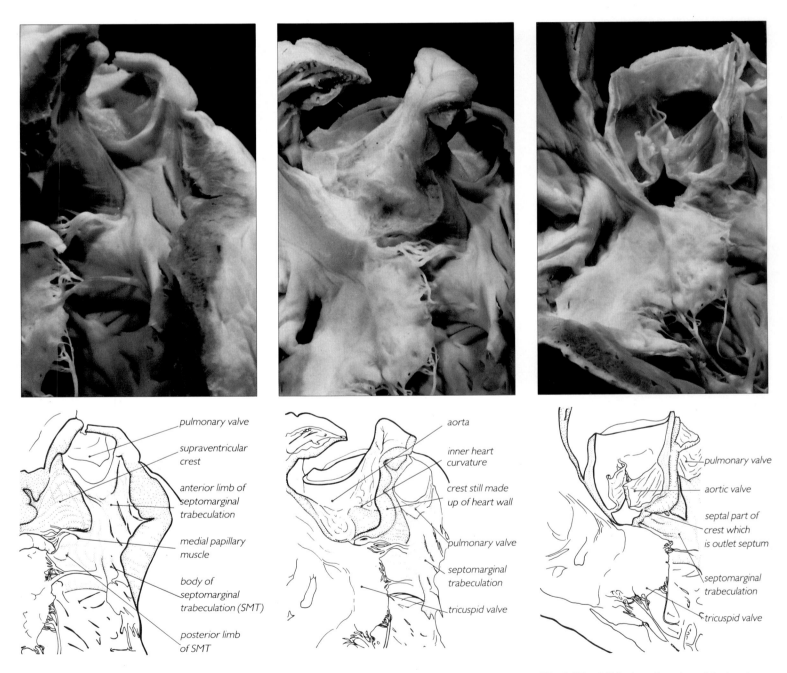

Fig. 1.35 This view of the septal aspect of the right ventricle shows the typical relationship of the supraventricular crest and the septomarginal trabeculation.

Fig. 1.36 As shown by this dissection of the heart seen in Fig. 1.35, the greater part of the supraventricular crest is made up of the inner curvature of the heart (the ventriculo–infundibular fold).

Fig. 1.37 Still further dissection of the heart shown in Figs 1.35 & 1.36 reveals that only a small part of the supraventricular crest separates the right and left ventricular outflow tracts.

the septal leaflet of the tricuspid valve. When traced towards the apex, the body of the trabeculation splits up to become continuous with the major papillary muscles supporting the anterosuperior and inferior leaflets of the tricuspid valve. One band passes prominently across the anterior papillary muscle and is known as the moderator band (Fig. 1.39). Several other prominent trabeculations, known as the septoparietal trabeculations (Fig. 1.38), take origin from the anterior margin of the septomarginal trabeculation and run round the parietal quadrant of the infundibulum.

The tricuspid and pulmonary valves

The three leaflets of the tricuspid valve occupy septal, anterosuperior, and inferior positions (Fig. 1.40). Consequently, the commissures between the leaflets are anteroseptal, anteroinferior, and inferior. The papillary muscles supporting the leaflets spring mostly from the septomarginal trabeculation and its apical ramification although, in the case of the septal and inferior leaflets, additional muscles or cords take direct origin from the superficial trabeculations of the ventricular septum. This is a most reliable feature for distinguishing the tricuspid from the mitral valve.

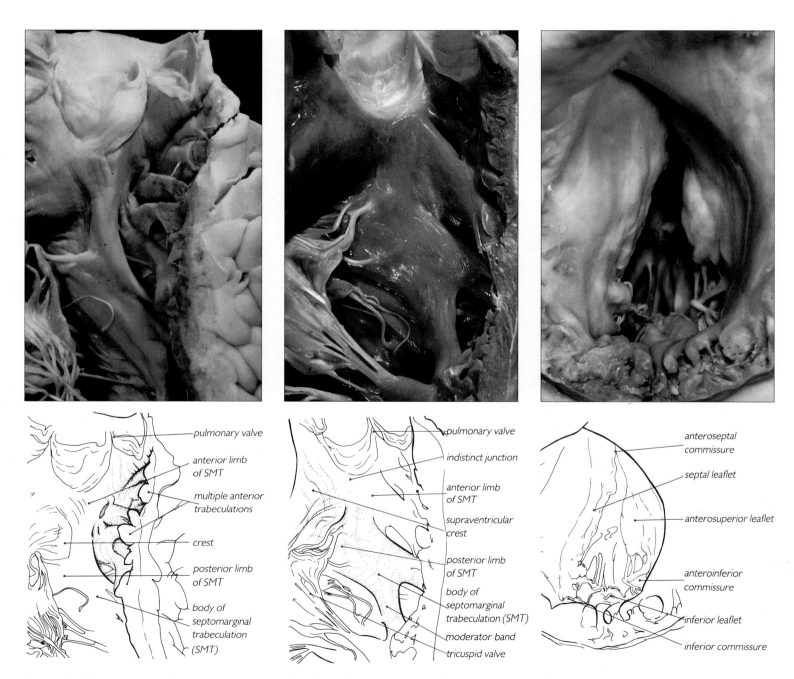

Fig. 1.38   This heart has well-formed septoparietal trabeculations springing from the anterior margin of the septomarginal trabeculation.

Fig. 1.39   This heart, with an indistinct junction between supraventricular crest and septomarginal trabeculation, shows the location of the moderator band and the anterior papillary muscle.

Fig. 1.40   This view of the unopened right atrioventricular junction, seen from the right atrium, shows the position of the leaflets of the tricuspid valve (compare with Fig. 1.31).

The leaflets of the pulmonary valve are seemingly supported throughout their circumference by the musculature of the infundibulum (Fig. 1.41) although, when studied carefully, it can be seen that the highest points of the semilunar attachments are adherent to the wall of the pulmonary trunk, while only the bases of the leaflets arise from the right ventricular musculature (Fig. 1.42). This arrangement of semilunar attachments is crucial when the arterial valves are considered in terms of possessing a ring or "annulus". The only true circular structure within the outflow tract is the area over which the fibrous wall of the pulmonary trunk is attached to the muscular wall of the infundibulum. This anatomic ventriculo–arterial junction is then crossed by the semilunar attachments of the leaflets. By virtue of this arrangement, three fibrous triangles of arterial wall are incorporated as part of the right ventricular outflow tract, while three crescents of infundibular musculature are incorporated within the sinuses of the pulmonary trunk (Fig. 1.43). Therefore the attachments of the leaflets constituting the haemodynamic ventriculo–arterial junction are arranged in semilunar fashion and have no resemblance to a ring or annulus. When naming the leaflets of the valve, advantage can be taken of the fact that

two of the leaflets "face" the corresponding leaflets of the aortic valve and, consequently, these can be termed right-facing and left-facing leaflets. This is in contrast to the third leaflet which is non-facing (Fig. 1.44).

The morphologically left ventricle

The morphologically left ventricle is a conical structure with tubular walls which narrow down to a rounded apex (Fig. 1.45). As with the right ventricle, it contains an inlet portion surrounding the mitral valve and its tension apparatus. There is an apical trabecular zone characterized by fine trabeculations and an outlet component supporting the aortic valve. Unlike the right ventricle, the outlet component is incomplete posteriorly so that the leaflets of the aortic and mitral valves are in fibrous continuity. There is, therefore, no structure in the left ventricle comparable to the supraventricular crest of the right ventricle, although a muscular fold (the ventriculo–infundibular fold) may occasionally interpose between the leaflets of the valves. The septal surface of the ventricle is smooth, so there is no structure corresponding to the septomarginal trabeculation in the left ventricle.

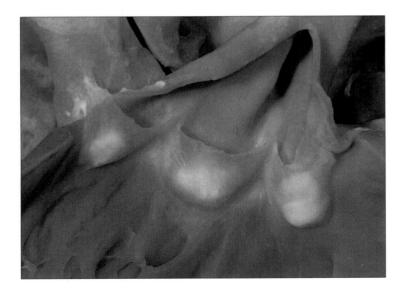

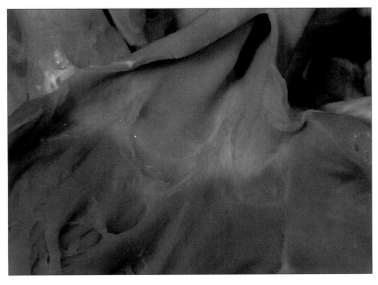

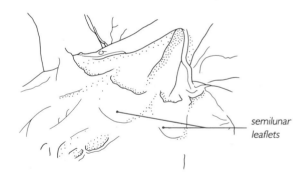

Fig. 1.41   This opened view of the ventriculo–pulmonary junction shows the typical semilunar attachments of the leaflets of the arterial valve.

semilunar leaflets

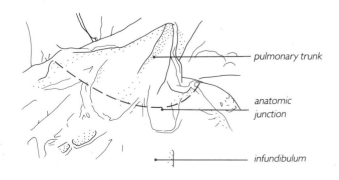

Fig. 1.42   Removal of the leaflets from the heart shown in Fig. 1.41 reveals how their attachment, marking the haemodynamic ventriculo–arterial junction, crosses the anatomic junction between the infundibular musculature and the wall of the pulmonary trunk.

pulmonary trunk

anatomic junction

infundibulum

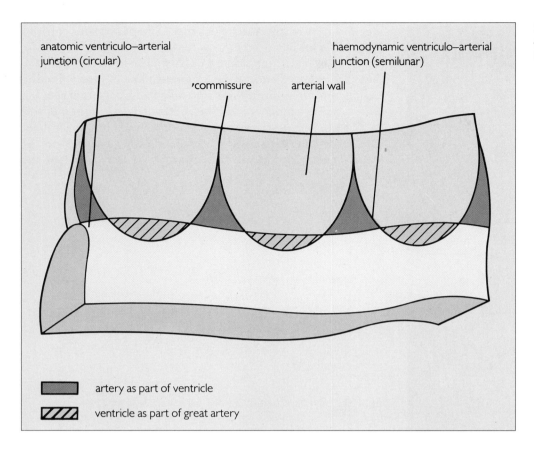

anatomic ventriculo–arterial junction (circular)

commissure

arterial wall

haemodynamic ventriculo–arterial junction (semilunar)

artery as part of ventricle

ventricle as part of great artery

Fig. 1.43 This diagram shows the consequences of the discrepancy between the anatomic and haemodynamic ventriculo–arterial junctions.

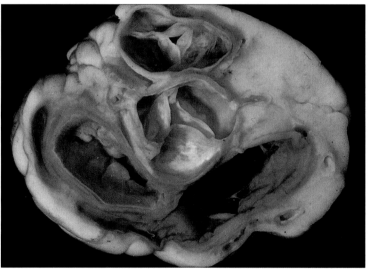

Fig. 1.44 This view of the short axis, seen from its atrial aspect, shows the central location of the aortic valve.

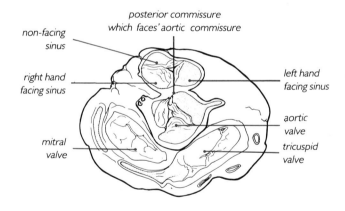

non-facing sinus

right hand facing sinus

mitral valve

posterior commissure which faces aortic commissure

left hand facing sinus

aortic valve

tricuspid valve

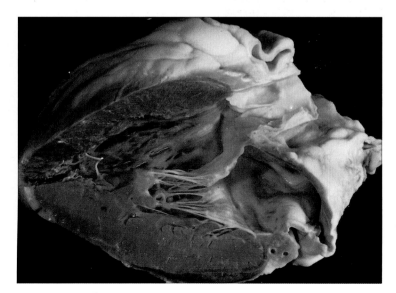

Fig. 1.45 This dissection shows the characteristic features of the morphologically left ventricle.

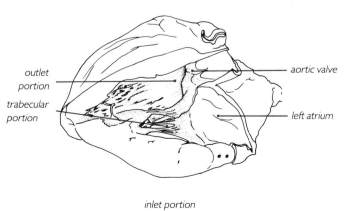

outlet portion

trabecular portion

aortic valve

left atrium

inlet portion

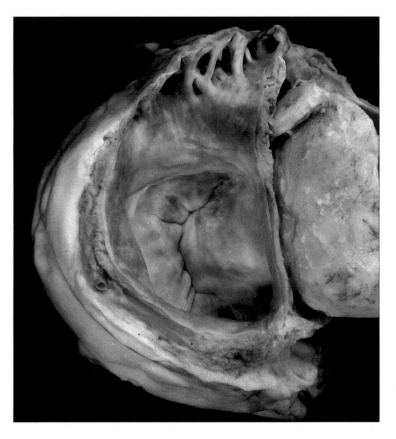

The mitral valve (the atrioventricular valve of the left ventricle) is characteristically described as having two leaflets (Fig. 1.46). Although it may often appear to have four leaflets (Fig. 1.47), there are only two ends to the prominent line of junction of the leaflets, and so we prefer to name only the two, considering the other units as components. The two leaflets recognized in this fashion are best described as being aortic and mural in location. The aortic leaflet, so named because of its continuity with the leaflets of the aortic valve, is attached to less than half the

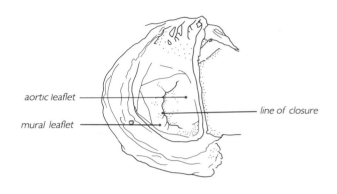

Fig. 1.46 This dissection, made after the left ventricle was perfused to ensure closure of the leaflets of the mitral valve, shows how there is a solitary line of closure with antero-lateral and postero-medial ends.

Fig. 1.48 This bisected mitral valve shows the aortic leaflet viewed from posteriorly. It is a semicircular leaflet with considerable depth.

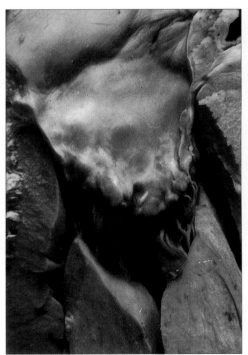

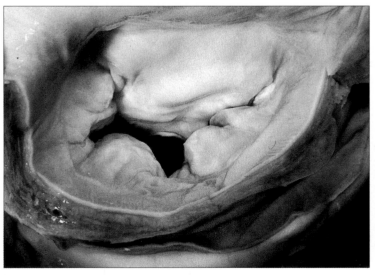

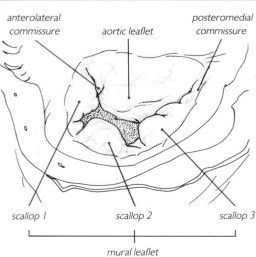

Fig. 1.47 This view of the atrial aspect of the mitral valve shows how the mural leaflet typically has three components, the so-called scallops.

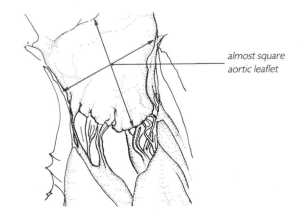

circumference of the left atrioventricular junction, but has considerable height and, consequently, presents as a large leaflet (Fig. 1.48). The mural leaflet, in contrast, is attached around two-thirds of the circumference of the junction but is shorter (Fig. 1.49), and occupies approximately the same area as the aortic leaflet. It is the mural leaflet which has a characteristic scalloped contour. Three scallops can usually be distinguished, and it is these three scallops which can be taken for discreet

leaflets (Fig. 1.47). Nonetheless, aberrations from this pattern are frequent, with two, five or even more scallops being seen in otherwise normal valves. Throughout its length, the mural leaflet is attached to the atrioventricular junction, whilst the aortic leaflet, in contrast, is in fibrous continuity with the leaflets of the aortic valve (Fig. 1.50). This fibrous continuity is further strengthened at each end by condensations of fibrous tissue known as the right and left fibrous trigones (Fig. 1.51).

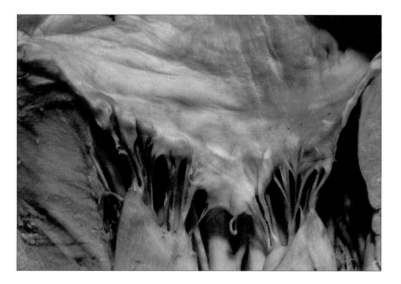

Fig. 1.49 This view of the posterior aspect of the bisected mitral valve seen in Fig. 1.48 shows how the mural leaflet has less depth but occupies considerably more of the overall circumference of the valvar orifice.

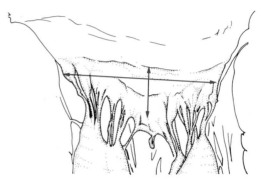

long and narrow mural leaflet

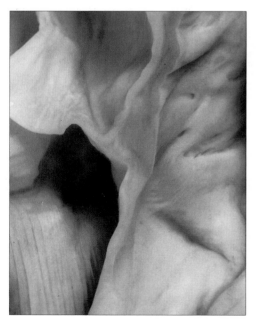

Fig. 1.50 This section across the aortic leaflet of the mitral valve shows its fibrous continuity with the leaflets of the aortic valve – hence its title as "aortic leaflet".

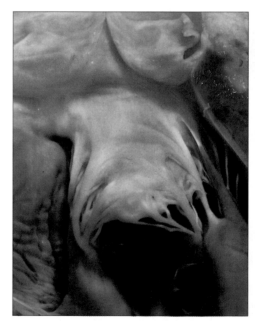

Fig. 1.51 This view of the outflow aspect of the aortic valve shows how the area of fibrous continuity with the leaflets of the aortic valve is strengthened at each end to form the fibrous trigones.

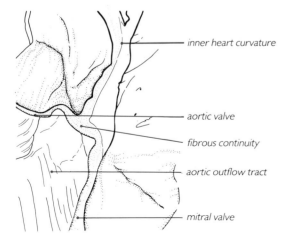

inner heart curvature

aortic valve

fibrous continuity

aortic outflow tract

mitral valve

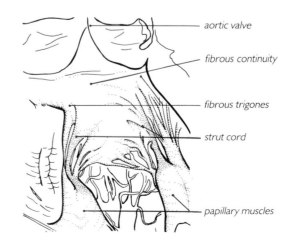

aortic valve

fibrous continuity

fibrous trigones

strut cord

papillary muscles

The tendinous cords supporting the leaflets of the mitral valve are themselves attached to two groups of papillary muscles situated underneath the ends of the commissural area in postero-medial and anterolateral positions. Their position is such that the cords between muscles and leaflets operate at maximal mechanical efficiency (Fig. 1.52), with each papillary muscle supporting the adjacent parts of both leaflets.

The apical trabecular portion of the left ventricle extends from the origin of the papillary muscles to the apex, its walls exhibiting fine trabeculations. The thickness of the ventricular wall diminishes markedly towards the apex where it may be no more than 1–2mm thick.

The outlet of the left ventricle supports the leaflets of the aortic valve, and is a partly muscular and partly fibrous structure (Fig. 1.53). The muscular part comprises the upper edge of the

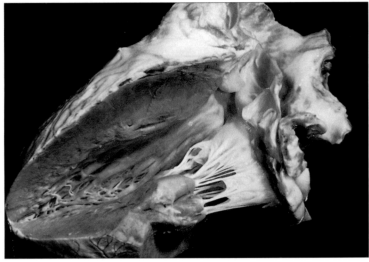

Fig. 1.52 This dissection, made by removing the parietal wall of the left ventricle, shows how the papillary muscles of the mitral valve are located close to each other, and at the point of maximal mechanical advantage relative to the cords of the valvar leaflets.

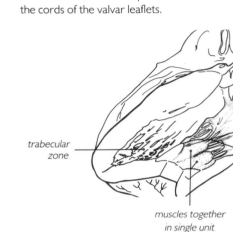

Fig. 1.53 The subaortic outflow tract is opened, showing its muscular and fibrous components.

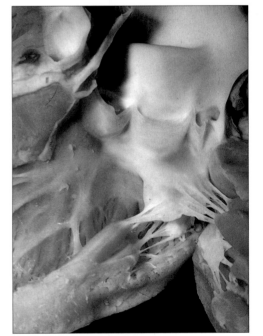

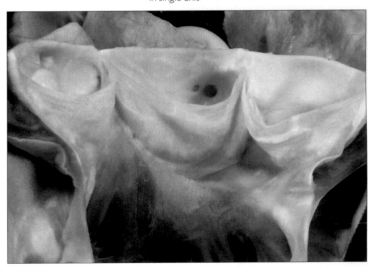

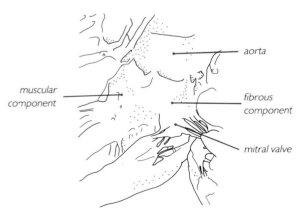

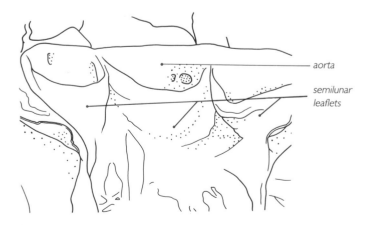

Fig. 1.54 This heart is opened across the ventriculo–aortic junction and spread to show the semilunar attachments of the leaflets of the aortic valve.

smooth trabecular septum medially and anteriorly, and the left margin of the ventriculo–infundibular fold laterally. The fibrous part consists of the area of continuity with the leaflets of the mitral valve. The extent of continuity varies in individual hearts, as do the precise proportions of the aortic leaflets contributing to this area of continuity as they continue from those of the mitral valve.

As in the right ventricle, the leaflets of the aortic valve are attached within the outlet in semilunar fashion, the semilunar

attachments crossing over the circular anatomic ventriculo–arterial junction (Figs 1.54 & 1.55). This anatomic junction is the only true "annulus" within the outflow tract. The apexes of the three triangles of aortic wall, which are incorporated into the outflow tract by the semilunar attachments, all point outside the heart. The one between the left coronary and non-coronary leaflets points into the transverse sinus (Fig. 1.56), whilst that between the non-coronary and right coronary leaflets opens above the supraventricular crest of the right ventricle (Fig. 1.57).

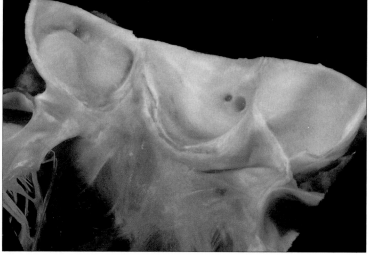

Fig. 1.55   Removal of the valvar leaflets from the heart shown in Fig. 1.54 reveals how the semilunar attachments are across the anatomic ventriculo–arterial junction (see Fig. 1.43).

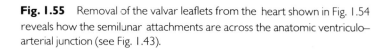

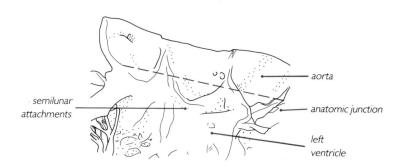

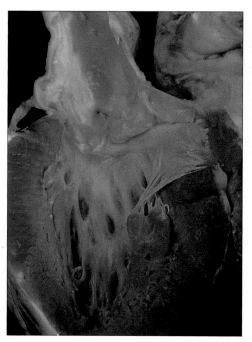

Fig. 1.56   The outflow tract of the left ventricle is opened so as to show how the fibrous triangle between the left coronary and non-coronary leaflets of the aortic valve points into the transverse sinus between the aorta and the left atrium.

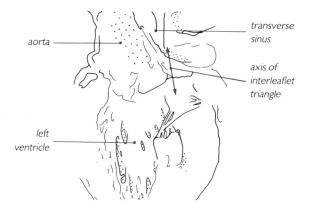

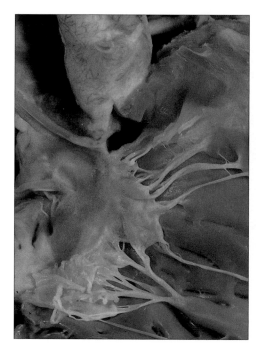

Fig. 1.57   In the heart shown in Fig. 1.56, removal of the fibrous triangle between the non-coronary and right coronary leaflets of the aortic valve shows how it points into and above the supraventricular crest of the right ventricle.

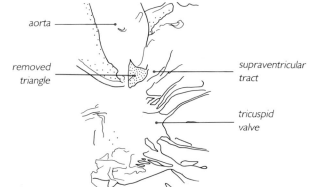

The third triangle, between the coronary leaflets, points to the base of the subpulmonary infundibulum (Fig. 1.58). The aortic valve has typical semilunar leaflets and is, therefore, a trifoliate structure (Fig. 1.59). There are various systems of naming the leaflets. Those using "anterior" and "posterior" in their titles give problems because of the oblique position of the aortic valve when the heart is in its usual location. This problem can be circumvented by taking account of the fact that two leaflets of the aortic valve always face the leaflets of the pulmonary valve (Fig. 1.60). As with the pulmonary valve, the leaflets can be named as right-facing, left-facing and non-facing. Account can also be taken, nonetheless, of the fact that, when two coronary arteries are present, they almost always arise from the sinuses related to the facing leaflet. The aortic leaflets, therefore, are also termed the right coronary, left coronary and non-coronary leaflets.

By virtue of its central position, the aortic valve is related to all other cardiac chambers. The right coronary leaflet is overlaid by the infundibulum of the right ventricle, its more posterior part being related to the anterior wall of the right atrium at its junction with the atrial appendage. The non-coronary leaflet is wedged in the interatrial fold and has a direct relationship to the right ventricle via the membranous septum, and an intimate relationship with the right atrium. The atrioventricular bundle penetrates the central fibrous body beneath the non-coronary leaflet. The left coronary leaflet has a relation to the left atrial cavity and also to the transverse sinus and a good portion of this leaflet forms part of the area of fibrous continuity with the mitral valve.

The ventricular septum

The septum between the ventricles is made up, for the most part, by muscle but is completed by a small fibrous component, the membranous septum (Fig. 1.61). In previous descriptions, we divided the muscular septum, like the ventricles, into inlet, apical trabecular, and outlet components. We now appreciate that this approach is an oversimplification. Because of the complex geometric interrelations of the ventricular components, the muscular septum separates most of the inlet of the right

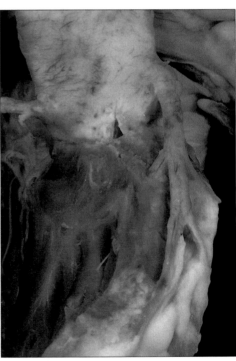

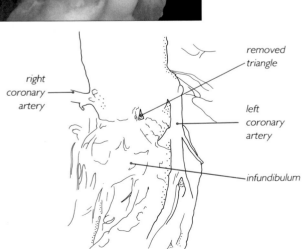

Fig. 1.58 In the same heart as shown in Fig. 1.56, removal of the fibrous triangle between the right and left coronary leaflets of the aortic valve shows how it points into the space between the aorta and the free-standing infundibulum of the right ventricle.

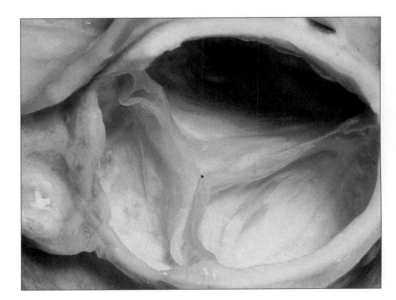

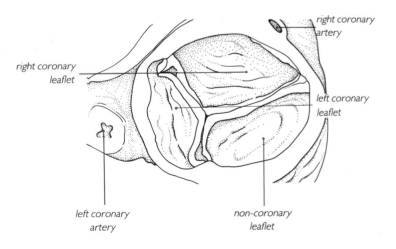

Fig. 1.59 This view of the aortic valve from above shows its typical trifoliate arrangement – note that all three leaflets are not of the same size.

ventricle from the outlet of the left. Furthermore, the sub-pulmonary infundibulum is free-standing, so the structure which we previously termed the "outlet septum" is, in reality, the posterior aspect of the muscular infundibulum. In the normal heart, therefore, we now distinguish simply the muscular and membranous components of the septum, differentiating also the ventricular from the atrioventricular septal structures (Figs 1.62 & 1.63).

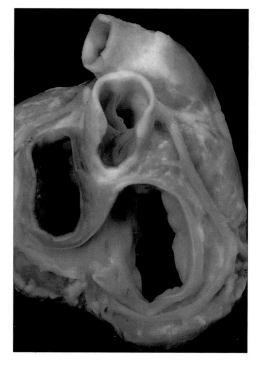

Fig. 1.60 This dissection shows how two of the sinuses of the aorta face the pulmonary trunk, and it is these sinuses which give rise to coronary arteries. The sinus which does not face (the non-facing sinus) does not give rise to a coronary artery.

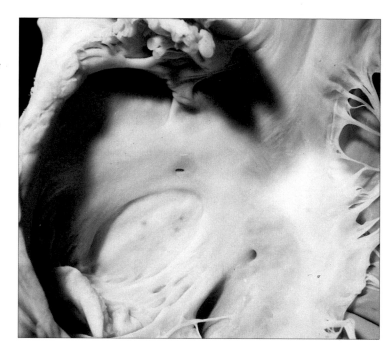

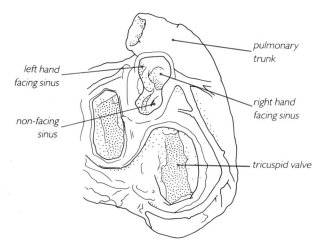

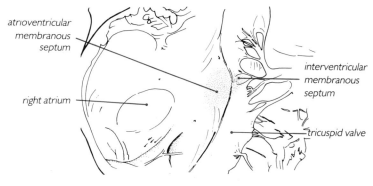

Fig. 1.61 This transilluminated specimen, seen from the right, shows the location of the membranous part of the septum, and reveals how the attachment of the leaflet of the tricuspid valve divides it into atrioventricular and interventricular components.

Fig. 1.62 This section through the aortic root shows how part of the membranous septum is located in atrioventricular position.

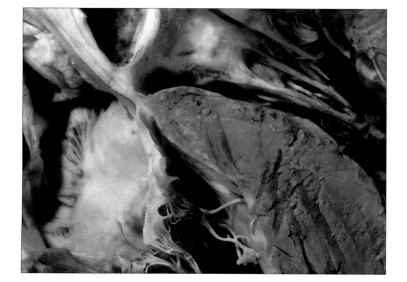

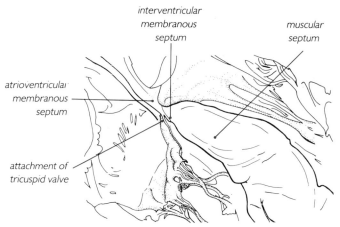

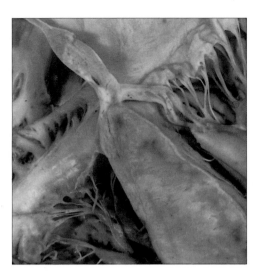

Fig. 1.63 This long axis section in "four-chamber" plane shows how the differential levels of attachment of the atrioventricular valves produce a muscular atrioventricular septum.

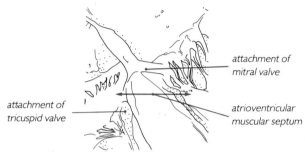

attachment of mitral valve

attachment of tricuspid valve

atrioventricular muscular septum

Fig. 1.64 This section through the right ventricle shows the aortic sinuses surrounding and supporting the leaflets of the aortic valve.

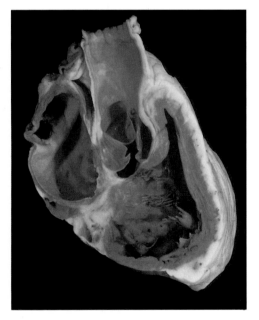

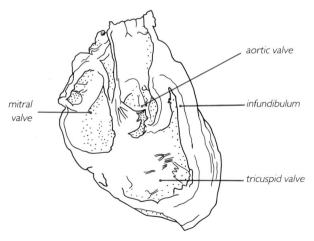

aortic valve

mitral valve

infundibulum

tricuspid valve

The aorta and its branches

As has been discussed above, the aorta commences at the anatomic ventriculo–arterial junction, rises into the upper mediastinum, and turns leftward as the brachiocephalic arteries take origin from its arch. It then descends through the thoracic cavity, lying to the left of the spine, to enter the abdomen through the diaphragm. The discordance between the anatomic and haemodynamic ventriculo–arterial junctions has also been discussed, this being the consequence of the semilunar arrangement of the leaflets of the aortic valve. These semilunar attachments are closely related to the sinuses of the aortic root and the fibrous extensions of the left ventricular outflow tract. The aortic sinuses (of Valsalva) themselves are the expanded areas of the aortic root which support and surround the leaflets of the aortic valve (Fig. 1.64). Inferiorly, the sinuses commence at the anatomic ventriculo–arterial junction whilst, superiorly, they form another obvious junction at the origin of the tubular ascending aorta. This second junction is variably described as the aortic bar, the aortic ridge, or simply the sinutubular junction. The peripheral attachments of the three commissures between the leaflets of the aortic valve are firmly anchored at this sinu-tubular junction, thickening it to accentuate a marked ring at the distal extent of the valvar apparatus (Fig. 1.65). Each of the fibrous extensions of the outflow tract is beneath the attachment of these commissures, and the extensions widen as the semilunar attachments of the leaflets extend down to the bases of the aortic sinuses, capturing a small crescent of the left ventricle within the proximal extent of each sinus (Fig. 1.55).

The coronary arteries arise within two of the sinuses of the aortic root (see below), and are the first branches from the aorta. In addition to the brachiocephalic arteries and the arterial duct, the intercostal, bronchial and oesophageal arteries also arise from the aorta within the thorax. The intercostal arteries are paired vessels that spring from the sides of the descending aorta to supply the musculature of the nine lowest intercostal spaces, the upper two spaces receiving their supply from the branches of the brachiocephalic arteries (the superior intercostal arteries). The bronchial and oesophageal arteries usually originate from the underside of the aortic arch, running forward to supply the visceral structures (Fig. 1.66). The variable number of bronchial arteries divide in concert with the bronchial tree. Their origin, however, can vary markedly and they often arise from behind the oesophagus.

The pulmonary trunk and its branches

The pulmonary trunk commences at the anatomic ventriculo–arterial junction with the infundibulum of the right ventricle. This arrangement is directly comparable with that of the origin of the aorta from the left ventricle, except that the infundibulum is exclusively muscular. Thus, the leaflets of the pulmonary valve are supported by the three sinuses of the pulmonary trunk, which interdigitate with the fibrous extensions of the outflow tract as a consequence of the semilunar attachments of the leaflets. As with the aorta, there is then a marked sinutubular junction at the commencement of the ascending component of the pulmonary trunk, with the upper extent of each of the commissures between the valvar leaflets being at this level. The trunk itself is then a relatively short structure which branches into the right and left pulmonary arteries, each of which extends to the hilum of its respective lung. During fetal life, the pulmonary arteries are side branches of the trunk, which continues directly as the arterial duct and conveys deoxygenated blood down the aorta and back to the placenta. It is often stated that the duct, during fetal life, is of much greater dimensions than the isthmus, and that the pulmonary arteries are of relatively small diameter. In contrast, our measurements show that, at least in the middle trimester, all of these structures are of comparable diameter (Fig. 1.67). The duct closes rapidly subse-

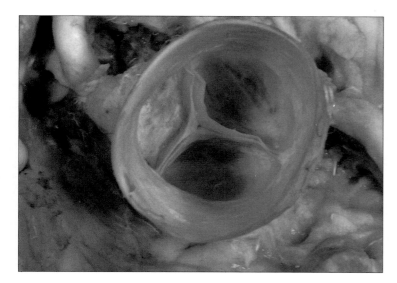

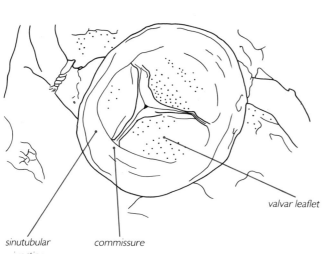

Fig. 1.65 This view of the aortic valve from above shows the prominant ring at the sinutubular junction.

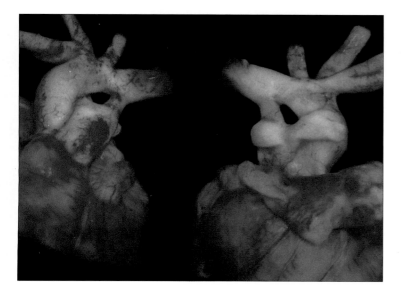

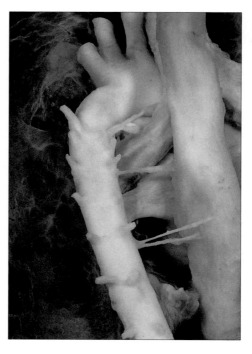

Fig. 1.66 This view of the descending aorta from behind shows the origin of the intercostal, bronchial and oesophageal arteries.

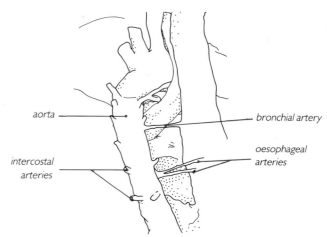

Fig. 1.67 These views of the great arteries of the midterm fetus, seen from in front (left) and behind (right) show how the diameter of the arterial duct is comparable to that of the pulmonary arteries and less than that of the isthmus of the aorta.

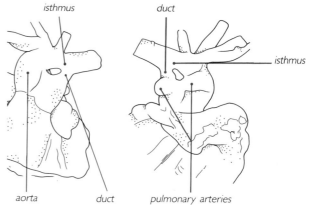

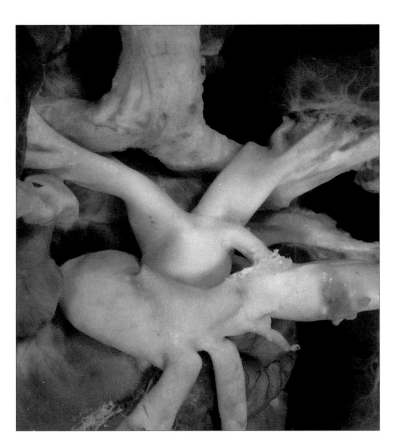

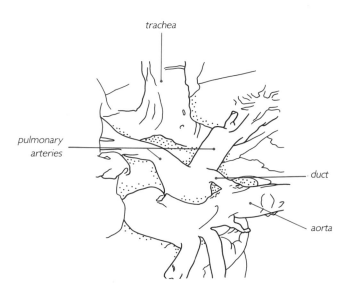

Fig. 1.68 This view of the great arteries of a neonate show how the arterial duct is in the process of becoming ligamentous.

trachea

pulmonary arteries

duct

aorta

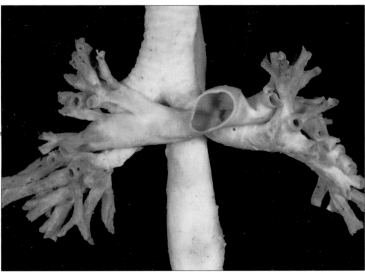

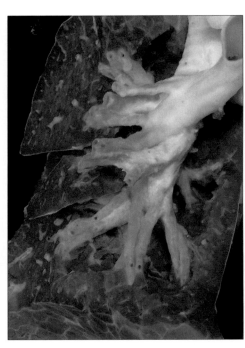

Fig. 1.70 This view is of the right lung of the bronchial tree shown in Fig. 1.69 prior to removal of the pulmonary parenchyma. It shows the segmental arteries to the front of the lung.

trachea

pulmonary trunk

oesophagus

Fig. 1.69 This dissection shows how the branches of the pulmonary arteries run in segmental fashion with the bronchial tree.

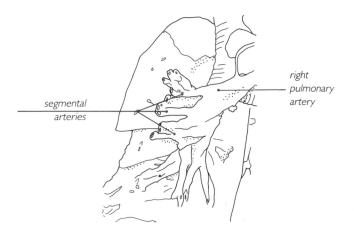

segmental arteries

right pulmonary artery

quent to birth and, within six weeks, is converted to the arterial ligament (Fig. 1.68).

Having reached the hila of the lungs, the pulmonary arteries themselves divide to supply the bronchopulmonary segments (Fig. 1.69), of which there are 10 in the right lung. One prominent branch of the right pulmonary artery supplies each segment (Fig. 1.70). Of the segments (Fig. 1.70), there are three in the upper lobe (apical, posterior and anterior); two in the middle lobe (lateral and medial); and five in the lower lobe (superior, medial basal, antero-basal, lateral basal and postero-basal). The left lung possesses only eight segments (Figs 1.71 & 1.72). Four of these are in the upper lobe (apico-posterior, anterior, supero-lingular and infero-lingular) and four are in the lower lobe (inferior, postero-basal, antero-basal and lateral basal).

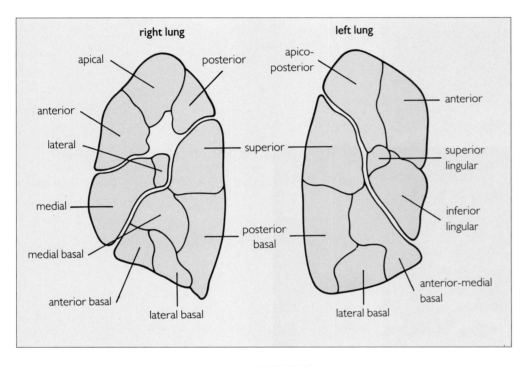

Fig. 1.71 This diagram of the mediastinal surfaces of the two lungs shows their division into bronchopulmonary segments – ten in the right lung but only eight in the left.

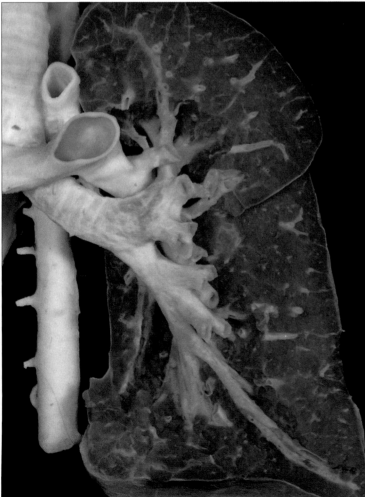

Fig. 1.72 This view of the left lung shown in Fig. 1.69 was taken prior to removal of the pulmonary parenchyma.

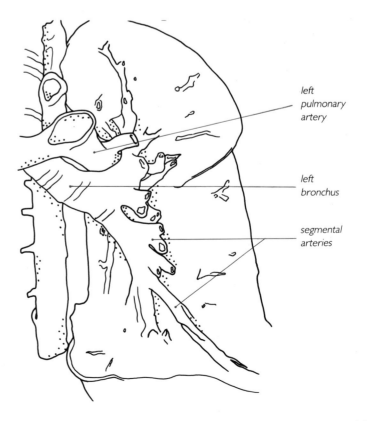

The fibrous skeleton of the heart

The cardiac skeleton has the function of separating the atrial and ventricular musculatures, as well as acting as an anchorage for insertion and origin of the ventricular myocardial fibres. When observing the bulk of myocardium present at the atrioventricular junction, it is hardly believable that all this musculature could be attached to the fibrous skeleton. Moreover, the skeleton itself is more pronounced in some parts of the atrioventricular junction than in others, the atrial and ventricular musculatures being, in many areas, separated by planes of adipose tissue rather than by firm collagenous rings. It seems to us that the major function of the skeleton is to support the leaflets of the atrioventricular valves and to anchor them to the ventricular mass. The skeleton includes the aortic root in its structure (Fig. 1.73), but has no direct relationships to the orifice of the

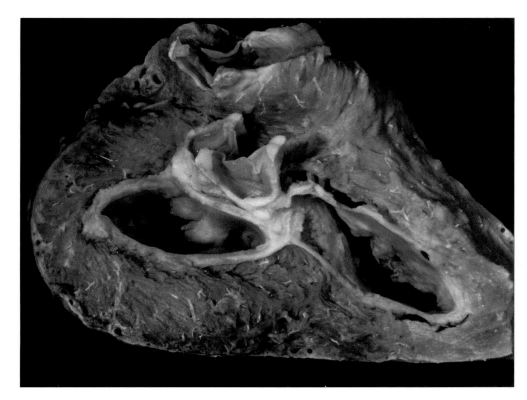

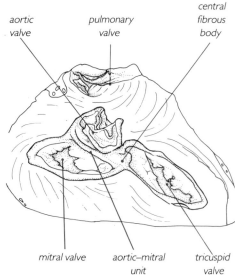

Fig. 1.73 The musculature of the atriums, together with the fibrous walls of the arterial trunks, has been removed to show the location of the fibrous skeleton.

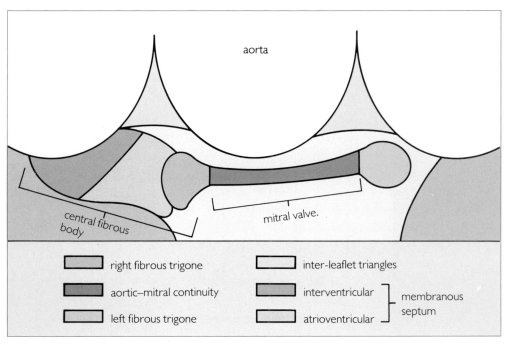

Fig. 1.74 This diagram, drawn from the left ventricular aspect, shows the components of the central fibrous body. Compare with Fig. 1.51.

pulmonary valve. Only the leaflets of the mitral, tricuspid and aortic valves, therefore, are set within the fibrous skeleton, although the dimensions of the fibrous structures are by no means uniform around the leaflets of the three valves. The strongest parts of the skeleton are found at the junctions between the leaflets of the mitral and aortic valves, the area of fibrous continuity being thickened to form the left and right fibrous trigones. The most prominent area is the central fibrous body, formed by the union of the right fibrous trigone and the membranous septum (Fig. 1.74). The attachment of the septal leaflet of the tricuspid valve crosses the membranous septal component of the body, dividing it into interventricular and atrioventricular components (Fig. 1.61). The attachments of the leaflets of the tricuspid and mitral valves diverge from the posterior margin of the central fibrous body. In this respect, the structures supporting the leaflets of the tricuspid valve are less well-formed than those supporting the mitral leaflets. In places, collagenous segments can be found reinforcing the attachment of the leaflets of the tricuspid valve, but there is rarely, if ever, a complete collagenous annulus. The skeleton supporting the leaflets of the mitral valve is better-formed, but this also tends to fade out around the midpoint of the mural leaflet.

The coronary circulation

The coronary circulation is derived from the coronary arteries, these being the first branches of the aorta. The circulation continues through a capillary network to reach the coronary veins which then drain, for the most part, into the coronary sinus and on in to the right atrium.

The coronary arteries

The two main coronary arteries (right and left) have, in the past, been considered to be end arteries, the belief being that the branches of the right coronary artery did not anastomose with those of the left. It has now been shown that, from birth onwards, collateral pathways exist which are not an expression of any pathological condition.

The two coronary arteries originate from the aortic sinuses which face the pulmonary valve (Fig. 1.60). These are best named as the right hand and left hand facing sinuses, this being judged from the stance of the observer standing, figuratively, within the non-facing sinus (Fig. 1.75). The coronary arteries usually arise within the sinus and below, or at the level of, the sinutubular junction (Fig. 1.76). There is usually only one orifice for the left coronary artery, although it is usual to find multiple orifices in the sinus giving rise to the right coronary artery. The major orifice supplies the main stem of the right coronary artery itself. Minor orifices, when present, supply the branches which, in the presence of a single orifice, originate from the initial part of the main arterial stem. The most frequent additional orifice supplies the infundibular (or conal) branch (Fig. 1.76). Although, usually, the arteries arise from within the aortic sinuses, they may arise above the level of the sinutubular junction, while the orifices may also be located close to a valvar commissure. In the latter situation, the coronary artery will tend to take an oblique course through the aortic wall, giving a so-called intramural arrangement.

The major branches of the coronary arteries all occupy a subepicardial position, being found in the atrioventricular

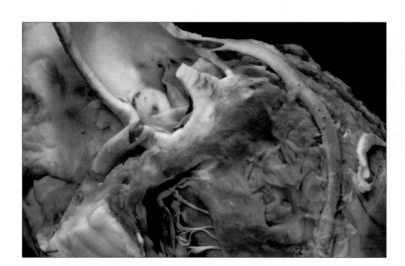

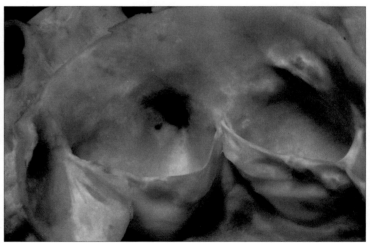

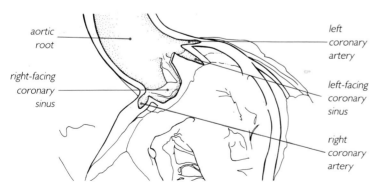

Fig. 1.75 This dissection, made by removing the subpulmonary infundibulum, shows the origin of the coronary arteries from the aortic root.

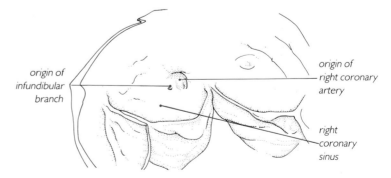

Fig. 1.76 This view of the right aortic sinus shows the origin of the right coronary artery within the sinus together with a separate origin for the infundibular artery.

and interventricular grooves. The extent of the myocardium supplied by the right and left arteries varies from heart to heart. The most frequent pattern is for the right coronary artery to encircle the tricuspid orifice and give rise to the posterior interventricular coronary artery whilst continuing to supply the diaphragmatic surface of the left ventricle. This arrangement, termed right dominance, is found in approximately 90% of hearts (Fig. 1.77). In most of the remaining hearts, the circumflex branch of the left coronary artery supplies the diaphragmatic surface of the left ventricle and the posterior interventricular artery, giving a left dominant pattern (Fig. 1.78). In a few hearts, branches of both the right coronary and the left circumflex artery give off parallel descending branches close to the interventricular groove, a so-called balanced pattern of coronary arterial supply.

In terms of its epicardial course, the right coronary artery emerges from the right coronary sinus directly into the atrioventricular groove (Fig. 1.79). It immediately gives off the infundibular artery (if this artery does not have a separate orifice from the sinus) which ramifies over the right ventricular outflow tract. The artery to the sinus node arises from the right coronary artery in much the same area in about 55% of individuals (Fig. 1.80), and ascends through the interatrial groove along the anteromedial wall of the right atrium. It may then run in front of or behind the caval vein, or branch to form a circle around the orifice of the vein prior to supplying the sinus node in the terminal groove. In approximately 1% of normal individuals the artery arises more laterally, and crosses the atrial appendage to reach the node whilst the right coronary artery itself continues in the anterior atrioventricular groove. The marginal branch is

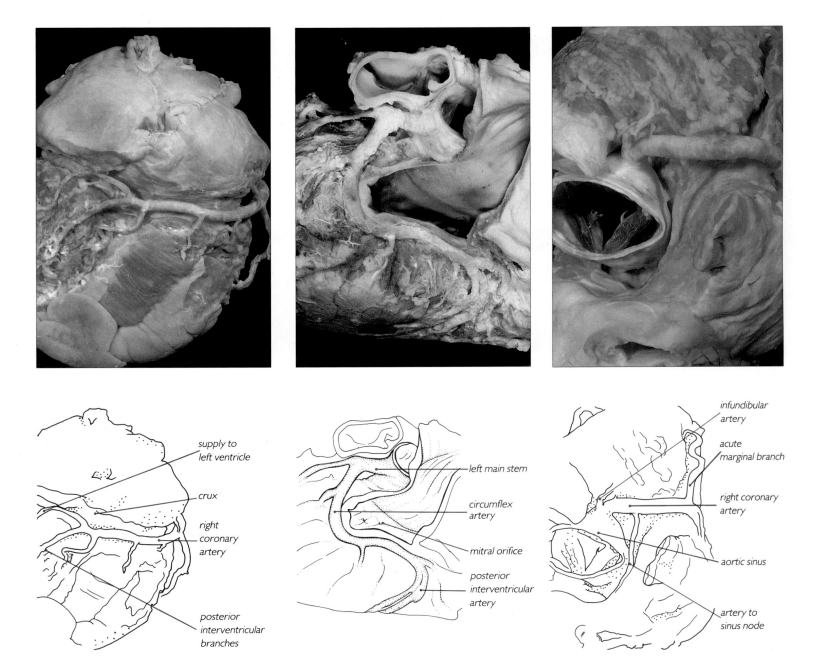

Fig. 1.77 This dissection shows a right dominant coronary artery extending across the crux to supply the diaphragmatic surface of the left ventricle.

Fig. 1.78 In this heart, the left coronary artery is dominant – compare with Fig. 1.77.

Fig. 1.79 This dissection shows the initial course of the right coronary artery.

its next major tributary and this runs along the acute margin of the heart towards the apex. Having entered the posterior atrioventricular groove, the right coronary artery runs to the crux of the heart. In those cases of right ventricular dominance, the posterior interventricular coronary artery, and the artery to the atrioventricular node, start at the crux. The terminal branches of the dominant right coronary artery beyond the crux usually supply the inferior wall of the left ventricle and part of the posteromedial papillary muscle group of the mitral valve. Throughout its course, the right coronary artery gives additional branches to both the right atrial and right ventricular walls, none of which have specific names.

The main stem of the left coronary artery emerges from the left aortic sinus into the left side of the atrioventricular groove (Fig. 1.81). The main stem of the artery is usually short, rarely exceeding 10mm before branching into the anterior descending and circumflex arteries. In approximately 30% of cases, there is a third branch at the site of division of the main stem which is termed the intermediate artery and which runs obliquely over the parietal ventricular wall. The anterior interventricular coronary artery (Fig. 1.82) gives rise to a diagonal branch close to its origin from the left main stem. This diagonal artery, or additional diagonal arteries, may also originate more distally from the anterior interventricular artery, passing backwards to supply

the obtuse margin of the heart. As the anterior interventricular artery passes towards the apex it gives off a series of branches which pass perpendicularly into the ventricular septum. These are the perforating branches (the first of which usually originates within 10mm of the origin of the anterior interventricular artery and is the largest artery), and they are intramyocardial rather than epicardial branches. The anterior interventricular artery itself, although usually an epicardial structure, can pass intramyocardially for some distance before returning to its epicardial position. This is called myocardial bridging (Fig. 1.83), and

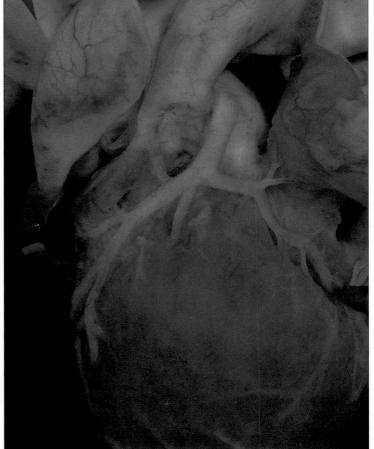

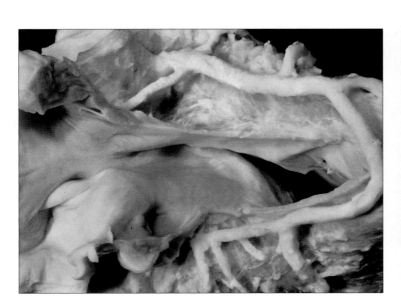

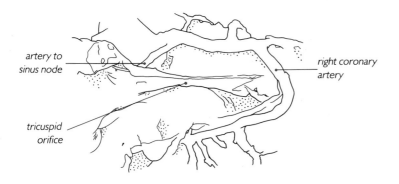

Fig. 1.80   This dissection shows how the right coronary artery encircles the orifice of the tricuspid valve. Note the course of the artery to the sinus node.

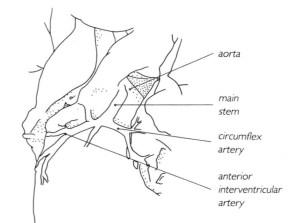

Fig. 1.81   There is a long initial course of the left coronary artery in this neonatal heart prior to its bifurcation.

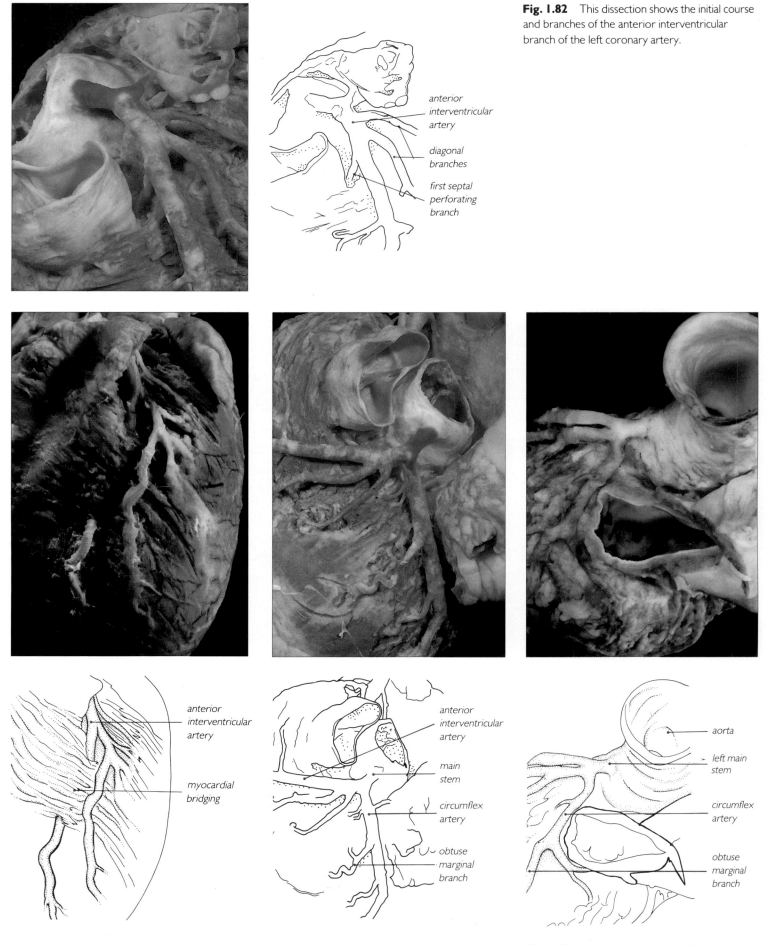

Fig. 1.82 This dissection shows the initial course and branches of the anterior interventricular branch of the left coronary artery.

anterior interventricular artery

diagonal branches

first septal perforating branch

anterior interventricular artery

myocardial bridging

anterior interventricular artery

main stem

circumflex artery

obtuse marginal branch

aorta

left main stem

circumflex artery

obtuse marginal branch

Fig. 1.83 There is marked myocardial bridging of the anterior interventricular coronary artery in this heart.

Fig. 1.84 This dissection of the heart shown in Fig. 1.82 shows the origin of the circumflex branch of the left coronary artery.

Fig. 1.85 In this heart, the circumflex branch supplies a very limited area of the left ventricle – compare with the arrangement seen in Fig. 1.78.

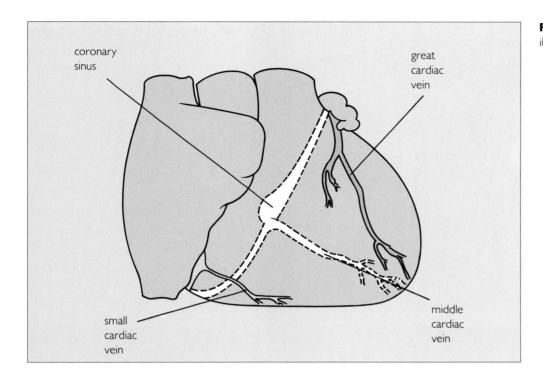

Fig. 1.86 This diagram, shown from the front, illustrates the arrangement of the coronary veins.

Labels on figure: coronary sinus; great cardiac vein; small cardiac vein; middle cardiac vein

certainly occurs in 33% of hearts, perhaps more. The distal part of the interventricular artery usually dips round the ventricular apex and continues in the posterior interventricular groove. The extent of the posterior supply depends upon the size of the posterior interventricular artery.

The circumflex branch of the left coronary artery is the other branch of the main arterial stem (Fig. 1.84). In approximately 45% of cases, it immediately gives rise to the artery to the sinus node which, having traversed the anterior interatrial furrow, takes a similar course to reach the node as that taken when it arises from the right coronary artery. In a small proportion of cases there can also be a lateral origin of the nodal artery from the circumflex artery. The circumflex artery itself continues along its course in the left atrioventricular groove, its extent depending upon whether the artery will become dominant. When not dominant, its area of supply depends upon the extent of the right coronary artery. A marginal branch usually originates from the proximal segment of the circumflex coronary artery. In cases of extreme right dominance, this branch may be the termination of the artery (Fig. 1.85). The proximity of the circumflex artery to the attachment of the mural leaflet of the mitral valve varies considerably, being much closer to the leaflet when the left coronary artery is dominant (compare Figs 1.78 & 1.85).

The myocardial supply from the epicardial coronary arteries is usually derived from perpendicular branches which penetrate the myocardium and run towards the endocardium. During their course, these arteries again branch off at right angles, and the branches themselves then ramify amongst the bundles of myocardial fibres, so causing an extensive intercommunicating network to be present within the subendocardium. Collateral networks always exist between the networks of the right and left coronary arteries. Some of these are present at precapillary level, while other pathways may use vessels of larger calibre. Among the latter category, two major pathways are recognized.

The first is the communication between perforating branches of the anterior and posterior ventricular arteries within the septum, whilst the second passes through atrial branches.

The coronary veins

The coronary arterial blood, having passed through the capillary network, is collected by venules which drain to the cardiac veins. Two major groups of veins exist: those draining to the coronary sinus, and those draining to the cardiac chambers, the latter being termed the Thebesian veins. A further group of larger veins, known as the anterior cardiac veins, runs over the anterior aspect of the heart, cross superficially over the right coronary artery, and drain blood directly to the right atrium.

The veins which drain to the coronary sinus run with the coronary arteries (Fig. 1.86). The great cardiac vein ascends along the anterior interventricular artery and through the left atrioventricular groove where it receives venous channels from the obtuse margin. It becomes the coronary sinus in the posterior atrioventricular groove. As it enters the right atrium, the coronary sinus receives the venous blood draining through the middle cardiac vein which ascends in the posterior interventricular groove, and that draining through the small cardiac vein which ascends alongside the marginal coronary artery and, with the right coronary artery, turns into the posterior atrioventricular groove. Veins from the atriums also drain into the coronary sinus. The oblique vein of the left atrium is the vestige of the left superior caval vein.

In addition to the arteries and veins, there is an extensive lymphatic network in the heart which is divided into a deep endocardial, a middle myocardial and a superficial epicardial network. Eventually, these channels all drain into collecting channels which follow an epicardial course, accompanying the major arterial stems. The primary lymph nodes draining the heart are found in the anterior mediastinum.

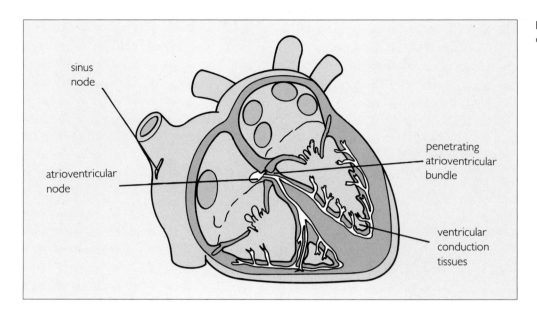

Fig. 1.87 This diagram shows the arrangement of the cardiac conduction tissues.

Labels in diagram:
- sinus node
- atrioventricular node
- penetrating atrioventricular bundle
- ventricular conduction tissues

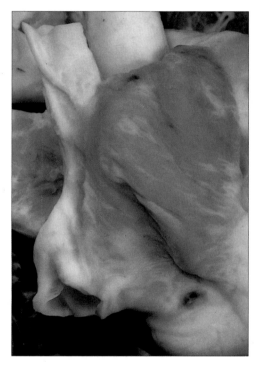

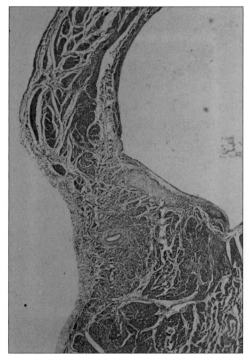

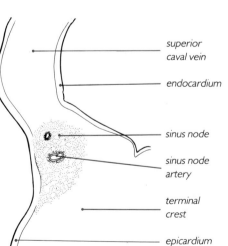

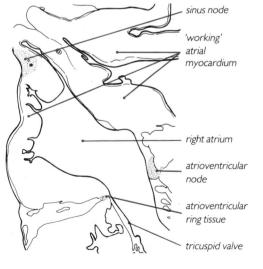

Labels (Fig. 1.88):
- superior caval vein
- sinus node
- appendage
- terminal groove
- inferior caval vein

Labels (Fig. 1.89):
- superior caval vein
- endocardium
- sinus node
- sinus node artery
- terminal crest
- epicardium

Labels (Fig. 1.90):
- sinus node
- 'working' atrial myocardium
- right atrium
- atrioventricular node
- atrioventricular ring tissue
- tricuspid valve

Fig. 1.88 In this heart, the location of the sinus node has been superimposed on the terminal groove of the right atrium.

Fig. 1.89 This section across the terminal groove, stained with the trichrome technique, shows the location of the sinus node.

Fig. 1.90 This section across the right atrium, stained with the trichrome technique, shows how the tissue between the nodes is composed of ordinary working atrial myocardium.

The conduction system

The conduction tissues are responsible for the initiation and conduction of the heart beat (Fig. 1.87). They are composed of myocardial tissues which are easily identified histologically from the atrial and ventricular myocardium and, for this reason, they are frequently described as the "specialized tissues" of the heart.

The sinus node, or pacemaker, is situated in the terminal groove at the lateral junction of the superior caval vein with the right atrium (Fig. 1.88). It is a spindle-shaped structure with a long tail running down the terminal groove towards the orifice of the inferior caval vein. Sometimes the node extends medially across the crest of the atrial appendage in horse-shoe fashion, and it is usually arranged around a prominent artery (Fig. 1.89). This nodal artery is a branch of the right coronary artery in 55% of individuals, and the circumflex artery in the remainder.

Although a single large artery usually passes through the sinus node, multiple small arteries may be observed.

The route of the sinus impulse to the atrioventricular node has been controversial. Although it was suggested that tracts of "specialized tissue" run between the nodes, our own studies have not substantiated this claim. We find the muscle bands and bundles which make up the wall of the right atrium and the interatrial septum to be composed of working myocardium (Fig. 1.90), and it is their geometric arrangement which provides the substrate for preferential conduction.

The atrioventricular node is found in the atrial component of the muscular atrioventricular septum at the apex of the triangle of Koch (Fig. 1.91). This triangle is delineated by the tendon of Todaro and the attachment of the septal leaflet of the tricuspid valve, the two meeting at the central fibrous body. The node is made up of a half oval of small densely-packed nodal cells set with its flat surface against the central fibrous body (Fig. 1.92).

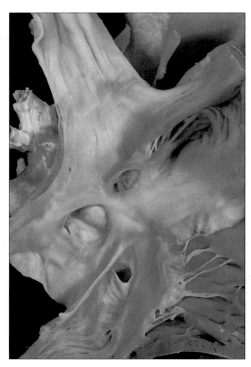

Fig. 1.91 This opened view of the right atrium shows the location of the landmarks of the triangle of Koch.

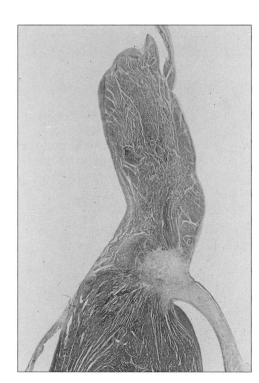

Fig. 1.92 This section through the triangle of Koch, stained with the trichrome technique, shows the site of the compact atrioventricular node.

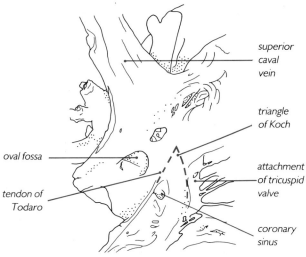

superior
caval
vein

triangle
of Koch

oval fossa

attachment
of tricuspid
valve

tendon of
Todaro

coronary
sinus

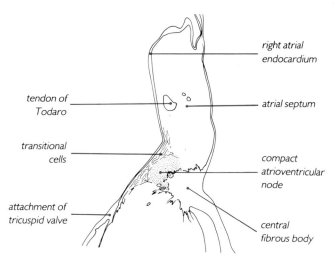

right atrial
endocardium

tendon of
Todaro

atrial septum

transitional
cells

compact
atrioventricular
node

attachment of
tricuspid valve

central
fibrous body

1.38

The axis of the compact node gathers at the apex of the triangle of Koch, and then runs into the central fibrous body to become the penetrating atrioventricular bundle (Fig. 1.93). Having penetrated the fibrous body, the axis of conduction tissue reaches the crest of the muscular ventricular septum beneath the membranous septum and begins to branch. This point, when viewed from the subaortic outflow tract, is beneath the commissure between the right and non-coronary leaflets of the aortic valve (Fig. 1.94) and the branching bundle is usually placed on the crest of the septum (Fig. 1.95). The fibres of the

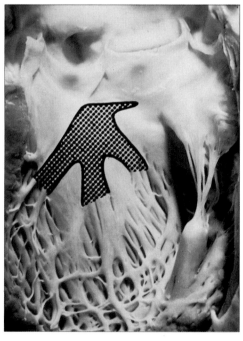

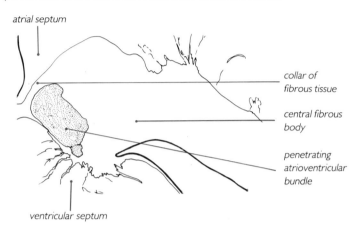

Fig. 1.93 This section, from the same heart as shown in Fig. 1.92, shows the penetration of the axis of atrioventricular conduction tissue.

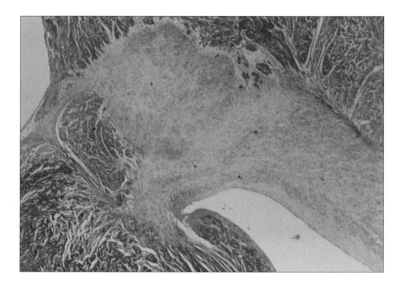

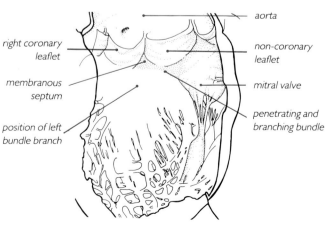

Fig. 1.94 This view of the left ventricular outflow tract has been marked to show the location of the branching bundle and the left bundle branch.

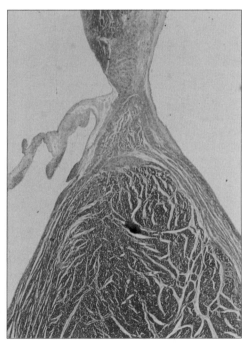

Fig. 1.95 This further section from the series shown in Figs 1.92 & 1.93 illustrates the branching atrioventricular bundle astride the ventricular septum.

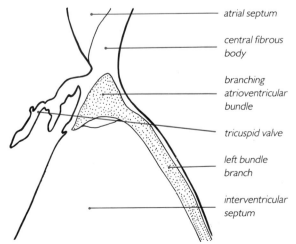

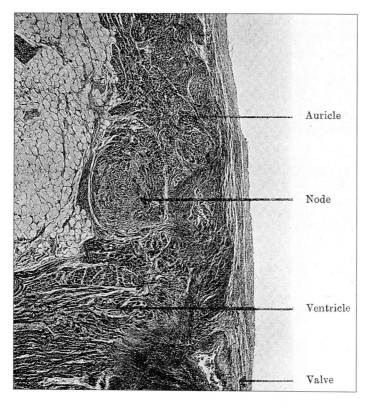

Auricle

Node

Ventricle

Valve

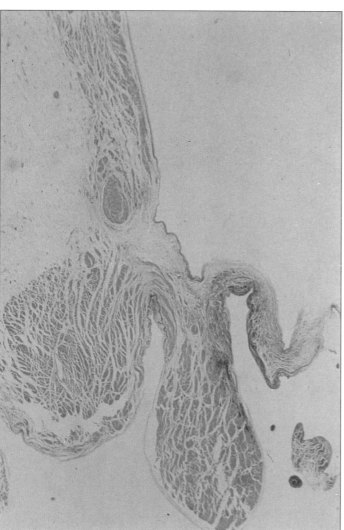

left bundle branch cascade down the septum as a continuous fan, forming an interweaving subendocardial sheet. The right bundle branch originates from the branching portion as a thin cord which enters the substance of the septomarginal trabeculation, tending to run beneath the medial papillary muscle complex. As they descend the ventricular septum, branches of both the right and left bundles are isolated by sheaths of fibrous tissue. They are composed of cells differentiated only minimally, in terms of size or staining affinities, from those of the ventricular myocardium. Consequently, when they lose their insulating fibrous sheath at the ventricular apices, it is not possible to trace the transitions which presumably occur between the conduction tissues and the working myocardium.

It is, however, possible to find remnants of conduction tissues elsewhere in the atrioventricular junction. These are present at the insertion of atrial myocardium into the anterosuperior and inferior leaflets of the tricuspid valve, particularly in the region of the aortic root (Fig. 1.96). Although bearing considerable resemblance to the tissues of the atrioventricular node, and to the tissues reported by Kent at the turn of the century, these remnants do not normally make contact with the ventricular myocardial tissues. It is also possible to find a continuation of the atrioventricular axis itself beyond its bifurcation. This becomes a dead-end tract in the subaortic outflow tract.

Nerves of the heart

The heart receives its supply of nerves from both the sympathetic and parasympathetic divisions of the autonomic nervous system. The precise supply of these different components to the various parts of the heart has yet to be fully determined, particularly in humans, as have the contributions of the so-called peptidergic system. Study of animal hearts shows a perplexing variability in patterns of innervation between different species, which highlights the danger of using results found in one species as the basis for conclusions drawn from experiments or results in another.

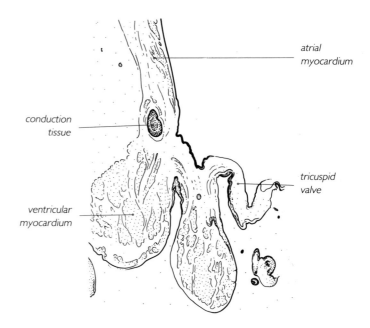

atrial myocardium

conduction tissue

tricuspid valve

ventricular myocardium

Fig. 1.96 This section, to the right, shows a remnant of atrioventricular ring conduction tissue, contrasting it with the structure illustrated by Kent (upper) at the turn of the century.

The parasympathetic nerves reach the heart through the large vagal nerves (Fig. 1.97) which carry both preganglionic fibres to the heart (their cell bodies being in the dorsal vagal nucleus), and sensory nerves from the heart (their cell bodies being in the nodose ganglions of the vagus). The nerves also carry fibres which supply many other organs. The fibres destined to supply the heart come from the nerves in both their cervical and thoracic course. The upper cervical branches of the vagus descend with cardiac branches of the sympathetic trunk to the deep part of the cardiac plexus. The lower cervical branches arise at the root of the neck and run along the branches of the aortic arch, and the arch itself, to the superficial part of the cardiac plexus. The thoracic cardiac branches arise from the vagus nerves as they descend alongside the trachea and are joined by cardiac branches from both recurrent laryngeal nerves to descend into the deep part of the cardiac plexus.

The sympathetic cardiac nerves originate from the superior, middle and inferior cervical ganglions of the sympathetic trunk, together with the upper five ganglions of the thoracic segment of the trunk (Fig. 1.98). They carry both efferent and afferent fibres, whilst the cervical and cardiac sympathetic branches descend through the mediastinum to join the cardiac plexus.

The cardiac plexus is the interconnecting network of nerves and ganglions found at the base of the heart, being formed by the cardiac branches of the vagal and sympathetic trunks. It is arbitrarily divided into superficial and deep parts, the two parts themselves being extensively linked. The superficial part of the plexus lies below the arch of the aorta in front of the right pulmonary artery and is mainly formed by branches from the left vagus and sympathetic trunks. The deep part of the plexus is found in front of the tracheal bifurcation, above the pulmonary bifurcation, but behind the aortic arch. The intrinsic cardiac plexuses run from the deep and superficial parts of the plexus to the coronary arteries, the conduction tissues, and to the musculature and covering membranes of the cardiac chambers themselves.

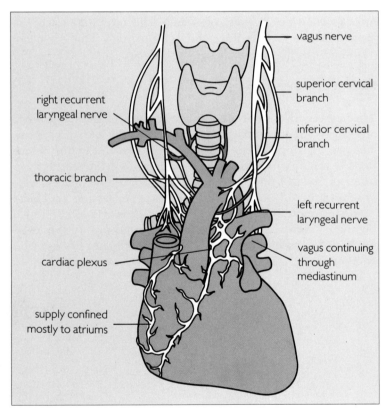

Fig. 1.97 This diagram shows how branches from the vagus nerves contribute to the cardiac plexus.

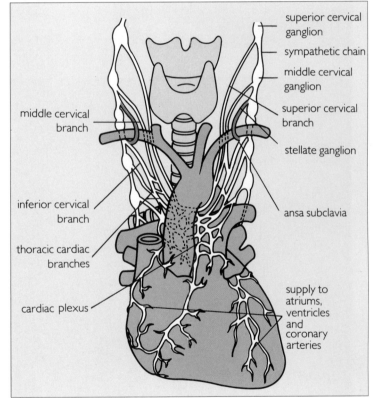

Fig. 1.98 This diagram shows the contributions of the sympathetic nerves to the cardiac plexus.

Structure, function and adaptation

2 STRUCTURE IN RELATION TO FUNCTION

The heart can be considered in terms of a mechanical pump, built of muscle and driven by electricity. Adequate function of the pump is guaranteed only by a balanced interaction between formation of the cardiac impulse, spread of excitation, excitation–contraction coupling and proper function of the cardiac valves (Fig. 2.1).

FORMATION OF THE IMPULSE AND SPREAD OF ACTIVATION

The sinus node (see Chapter 1) is the site of formation of the cardiac impulse. The discharge originates from a small cluster of cells, characterized by rhythmic spontaneous depolarization and composed of pacemaker cells (or typical nodal cells), which are poor in myofibrils but rich in glycogen. The impulse spreads from its site of initiation within the node towards the periphery. Within the node itself, the cellular characteristics change gradually from those of typical pacemaker cells, through so-called transitional cells, to those of typical working myocardial cells. The latter show a predominance of myofibrils and associated mitochondria, while transitional cells are made up of intracellular components which are truly transitional between pacemaker and working myocardial cells.

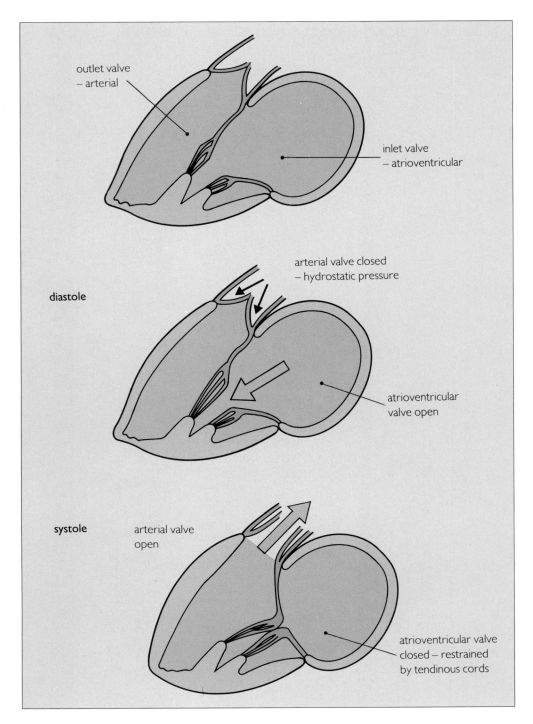

Fig. 2.1 These diagrams show how the heart can be considered in terms of a mechanical pump with inlet and outlet valves which alternate their opening and closing in systole and diastole.

outlet valve – arterial

inlet valve – atrioventricular

diastole

arterial valve closed – hydrostatic pressure

atrioventricular valve open

systole

arterial valve open

atrioventricular valve closed – restrained by tendinous cords

The predominant route of exit from the sinus node is to the terminal crest (see Chapter 1). The orientation of the muscle fibres within the crest, and its continuation with the atrial septal structures, is responsible for rapid spread of activation to the atrioventricular node (Fig. 2.2). Hence, so-called preferential conduction through the atrial musculature is a consequence of geometry rather than the presence of specialized and insulated tracts (such as exist for conduction to the ventricular myocardium).

The sinus node is richly innervated, and abnormalities in the input of the autonomic nervous system may be reflected as abnormal function of the sinus node. Likewise, there is rich vascular supply via atrial branches of the main coronary arteries, one of which is particularly prominent and designated as the 'sinus nodal artery'. The peripheral position of the sinus node, nevertheless, renders the tissues vulnerable to ischaemia in cases of obstructive coronary arterial disease (Fig. 2.3), or because of a steal phenomenon via collateral arteries (Fig. 2.4).

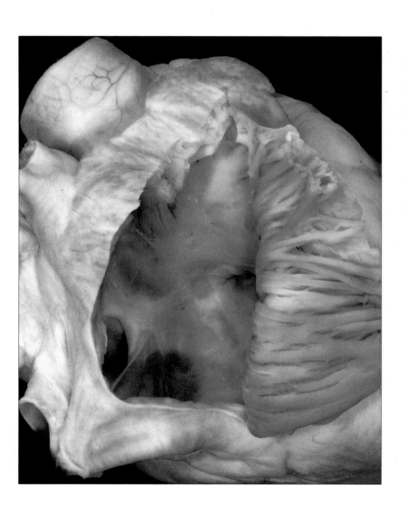

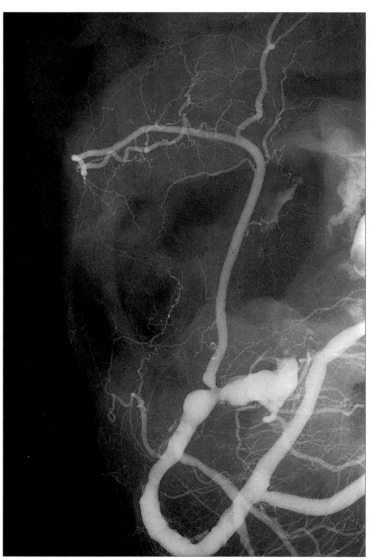

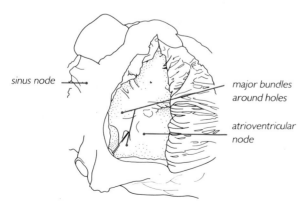

Fig. 2.2 This gross view of the right atrium, with a window created in the appendage, shows the position of the sinus node and the anatomy dictating preferential spread of activation towards the atrioventricular node.

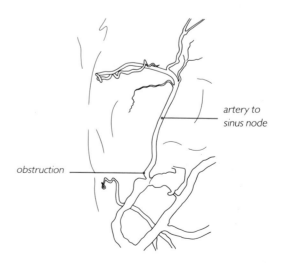

Fig. 2.3 This post-mortem coronary angiogram shows obstruction at the site of origin of the main atrial coronary artery that supplies the sinus node.

The atrioventricular node is located in the apex of the triangle of Koch (see Chapter 1). The architecture of the fibres within the central part of the atrioventricular node shows an interweaving pattern, which changes gradually towards a more longitudinal orientation within the penetrating atrioventricular bundle (Fig. 2.5). The architectural characteristics most likely underly the differences in conduction velocity between node and bundle. The precise relationships within the nodal area are variable, and largely dependant on the degree of development of the central fibrous body and its interaction with the nodal tissues. Deficiencies in the central fibrous body may create the potential for atriofascicular connections, which may interfere with regular ventricular excitation. Similarly, strands of nodal tissue dispersed within the central fibrous body (so-called fetal dispersion: Fig. 2.6), may create connections between node and bundle (so-called nodo-fascicular tracts), or between the axis of atrioventricular conduction tissue, on the one side, and ventricular myocardium on the other (so-called Mahaim connexions: Fig. 2.7).

Excitation–contraction coupling

The structure of working myocardial cells is tailored towards the transformation of chemical energy into mechanical processes. The sarcolemma shows invaginations into the cell, the so-called transverse tubular system (or T system), thus ensuring a large area of surface for interaction between extracellular substances and intracellular organelles. The sarcoplasmic reticulum forms a longitudinal system of branching tubers in close contact with the contractile proteins, and also has several sites of contact with the sarcolemma and the T-system. The contractile apparatus itself is composed of actin and myosin proteins, bundled in myofibrils, closely associated with mitochondria to provide the energy necessary for contraction.

Excitation–contraction coupling is essentially a reversal of the membrane potential, accompanied by ion exchanges across the membrane. An initial influx of calcium ions across the sarcolemma occurs by way of voltage dependent calcium

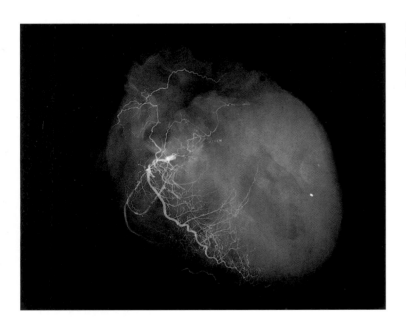

Fig. 2.4 This post-mortem coronary angiogram in the right coronary artery shows extensive obstructive disease of the main coronary arteries with filling of the left coronary arterial system through the network of atrial coronary arteries. This phenomenon could be responsible for a 'steal', thus underlying myocardial ischaemia and fibrosis.

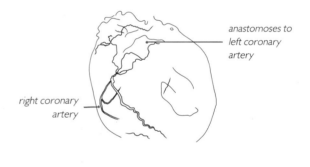

anastomoses to left coronary artery

right coronary artery

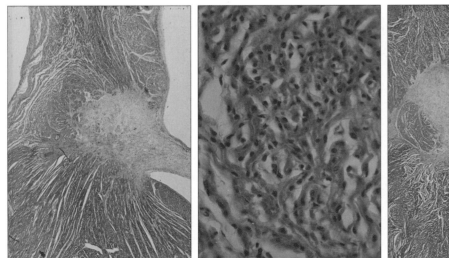

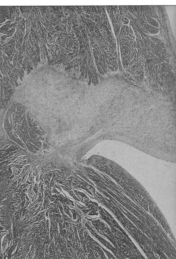

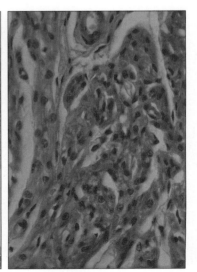

Fig. 2.5 These histological sections through the atrioventricular node (left hand pair) and the penetrating atrioventricular bundle (right hand pair) show the differences in orientation of the muscular fibres.

channels. These calcium ions function as a 'trigger' that releases further calcium ions from sub-sarcolemmal cisterns (dilatations of the sarcoplasmic reticulum). Free calcium ions in the cytosol then bind with a regulatory protein, a complex of troponin and tropomyosin, which is itself bound to actin. This induces a change in the sites of binding between troponin and tropomyosin, which then results in a sliding of the actin filaments between the myosin filaments and, hence, contraction. Relaxation occurs when calcium ions dissociate from the contractile apparatus. The mechanism of excitation–contraction coupling is modulated by calcium channels dependent upon receptors, of which the adrenergic receptors (ß-receptors), themselves dependent upon catecholamines, are the most important. Stimulation of these receptors enhances the release of activator calcium ions, thereby causing an increase in contractility of heart muscle.

The energy necessary for the interaction between actin and myosin is provided by adenosine triphosphate, regenerated in mitochondria from adenosine diphosphate. Phosphates rich in energy are stored mainly in the form of creatine phosphate.

A dysfunction in the chain of events underlying excitation–contraction coupling may eventually cause heart failure (see Chapter 3).

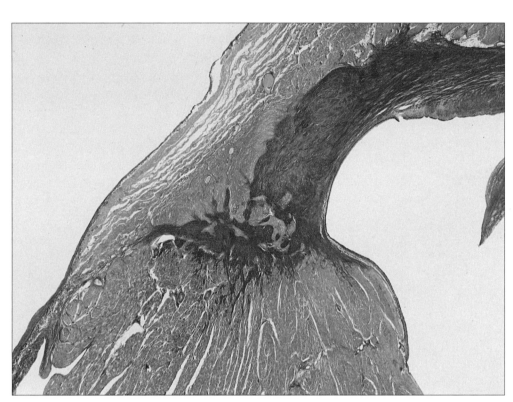

Fig. 2.6 This section through the atrioventricular node shows extensive dispersion of nodal tissue within the central fibrous body (so-called fetal dispersion).

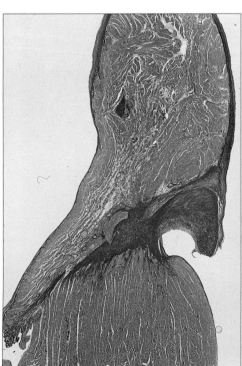 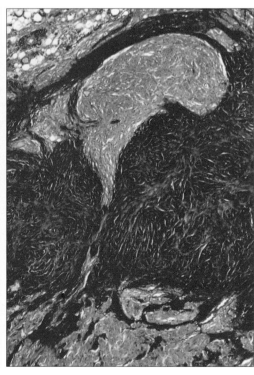

Fig. 2.7 This section, through the posterior aspect of the atrioventricular node, shows a narrow but prominent nodofascicular (or Mahaim) tract connecting the axis of atrioventricular conducton tissue to the ventricular myocardium. The left hand panel provides an overall view; the right hand panel shows the tract in more detail.

Myocardial integrity

The integrity of the myocardium to a large extent depends on a fine fibrillar meshwork of connective tissue that embraces individual myocytes. This extracellular matrix constitutes a tensile element that resists stretch and provides a restoring force that allows individual myocardial cells to return to their original length after contraction. A distinction is made between the endomysium, the perimysium and the epimysium (Fig. 2.8). The endomysium surrounds individual cells and is composed of meshwork of collagen fibres (weaves) which are connected by struts to the basal lamina of the myocytes. Neighbouring weaves are interconnected through single strands of collagen. Weaves and struts play an important role in safeguarding the integrity of the myocardium during myocardial diastole. The weaves are anchored in the perimysium, which connects groups of myocytes and is composed of coiled fibres of collagen which are arranged along the length of small groups of myocytes and are interconnected so as to inhibit myocardial overstretching during the phase of end-diastole. The coils also store energy during systole, providing, in this way, the basis for considering the heart as a suction pump. The epimysium then enwraps several of the bundles of myocardial cells grouped by the perimysium and is oriented parallel to the long axis of the muscle fibres. The overall extracellular matrix provides considerable strength to resist overdistension of the myocardium (see Chapter 3).

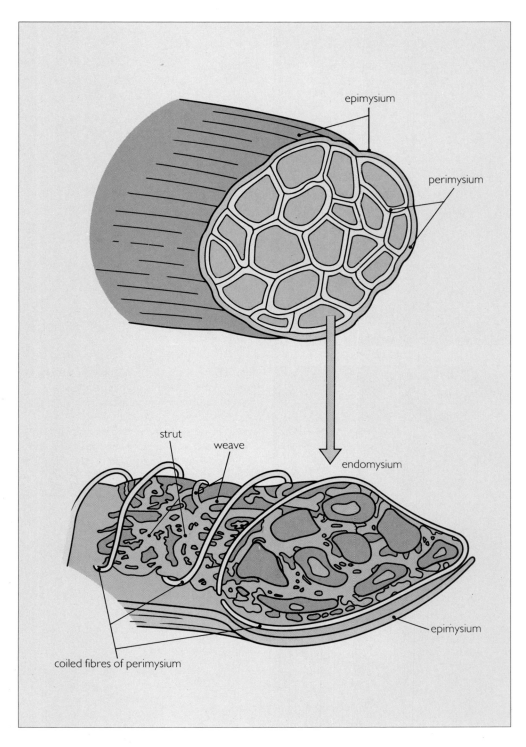

Fig. 2.8   This drawing highlights the relationship between the endomysium, the perimysium and the epimysium.

Function of cardiac valves

The function of the heart as a mechanical pump depends heavily on proper functioning of the valves (Fig. 2.1). From a functional view point, both the atrioventricular valves should be considered in terms of a valvar apparatus, composed of ventricular myocardium, papillary muscles, tendinous cords, valvar leaflets, valvar annulus (or atrioventricular junction), and atrial wall. Part, but not all, of the apparatus is dependent on adequate blood supply (the ventricular myocardium and papillary muscles) and this has important clinical relevance in cases of impaired myocardial perfusion (see Chapter 3).

The functioning of the arterial valves is far more simple (see Section 4), despite the rather complicated architecture, with a semilunar attachment of the valvar leaflets within the interlocking outflow tracts and arterial sinuses. Dilatation of the proximal parts of either the aorta or pulmonary trunk may affect valvar function, causing regurgitation, while the leaflets themselves may, initially, be unaffected (Fig. 2.9). From this point of view, therefore, arterial (semilunar) valves should also be considered in a broader sense than that dictated by the simple anatomy of the semilunar leaflets.

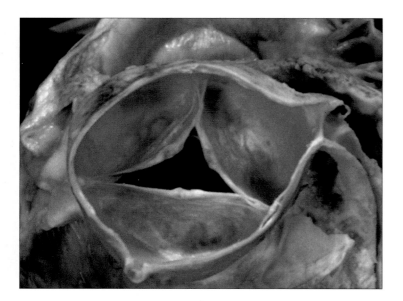

Fig. 2.9 This view of an aortic valve from above in a hypertensive patient shows how simple dilatation of the aortic root produces the substrate for regurgitation despite normal structure of the valvar leaflets.

3 ADAPTATION AND ITS COMPLICATIONS

Changes in the working conditions of the heart always evoke a response known as adaptation. Since, as we discussed in the previous section, the heart can be conceptualized in terms of a muscular pump driven by electricity, adaptive mechanisms must be anticipated to occur from the electrical side as well as from the mechanical side. The heart can adapt either its frequency of

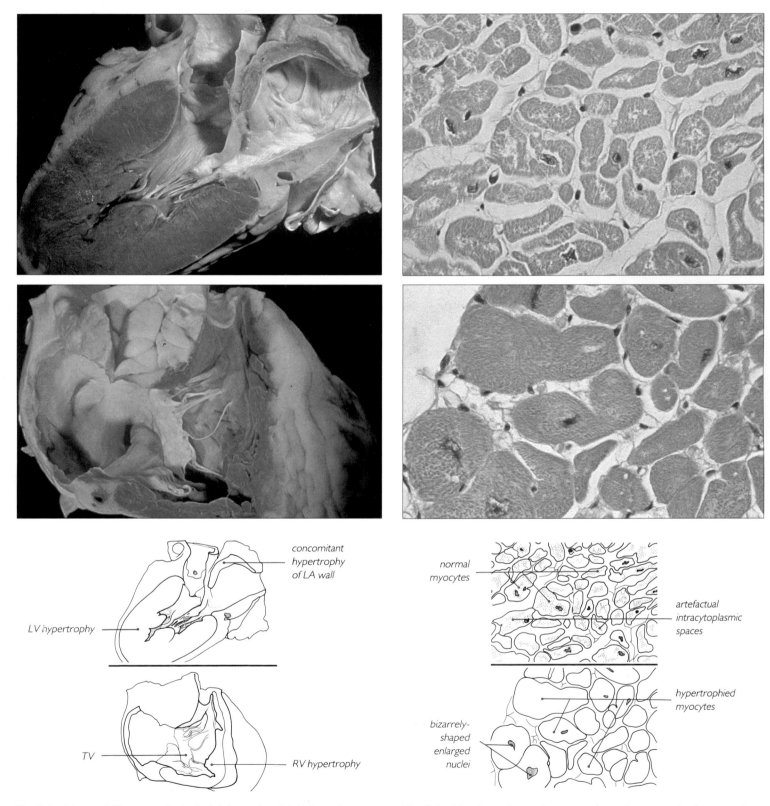

Fig. 3.1 Myocardial hypertrophy in the left (upper) and right (lower) ventricles.

Fig. 3.2 Histology of normal myocytes (upper) compared to hypertrophy (lower) at the same magnification. H&E stains.

contraction or its stroke volume and these adaptive phenomena are basically physiological in nature. Morphological changes come afterwards and consist of either hypertrophy of myocytes or dilatation of the chambers. The clinical significance of these morphological changes is determined largely by secondary consequences, which render the heart muscle vulnerable to ischaemia.

HYPERTROPHY

Hypertrophy of the heart is defined as an increase in the myocardial mass due to enlargement of the myocytes (Fig. 3.1), a process which is potentially reversible. The increase in volume of myocytes is mainly due to an increase in the amount of contractile proteins in the myofibrils (Fig. 3.2), together with an increased volume of the mitochondria providing the energy for contraction (Fig. 3.3). These adaptive changes produce an increased total demand for oxygen by the myocardium. Indeed, dilatation of the main coronary arteries (Fig. 3.4) occurs together with expansion of the capillary network, thus accommodating the increased demand for oxygen.

Hypertrophy may affect one, two, three or all four chambers, depending on the underlying cause. The mechanisms that initially lead to primary left ventricular hypertrophy may also, in time, cause hypertrophy of the right ventricle (see also Chapter 7), although the mechanisms by which isolated right ventricular hypertrophy may subsequently lead to left ventricular hypertrophy remain uncertain as yet. Hypertrophy of both right and left ventricles has a profound effect on the shape of the ventricular septum and, hence, on the geometry of the ventricular mass. Left ventricular hypertrophy causes a rightward convexity of the septum, accentuating the usual configuration and com-

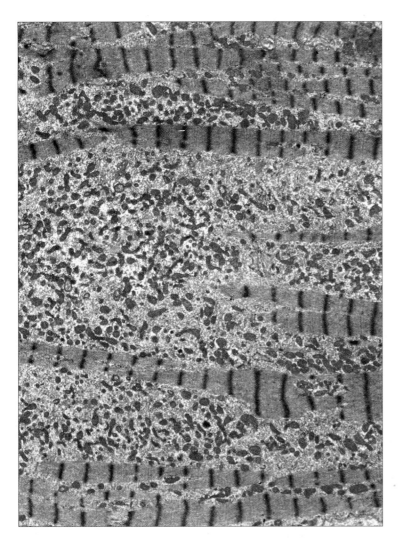

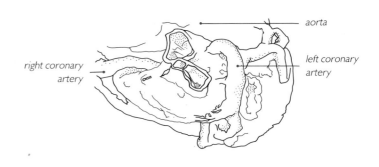

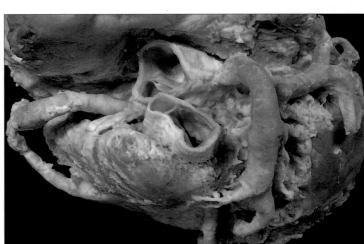

Fig. 3.3 Hypertrophied myocyte showing an increased number of mitochondria. EM, ×8500. By courtesy of Dr. K.P. Dingemans.

Fig. 3.4 Superior view of a heart shows the aorta and proximal parts of the main coronary arteries. These are dilated as an adaptive phenomenon to accommodate for an increased myocardial demand for oxygen consequent to myocardial hypertrophy.

promising the right ventricular cavity (Fig. 3.5). Right ventricular hypertrophy, in contrast, particularly when associated with dilatation, transforms the shape of the septum from its convex configuration to more of a straight shelf. This process, of necessity, has a marked effect on the geometry of the left ventricle (Fig. 3.6). A categorization of myocardial hypertrophy has been suggested on the basis of the condition which underscores the muscular changes.

Pressure load hypertrophy

This form occurs in response to exercise, particularly isometric exercise such as weight lifting. The commonest pathological conditions producing hypertrophy secondary to imposition of pressure load are, as far as the left ventricle is concerned, systemic hypertension, aortic valvar stenosis and aortic coarctation. The comparable lesions of the right ventricle are diseases

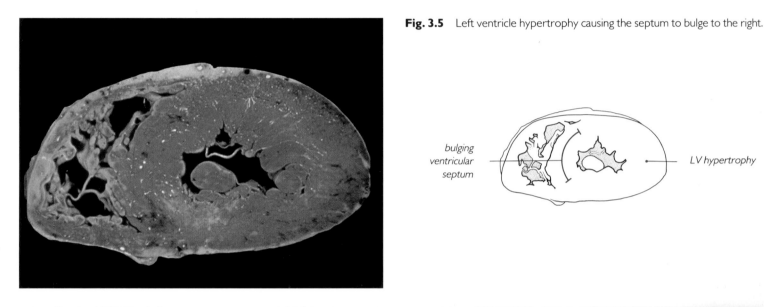

Fig. 3.5   Left ventricle hypertrophy causing the septum to bulge to the right.

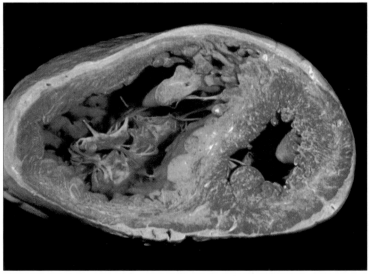

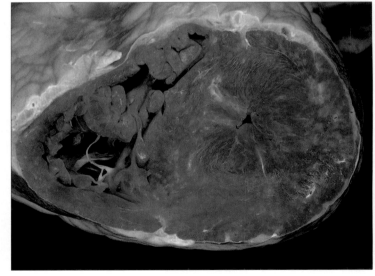

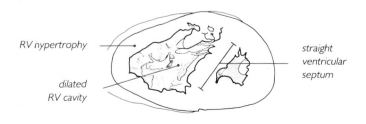

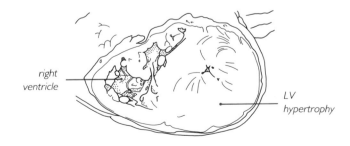

Fig. 3.6   Right ventricle hypertrophy causing the septum to assume an almost straight configuration.

Fig. 3.7   Cross section through a heart with marked left ventricular hypertrophy without enlargement of the chamber, known as 'concentric hypertrophy' and, in this instance, due to aortic stenosis.

of the left side of the heart with left heart failure, pulmonary disease causing an increase in pulmonary vascular resistance and pulmonary valvar stenosis.

The morphology of pressure load hypertrophy is characterized by an increase in the thickness of the wall without enlargement of the affected chamber (Fig. 3.7). This morphology, somewhat confusingly, has become known as 'concentric hypertrophy' although it is better considered as hypertrophy without dilatation. The thickness of the ventricular wall increases, thus increasing the volume of the myocytes. This counteracts the elevated systolic pressures and compensates, according to the law of Laplace, for the high stress within the wall during peak systole (Fig. 3.8).

Fig. 3.8 Laplace's law, when both hypertrophy and dilatation occur.

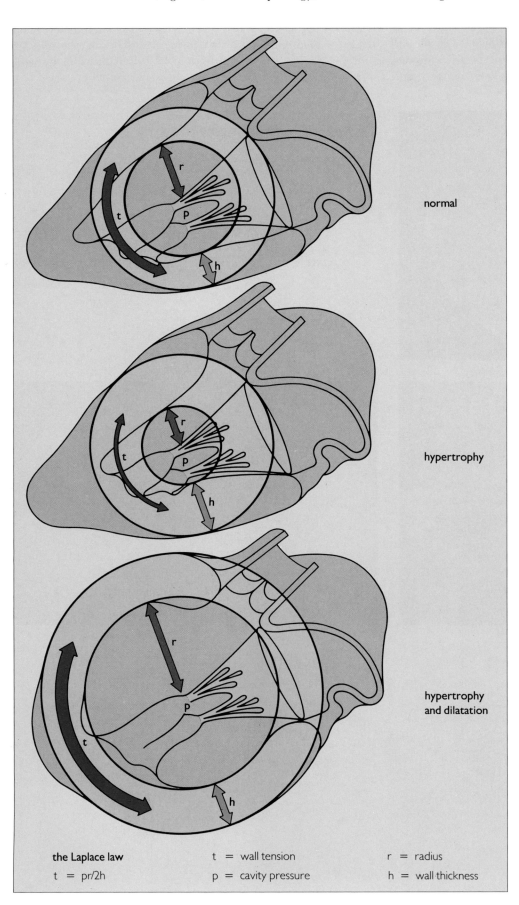

normal

hypertrophy

hypertrophy and dilatation

the Laplace law	t = wall tension	r = radius
t = pr/2h	p = cavity pressure	h = wall thickness

3.4

Volume load hypertrophy

This form of adaptive hypertrophy occurs in response to exercise, particularly in dynamic forms of conditioning as seen in athletes undertaking endurance sports. It also occurs under pathological circumstances, such as aortic and mitral valvar regurgitation with regard to the left ventricle, and pulmonary or tricuspid valvar insufficiency for the right.

The morphology of hypertrophy produced by a volume load is that of a thickened wall associated with an increase in volume of the chamber such that the overall ratio between volume and wall thickness remains unaltered (Fig. 3.9). The term 'eccentric hypertrophy' has been introduced for this morphology, in contrast to the concentric hypertrophy produced by pressure loading. The concept of eccentric hypertrophy is extremely confusing, since it can easily be confused with the asymmetrical variant of hypertrophy observed in hypertrophic cardiomyopathy. Indeed, the hypertrophy due to volume loading is itself symmetrical and, from this point of view, is just as concentric as that produced by pressure loading. It is much simpler, and more accurate, to describe the hypertrophy produced by volume loading as being associated with dilatation of the ventricular chamber.

Fig. 3.9 Cross section through a heart with marked left ventricular hypertrophy with some dilatation of the chamber to the extent that the overall ratio between volume and wall thickness remains unaltered, known as 'eccentric hypertrophy'.

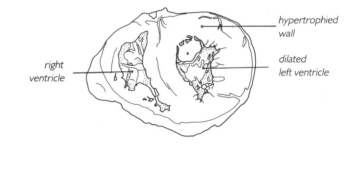

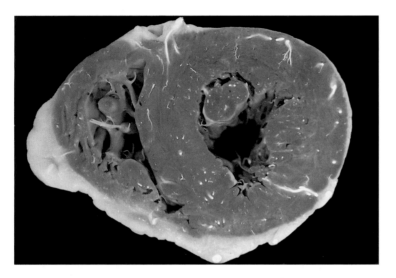

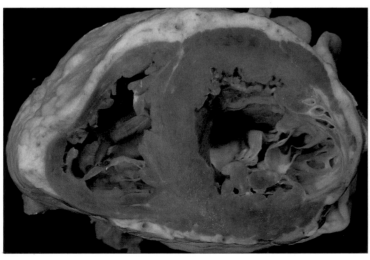

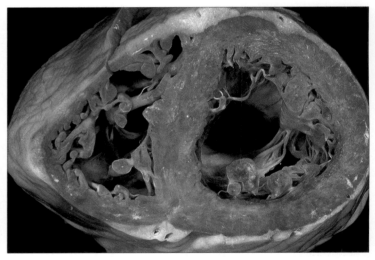

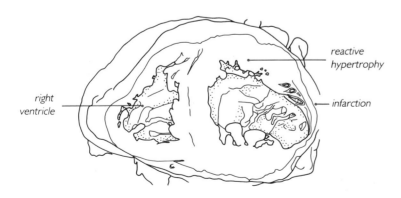

Fig. 3.10 Cross section through a heart shows reactive hypertrophy of left ventricular myocardium following infarction of the left ventricular lateral wall.

Fig. 3.11 An acutely dilated left ventricle.

The myocytes show an increase in volume, mainly due to an increase in their length, which counteracts the increased wall stress produced during end diastole and thus allows for the essential volume increase (Fig. 3.8). The integrity of the extracellular matrix is also essential to prevent spatial disorganization of the myocardial cells.

Reactive hypertrophy

This form of hypertrophy, also known as 'remodelling', is seen after myocardial infarction (Fig. 3.10). Hypertrophy of the remaining viable myocardium compensates for the loss of the infarcted area, if at all possible, in a fashion proportional to the amount of loss of myocardium in the infarcted zone. The ability to hypertrophy, however, is largely determined by the effects of the underlying coronary arterial vascular obstructive disease and, depending on the extent of the myocardial infarction, the ventricle may have to cope with chronic volume overload.

DILATATION

In cases of a sudden volume overload, the heart will dilate instantly (Fig. 3.11). Depending on the cause of the volume overload, the initial dilatation may resolve, may remain in the setting of an adjusted haemodynamic level or, ultimately, may end up as volume overload with impaired haemodynamics. The combination of overload with impaired haemodynamics corresponds with the clinical condition of 'heart failure'.

Heart failure in clinical terms can be defined as the situation in which the heart is no longer capable of maintaining an adequate circulation. Such failure ensues as soon as parts of the pump are damaged, or once the balance between the various functional processes is disturbed, and the adaptive mechanisms discussed above are no longer capable of compensating for the damaging effects. Many diseases may lead to failure of the heart. These include abnormal formation and conduction of the cardiac impulse (such as ventricular extrasytoles and tachycardias); diseases of the heart muscle itself (such as myocardial infarction and myocarditis); and abnormalities of the heart valves (such as valvar stenosis or insufficiency). Whatever the disease, the basic mechanism causing inadequate myocardial function occurs at the molecular level. The brief outline of the various biochemical processes associated with excitation–contraction coupling (see Chapter 2) shows that a variety of mishaps may disturb the chain of events that should lead to contraction. Of all the possibilities, abnormal handling of intracellular calcium ions is of most significance (Fig. 3.12). The evidence in favour of this mechanism is based mainly on animal experiments, which have shown that a reduction in the quantity of calcium ions available for activation of the contractile proteins plays an important role in a condition known as the 'stunned myocardium'. 'Stunning' is defined as an acute depression of contraction of the myocardium, lasting at least for a few hours to days, following temporary occlusion of the coronary artery. Several observations in man endorse the concept of an abnormal handling of intracellular calcium ions as a major feature in heart failure. A deficiency in the production of cyclic adenosine monophosphate has been demonstrated, which could indicate a change in those calcium channels in the membranes which are dependent upon receptors. Moreover, in heart failure, the β_1-adrenergic receptors are 'down regulated', while the density of a-adrenergic receptors does not change significantly. This has led to the assumption that a positive inotropic response mediated by a-receptors plays an important role in maintaining contractility of the failing heart.

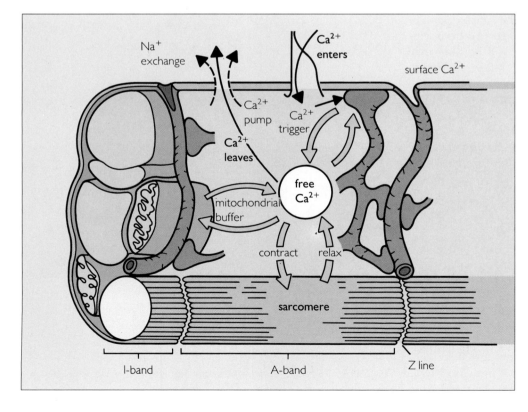

Fig. 3.12 This drawing shows the potential sites of abnormal handling of intracellular calcium which may underscore heart failure.

ADAPTATION TO HEART FAILURE

Once heart failure occurs, a chain of events is initiated which should be considered in terms of adaptive or compensatory mechanisms of the circulatory system. Indeed, these effects will dominate the clinical picture of heart failure, particularly since the mechanisms initiated will, eventually, lose their beneficial effects and become harmful.

Several systems are involved in the adaptive mechanisms. The heart will show dilatation of chambers, thus accounting for an increased volume (Fig. 3.13). This will enhance the stroke volume so that, at rest, cardiac output is not necessarily diminished. The heart muscle will adapt by hypertrophy in order to counteract the increase in end-diastolic pressure. This adaptive phenomenon, nevertheless, induces an increase in the total demand for oxygen by the heart muscle. This enhances the risk of myocardial ischaemia in a setting where maintenance of an adequate circulation is compromised because of the failing pump.

Heart failure will also stimulate the cardiopulmonary baroreceptors, thus introducing adaptive mechanisms initiated through the sympathetic and parasympathetic nervous systems. In longlasting situations of heart failure, the level of response of the baroreceptors, and the activities of the autonomic nerves with respect to changes in pressure and volume, will be upregulated, thereby diminishing the intended modulating effects.

The most important adaptive changes occur outside the heart, and are all part of the essential homeostatic mechanisms that regulate perfusion of vital organs (Fig. 3.14). Early in the process of heart failure, the kidneys will diminish the excretion of sodium and water, most likely as a response to diminished cardiac output. Activation of the adrenergic system causes vasoconstriction at several peripheral sites, such as the kidneys and the intestines. The renin-angiotensin system is also activated, most likely because of arterial hypotension.

At the basis of these secondary compensatory mechanisms is the fact that the failing heart is unable to maintain an adequate circulation and, therefore, to meet the demand for energy imposed by the tissues and organs. The circulation becomes insufficient in latent heart failure only when the consumption of energy is increased, for instance during stress. In all other forms of heart failure, the functional parameters will be abnormal under all circumstances. Inadequacies in circulation will lead to processes which may become evident clinically as congestion of the venous system (backward failure) or insufficient filling of the arterial system (forward failure). Both will lead to adaptation, which will mask for as long as possible the effect of the underlying heart failure on the vital organs. Eventually, however, the heart will no longer be able to cope with the 'compensatory' expansion of volume. Progressive and irreversible heart failure will then ensue (Fig. 3.15).

COMPLICATIONS CONSEQUENT TO MYOCARDIAL ADAPTATION

As previously discussed, the increase in muscle mass of the heart translates into an increase in demand for oxygen. Once other mechanisms occur that may jeopardize the supply of oxygen or, otherwise, may lead to a further increase in oxygen demand, the scene is set for ischaemic complications. This is particularly so in cases of the combined occurrence of hypertrophy and dilatation, especially when associated with an increase in volume no longer proportional to the increase in mural thickness. The transmural

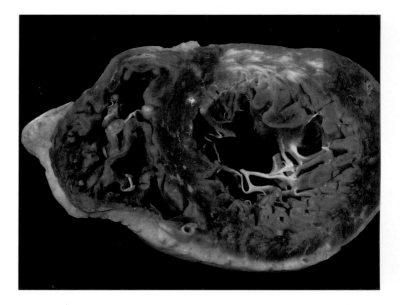

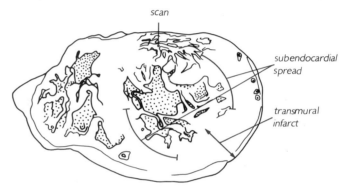

Fig. 3.13 Cross section through a heart shows a regional transmural infarct with subendocardial spread, consequent to dilatation of the left ventricular cavity and impaired transmural coronary arterial perfusion.

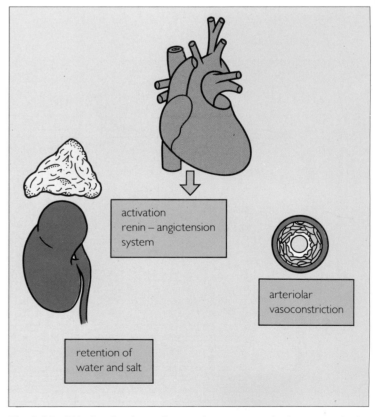

Fig. 3.14 This drawing shows the most important mechanisms operative in regulating perfusion of vital organs as a consequence of chronic heart failure.

perfusion pressure in these circumstances may be affected significantly, leading to potentially impaired perfusion of the subendocardial myocardial layers. This phenomenon becomes prevalent once volume overload and hypertrophy coexist with obstructive coronary arterial disease (Fig. 3.16). Once ischaemia of the subendocardial myocardial layers is present, this may further impair the effectiveness of the myocardial pump, hence introducing a vicious cycle leading to further myocardial damage. It is not uncommon for this train of events to end in a rapidly spreading and circumferential subendocardial myo-

cardial infarction which irrevocably terminates in irreversible and rapidly progressive left heart failure. The whole process may be aggravated by other secondary consequences of ventricular dilatation, such as atrioventricular valve dysfunction. Once dilatation of a ventricle has occurred, whether diffusely or focally, the integrity of the valvar apparatus may be distorted. Such dysfunction of the papillary muscles then leads to further accentuation of the ventricular dilatation, and further impairment of effective cardiac output.

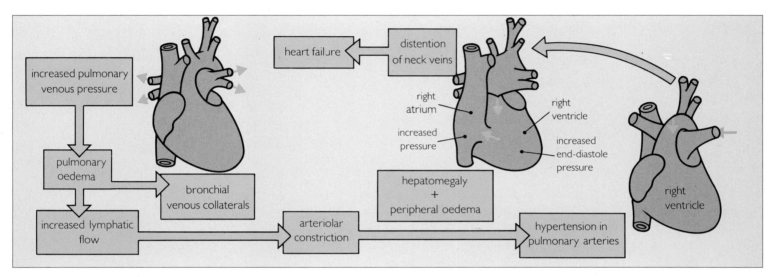

Fig. 3.15 This drawing demonstrates the effects of failure of the left heart as they become clinically evident.

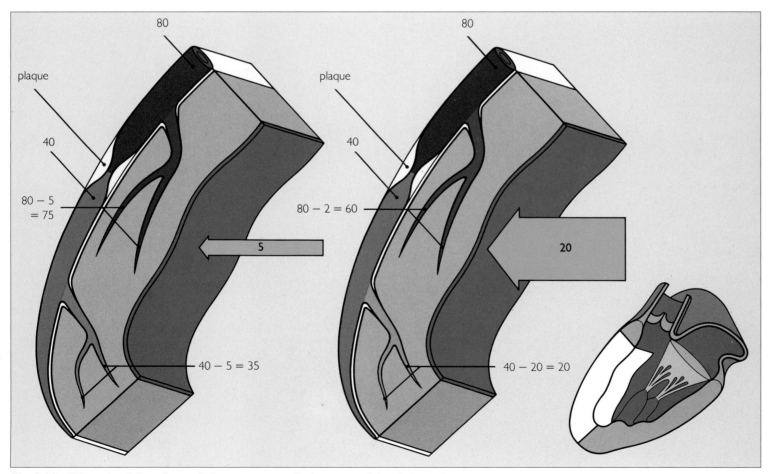

Fig. 3.16 Effects of end-diastolic ventricular pressure on effective myocardial perfusion in the presence of an obstructive coronary arterial lesion. A rise of cavity pressure from 5 to 20mmHg reduces perfusion pressure distal to the obstruction from 35 to 20mmHg.

The pulmonary vasculature

INTERACTION BETWEEN HEART AND LUNGS   **4**

4   INTERACTION BETWEEN HEART AND LUNGS

Cardiac pathology cannot be studied without consideration of the lungs. Like all other organs, the lungs receive a systemic arterial supply through the bronchial arteries for their own nutrition, but the main vascular circuit is that supplied by the pulmonary arteries for the purpose of oxygenation of the blood. In this respect, the lungs are unique in receiving, at least in the postmature state, the total volume of blood ejected by one ventricle. Desaturated blood is conveyed through an extensive network of arteries and arterioles into capillaries which are intimately related to the alveolar spaces. It is in the alveoli that the necessary exchange of oxygen and carbon dioxide takes place. The oxygenated and purified blood is recollected in pulmonary venules and veins which eventually drain into the left atrium (Fig. 4.1), and it is because of the position of the pulmonary vascular circuit, which is interposed between the right and left sides of the heart, that one cannot be studied without the other.

The pulmonary vasculature is usually confronted with a flow of blood far in excess of that in comparative segments of the systemic circulation although the pressures are much lower. Consequently, the pulmonary vessels tend to be wider in diameter but are thin-walled compared to similar-sized systemic arteries. Normal post-mortem pulmonary angiograms show extensive arborization of the arterial tree (Fig. 4.2, left).

Cardiac abnormalities, be they acquired or congenital, whether they affect contractility or result in primary volume or pressure overload, all have an impact on the pulmonary circulation. On the other hand, primary parenchymal lung diseases, such as chronic bronchitis, emphysema and interstitial fibrosis, also alter the pulmonary vascular bed and, hence, may affect the heart.

In general, the pulmonary vasculature responds by either increasing or decreasing the pulmonary vascular resistance. Such functional alterations may initially be part of a general adaptive mechanism and, as such, are potentially reversible although morphological changes may eventually ensue, some of which may then progress to irreversible pulmonary vascular obstructive disease.

CARDIAC DISEASE AFFECTING THE LUNG

Many cardiac abnormalities affect the pulmonary vasculature, either directly or indirectly. Typical of this are the pulmonary vascular changes evoked by congenital heart disease. An initial increase in flow can occur, and is occasionally accompanied by a rise in pressure, and sometimes the flow may decrease. This mainly affects the arterial segment of the pulmonary circuit, although venous congestion may also occur in congenital heart disease, as well as in many different types of acquired pathology of the left heart. Almost all conditions that primarily affect either contractility or pressure/volume load of the chambers of the left heart may lead to pulmonary venous congestion and, eventually, to secondary abnormalities in both the veins and the arteries.

thin-walled
muscular PA

Fig. 4.1 Diagram of the pulmonary vascular bed interposed between the right and left heart.

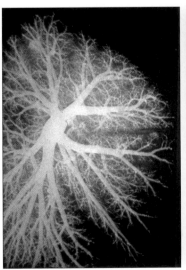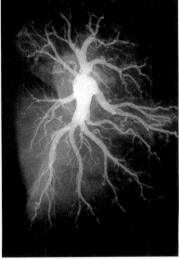

Fig. 4.2 Postmortem angiogram showing usual filling of vessels; (right) 'winter tree' indicative of obstructive pulmonary vascular disease.

Primarily increased pulmonary flow

Left-to-right shunts can occur within the heart, through atrial or ventricular septal defects, for example, as well as outside the heart through a patent arterial duct, a common arterial trunk, an aortopulmonary window or via anomalous pulmonary venous connexions. Shunts at the 'pre-tricuspid' level lead primarily to a volume load of the circuit through the right ventricle and pulmonary arteries, whereas post-tricuspid shunts add to this high left ventricular pressures. As a consequence, structural changes of the pulmonary vascular bed occur more frequently, and at an earlier age, in post- rather than in pre-tricuspid shunts (Fig. 4.3).

The pulmonary vascular changes thus initiated are collectively termed 'plexogenic pulmonary arteriopathy'. This term encompasses a spectrum of the structural alterations of pulmonary arteries that share the plexiform lesion as their end point. Plexogenic pulmonary arteriopathy occurs not only in congenital heart disease with left-to-right shunts, but also in patients with so-called primary pulmonary hypertension.

Post-mortem pulmonary angiograms show that blockage in the pulmonary vascular bed mainly occurs because of occlusion of the medium and small-sized pulmonary arteries. This feature underlies the classical 'winter tree' appearance of the pulmonary arterial vasculature (Fig. 4.2, right).

Early changes

The early change is usually described as medial hypertrophy of muscular pulmonary arteries (Fig. 4.4, left), although in the early phase of pulmonary hypertension, due to a left-to-right shunt, the muscular coat may extend peripherally onto arterioles which, under normal circumstances, do not contain an appreciable muscular layer. This phenomenon is known as muscularization, and is probably due to increased flow (Fig. 4.4, right). The changes of muscularization and medial hypertrophy are both considered to be reversible.

When analyzing these early changes in the setting of congenital heart disease, it is also necessary to take account of the number of pulmonary arteries, as some congenital cardiac malformations, such as ventricular and atrioventricular septal defects, are associated with a decreased number of arteries accompanying the alveolar ducts. This finding could explain why, in some instances, successful surgical repair is not accompanied by the anticipated drop in pulmonary vascular resistance.

Although the early changes have been described as occurring in the intra-acinar arteries, it has been shown that, in some instances, early obstructive lesions occur more proximally, affecting arteries at the pre-acinar level. This should be noted when lung biopsies are evaluated.

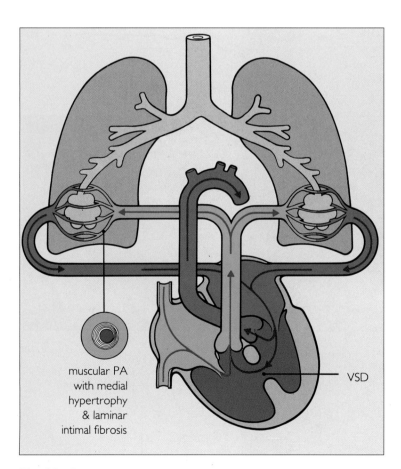

Fig. 4.3   Diagram of the relationship between heart and lungs in the presence of septal defect.

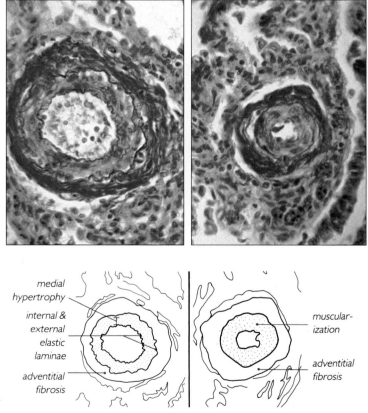

Fig. 4.4   Histology of medial hypertrophy of a muscular pulmonary artery (left). The abnormal musculature extends into the pulmonary arterioles (right). E-VG stain.

Cellular intimal proliferation

This change affects the intimal layers of muscular arteries and arterioles, narrowing the lumen (Fig. 4.5) by proliferation of smooth muscle cells (Fig. 4.6). The degree and extent of cellular intimal proliferation may vary from site to site. The change is potentially reversible, and should not be used as an argument against surgical repair, despite the fact that a fair proportion of arteries thus affected may show virtual obliteration of their lumens. Indeed, there is good evidence that these early proliferative lesions, even when they contain some collagen, may regress to a stage where they have no clinical significance.

Intimal fibrosis

Fibrosis of the intima is generally considered as a more advanced form of cellular intimal proliferation. It consists of deposition of collagen, among which cellular elements can often still be recognized (Fig. 4.7). In 'older' lesions, the deposition of collagen may predominate, often taking on a concentric appearance (Fig.

4.8). On occasions, particularly in patients with congenital left-to-right shunts, the intimal proliferation may also contain condensed elastic fibres (Fig. 4.9).

In general, intimal fibrosis tends to develop in concentric fashion, often showing centripetal stages of maturation (Fig. 4.10). In other instances, a concentric layering of collagen may lead to so-called 'onion-skinning' (Fig. 4.11), a clinically important phenomenon which seems to reflect a rapidly progressive change and which occurs predominantly in patients with so-called primary pulmonary hypertension.

Intimal fibrosis may vary considerably in degree and extent. In some areas, arteries may be almost completely occluded whereas, at other sites, the changes may be minimal or even absent. When making a functional evaluation, therefore, it is necessary to examine the overall picture. This is particularly important since intimal fibrosis is considered to be basically irreversible, although there is strong evidence that further progression of such lesions may be arrested following the repair of the underlying cardiac anomaly.

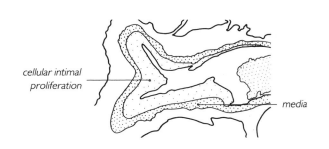

Fig. 4.5 Histological sections showing cellular intimal proliferation at a site of dichotomy in a muscular artery. E-VG stain.

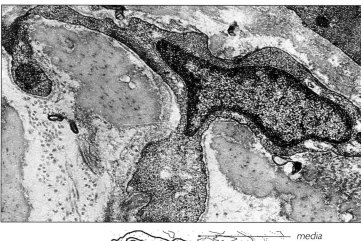

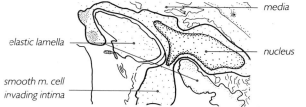

Fig. 4.6 Smooth muscle cell invading the intima through a gap in the inner elastic lamella, EM, × 15,900. By courtesy of Dr A.G. Balk, from *Virchows Archiv, A Pathological Anatomy and Histology*, **382**, 139–150, 1979 (Heidelberg: Springer-Verlag).

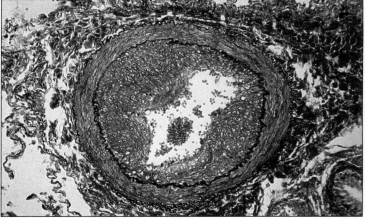

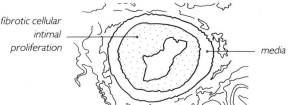

Fig. 4.7 Histological section showing intimal fibrosis intermingling with cellular proliferation. E-VG stain.

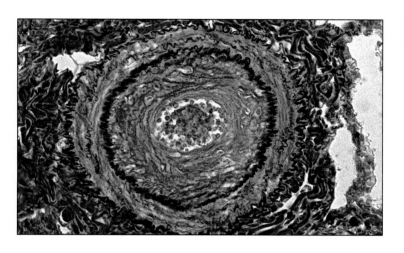

Fig. 4.8 Histological section showing intimal fibrosis composed of concentric layers of dense collagen. E-VG stain.

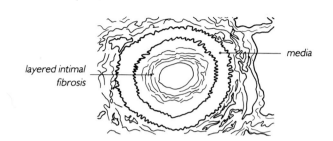

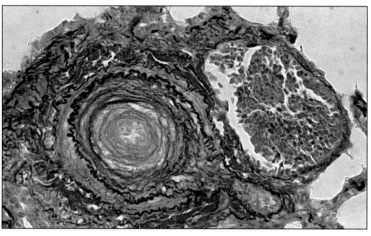

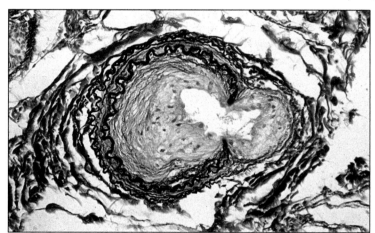

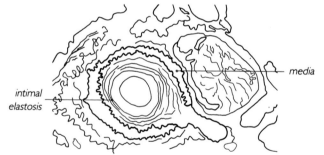

Fig. 4.9 Histological section showing intimal elastosis. E-VG stain.

Fig. 4.10 Histological section showing intimal fibrosis with centripetal maturation. E-VG stain.

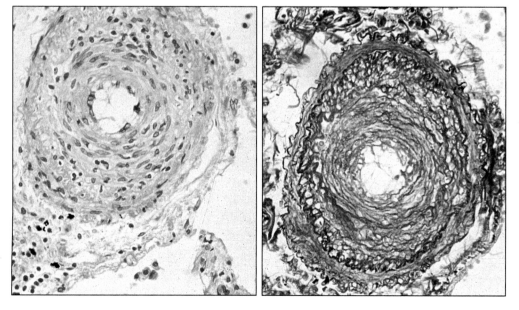

Fig. 4.11 Histological sections of a muscular artery with 'onion-skinning', demonstrating cellularity (left) and concentric fibrotic layers (right). H&E (left), E-VG (right) stains.

'Cushion-like' intimal fibrosis may occur as a feature of plexogenic pulmonary arteriopathy, although it is usually limited to the branching points of arteries (Fig. 4.12) and consequently must be distinguished from organized thrombosis (see Fig. 4.26).

Plexiform lesions

Plexiform lesions consist of a widely dilated segment of a pulmonary artery, usually found just beyond a branching point. The arterial wall is thinner at this point, and the cavity is occupied by proliferating cells packed around slit-like luminal spaces (Fig. 4.13). The proliferating cells resemble those present in early cellular intimal lesions. Often they are glued together with fibrinoid material, which adds to the complexity of the histological picture. The artery continues beyond the plexus as a widely dilated, tortuous and extremely thin-walled channel. The lesion probably develops on the basis of fibrinoid necrosis. Plexiform lesions are considered irreversible and, when found, indicate a grave prognosis.

Dilatation lesions

These changes are characterized by the presence of thin-walled tortuous and dilated vessels as in the plexiform lesion, but the intraluminal plexus is absent (Fig. 4.14). The lesions are indicative of a well advanced and irreversible state of plexogenic pulmonary arteriopathy, although care is needed if they are not to be misinterpreted as congested veins.

Fibrinoid arteritis

This change is characterized by fibrinoid necrosis of a segment of an arterial wall and is usually accompanied by a cellular intimal proliferation as described above. Occasionally, however, fibrinoid necrosis may be accompanied by an inflammatory cellular infiltrate (Fig. 4.15), and under these circumstances, the fibrinoid lesion must be distinguished from septic emboli. The distinction is usually easy, since fibrinoid arteritis represents a well-advanced state of plexogenic pulmonary arteriopathy and,

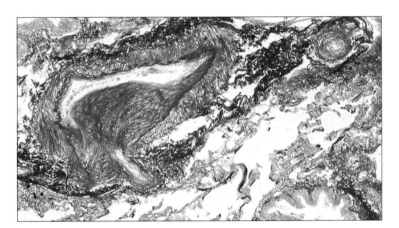

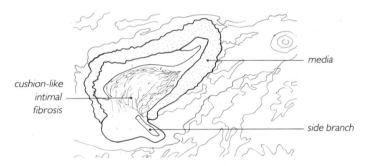

Fig. 4.12 Histological section showing cushion-like intimal fibrosis at the site of a branching point. E-VG stain.

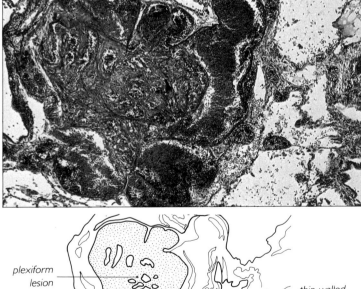

Fig. 4.13 Histological section showing a plexiform lesion. E-VG stain.

Fig. 4.14 Histological section showing a dilatation lesion in the absence of any plexiform change. E-VG stain. By courtesy of Prof C.A. Wagenvoort.

hence, is nearly always associated with various other advanced obliterative changes. Indeed, fibrinoid arteritis is considered the forerunner of the plexiform lesion (see above).

Bronchial compression

The congenital cardiac malformations which permit a significant left-to-right shunt may also produce dilatation of pulmonary arteries under such markedly increased pressures that they induce bronchial compression. Bronchial compression may also complicate anomalies which have unusual vascular relations, or those which produce widely dilated pulmonary arteries with low pressures, such as occur when tetralogy of Fallot is associated with the absence of the leaflets of the pulmonary valve.

The normal anatomy of the pulmonary arteries relative to the tracheobronchial tree is such that the right pulmonary artery, beyond its ramification into the right upper lobar artery, crosses over the intermediate bronchial segment and descends posteriorly to the right middle lobar branches (Fig. 4.16, lower left). Consequently, the intermediate segment and the right middle lobar bronchus may become compressed by dilatation of the right pulmonary artery (Fig. 4.17). On the left side, the main pulmonary artery itself crosses over the main stem of the left bronchus, using the base of the left upper lobe as a hinge (Fig. 4.16, lower right). Dilatation of the left pulmonary artery, therefore, may thus compromise the main stem of the left bronchus as well as the origin of the left upper lobe (Fig. 4.17). Bronchial compression may lead to dyspnoea, and may also be accompanied by either hyperinflation or atelectasis of the affected lung segments.

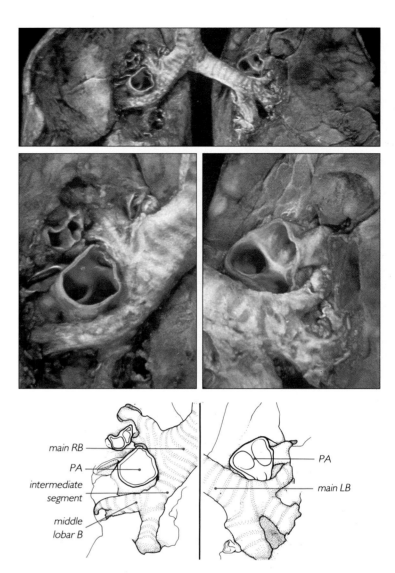

Fig. 4.16 Topography of the right and left branches of the pulmonary trunk with respect to the tracheobronchial tree. Overall view (upper); details of right and left bronchial anatomy (lower, left & right).

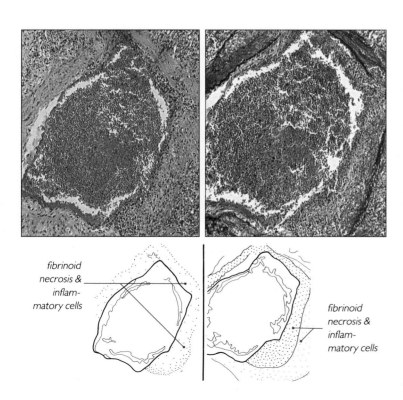

Fig. 4.15 Histological sections of a muscular artery with fibrinoid necrosis. H&E (left), E-VG (right) stains.

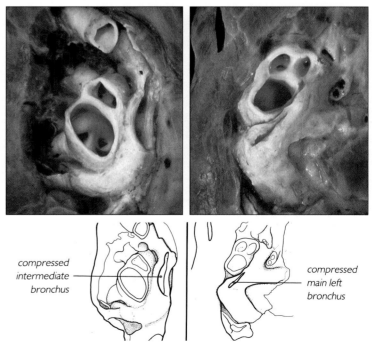

Fig. 4.17 Bronchial compression of the morphologically right (left) and morphologically left bronchus (right) due to dilatation of the pulmonary arteries.

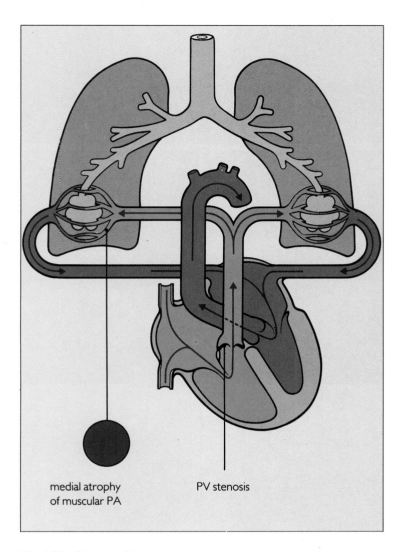

Fig. 4.18 Diagram of the pulmonary vascular consequences of decreased pulmonary flow in valvar pulmonary stenosis.

Primary decreased pulmonary flow

The conditions that produce a decrease in pulmonary flow are also usually congenital in nature (Fig. 4.18), with Fallot's tetralogy as the paradigm (see Chapter 6). The pulmonary vascular bed shows generalized atrophy of the vessel walls (Fig. 4.19). Elastic-type arteries take a tortuous course and have thin walls containing wavy elastic lamellae. The muscular pulmonary arteries are extremely thin-walled and often have no media (Fig. 4.20).

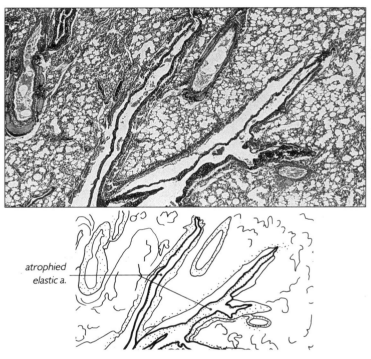

Fig. 4.19 Histology of lung showing generalized atrophy of vessel walls due to decreased pulmonary flow. E-VG stain.

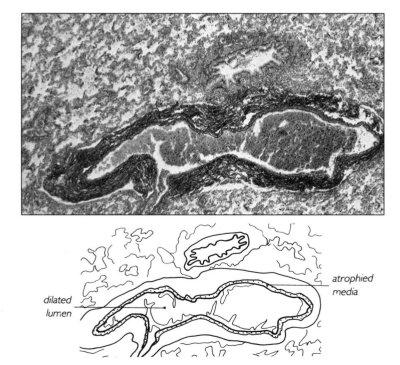

Fig. 4.20 Histological section of a muscular artery which is extremely dilated and thin-walled. E-VG stain.

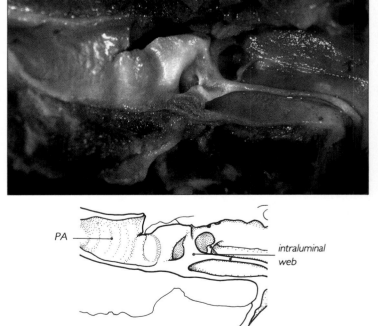

Fig. 4.21 Pulmonary artery containing a fibrous intraluminal web.

The condition of decreased pulmonary flow, often aggravated by an increased haemotocrit, enhances spontaneous intravascular thrombosis which, through a process of organization, may eventually lead to production of fibrous bands or webs within the arterial lumens. These can be detected with the naked eye in the vessels of larger calibre (Fig. 4.21), but microscopical examination is needed in the smaller-sized arteries (Fig. 4.22). Only rarely will these webs impede pulmonary flow.

Pulmonary venous congestion

Almost all conditions that affect the systemic side of the heart, either congenital or acquired, may eventually lead to pulmonary venous congestion. The changes set in motion by either mitral stenosis or insufficiency serve as an example (Fig. 4.23). The lung shows congested and dilated veins, often accompanied by dilated lymphatics and oedema of intralobular septums (Fig. 4.24). The flow through bronchial veins is particularly increased

Fig. 4.22 Section through a small pulmonary artery containing a fibrous web. E-VG stain.

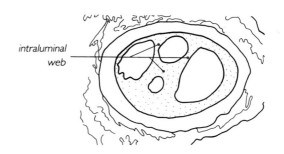

intraluminal web

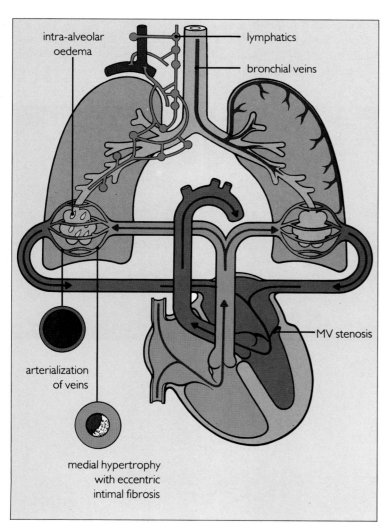

intra-alveolar oedema

lymphatics

bronchial veins

arterialization of veins

MV stenosis

medial hypertrophy with eccentric intimal fibrosis

Fig. 4.23 Diagram of the haemodynamic consequence of pulmonary venous hypertension in a case of mitral stenosis. The enlarged lymphatics are shown in the right lung and the dilated bronchial veins in the left lung.

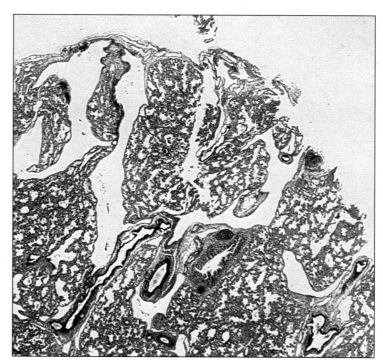

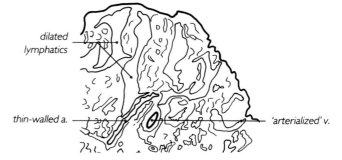

dilated lymphatics

thin-walled a.

'arterialized' v.

Fig. 4.24 Histological section of lung showing dilated veins and lymphatics with oedema of intralobular septa. E-VG stain.

in diseases of the mitral valve, probably as an expression of bronchopulmonary venous anastomoses. It is bleeding from these structures into the bronchioles which explains the haemoptysis that may occur in these patients. In longstanding cases, fibrosis of alveolar septums may occur.

If unchecked, the congestion can progress to produce intra-alveolar oedema, which then leads to the classical clinical signs and symptoms of left heart failure, with structural alterations appearing in longstanding cases. Pulmonary veins and venules develop hypertrophy of the media, suggesting an adaptation to the elevated venous pressures. Medial hypertrophy is often accompanied by a reduplication and reorientation of the elastic fibres. These changes give the veins a superficial resemblance to pulmonary arteries, hence the term 'arterialization' (Fig. 4.25). Intimal fibrosis of veins is common and should be distinguished from naturally occurring age-dependent intimal fibrosis.

The pulmonary arterial bed is also changed in cases with longstanding pulmonary venous hypertension. The muscular pulmonary arteries show medial hypertrophy, with muscularization of arterioles. This process is further complicated by intimal fibrosis, often eccentric (Fig. 4.26) but occasionally concentric in nature, and usually mild to moderate in extent. These intimal lesions show neither the characteristic 'onion-skinning' nor the cellular intimal hyperplasia seen in patients with plexogenic pulmonary arteriopathy (see Fig. 4.11).

In contrast to other types of pulmonary hypertension, the vascular lesions in chronic venous congestion have a regional distribution, with the lower parts of the lungs being more severely affected than the upper parts, probably an effect of superimposed hydrostatic pressures. As a consequence of chronic venous congestion, the lungs may become 'stiff' and, eventually,

may develop interstitial and subpleural fibrosis. Fibrosis of the alveolar walls is a particularly important complication. Hypoxic pulmonary vascular disease may develop as a consequence of longstanding raised pulmonary arterial pressure and this is characterized by the finding of longitudinally oriented smooth muscle cells in the intima of small muscular pulmonary arteries (Fig. 4.27). The pulmonary trunk and main pulmonary arteries may exhibit advanced ageing changes, including not only excessive pooling of mucopolysaccharides and extensive loss of elastic fibres, but also marked degrees of atherosclerosis (Fig. 4.28).

DISEASES OF THE LUNGS AFFECTING THE HEART

Many diseases of the lung may cause increased pulmonary arterial resistance and pressure, although the aetiology of the diseases and the pathogenesis of the vascular changes may vary considerably. The most commonly encountered conditions with a clinically relevant effect on the heart are chronic bronchitis, pulmonary emphysema, bronchial asthma and the vast number of diseases that result in interstitial fibrosis.

In general terms these conditions, probably because of an impairment in gas exchange at the alveolar capillary level, lead to arteriolar hypoxia and, eventually, to pulmonary vascular pathology. The changes that occur are located predominantly in the arterioles and small muscular pulmonary arteries. There is hypertrophy of medial smooth muscle cells, and the development within the intima of such smooth muscle cells which are oriented longitudinally (see Fig. 4.27). As in chronic pulmonary venous congestion, longstanding pulmonary hypertension results in the development of atheroma in the pulmonary trunk and major pulmonary arteries.

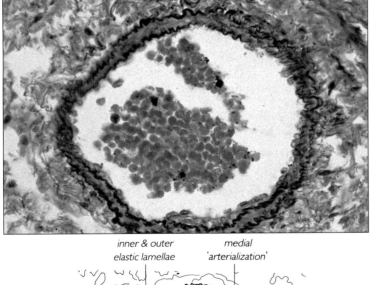
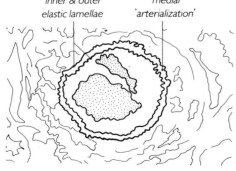

Fig. 4.25 Pulmonary vein with medial hypertrophy and 'arterialization'. E-VG stain.

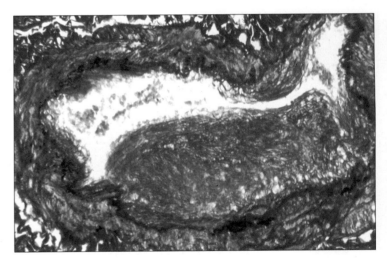
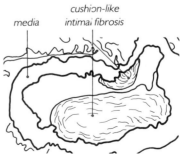

Fig. 4.26 Histological section of a muscular artery showing eccentric cushion-like intimal fibrosis due to organized thrombosis in a case of mitral stenosis. E-VG stain.

Among the diseases of the lung that affect the heart are those cases of pulmonary hypertension which have no immediately obvious cause. There are three such major conditions. The first, thromboembolic pulmonary hypertension, is particularly evident in cases with chronic, and clinically 'silent', emboli over many years. The pathology is that of organized thrombosis (see Fig. 4.22). The second is pulmonary venous occlusive disease, where there is obliteration of pulmonary veins and venules by fibrous

tissue, and the third is so-called primary (or idiopathic) pulmonary hypertension, characterized by plexogenic pulmonary arteriopathy (see above).

Regardless of the underlying cause, any longstanding rise in pulmonary arterial pressure will affect the right side of the heart, with the right ventricular wall becoming hypertrophied and the chamber dilated (Fig. 4.29). This process changes the shape of the ventricular septum and, hence, that of the left

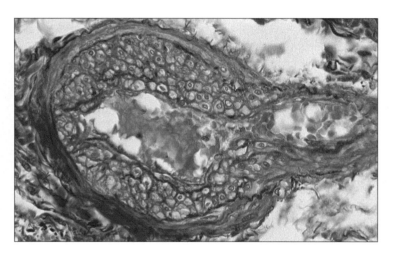

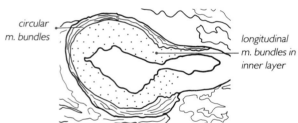

Fig. 4.27 Histological section of muscular artery with extensive longitudinal smooth muscle bundles in the inner layers. E-VG stain.

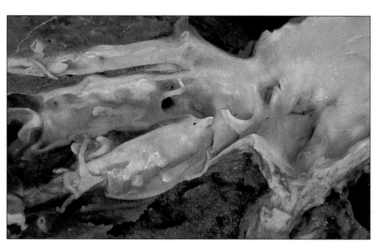

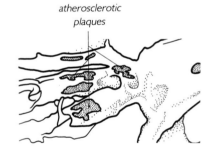

Fig. 4.28 Atherosclerosis of hilar pulmonary arteries.

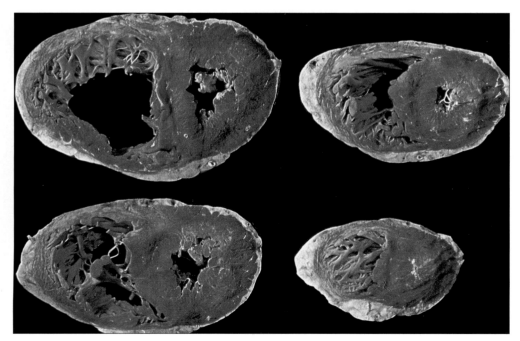

Fig. 4.29 Transverse slices of heart with marked right ventricular hypertrophy and dilatation in a case of chronic emphysema.

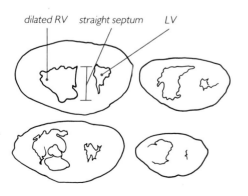

ventricle (see Chapter 3). These alterations may play a role in the pathogenesis of 'pure' right ventricular infarction (see Chapter 7). A chronic overload of the right ventricle produced by increased pressure and volume may, eventually, lead to right atrial dilatation and hypertrophy. Atrial fibrillation is common in this setting, and may contribute to the eventual development of right heart failure.

GRADING OF PULMONARY VASCULAR DISEASE

Among cardiologists and pathologists alike, it is common practice to express the severity of pulmonary vascular disease according to the grading system proposed by Heath and Edwards. The system progresses from grades one through six, and was devised to distinguish potentially reversible from irreversible pulmonary vascular diseases. In the past decade, however, important deficiencies in this grading system have been identified, the main one being that it does not account for the different types of intimal fibrosis. The significance, for example, of finding occlusive intimal fibrosis in an occasional pulmonary artery amidst other arteries with only medial hypertrophy, or sparse cellular intimal proliferation, is markedly different from the finding of such occlusive intimal fibrosis in almost all the pulmonary arteries.

Likewise, eccentric intimal fibrosis is often an expression of organized thrombosis, while concentric fibrosis is usually an expression of plexogenic pulmonary arteriopathy. Hence, a descriptive approach to evaluation is preferred, particularly since examination of lung biopsies is gaining increasing significance as a preoperative diagnostic tool.

Diagnostic evaluations are particularly directed, at present, to the very young and therefore it is necessary to concentrate on changes which occur within the first two grades of the traditional system. Consequently, evaluation of lung biopsies should include the evaluation of muscularization with or without medial hypertrophy of the small muscular pulmonary arteries. It should also take into account the ratio of alveoli to arteries, although this ratio may be increased, in some cases of congenital heart disease, due to a reduction in the number of arteries. If these aspects are to be properly studied, the biopsy must be adequate, and should include intra-acinar as well as pre-acinar structures. As previously outlined, some of the early changes (see above) may occur in the pre-acinar arteries, leaving the intra-acinar arteries and arterioles unaffected or only slightly changed. Taken together, these considerations indicate that the classical grading system of Heath and Edwards forms only the basis of modern day evaluation.

Congenital malformations

5   THE CONGENITALLY MALFORMED HEART

RECOGNITION OF CHAMBERS AND ARTERIAL TRUNKS: THE MORPHOLOGICAL METHOD

The criteria used for identification of any given cardiac chamber must be derived from features that are universally present in the chamber, however malformed or rudimentary it may be. When viewed in this light, the criterion of most value in distinguishing the morphologically right from the morphologically left atrium is the structure of the appendage and the nature of its junction with the venous component.

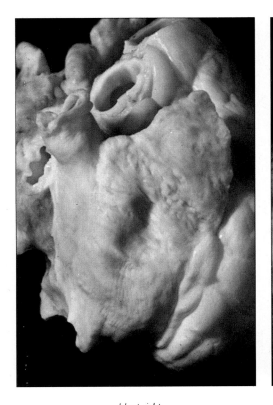

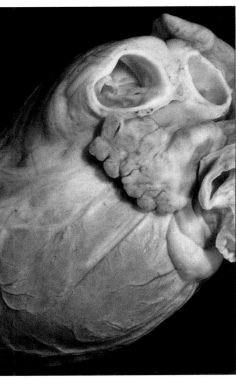

Fig. 5.1   These figures compare and contrast the shape of the morphologically right appendage (left) with that of the morphologically left appendage (right).

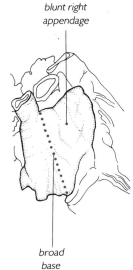

blunt right appendage

broad base

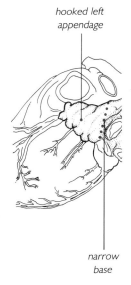

hooked left appendage

narrow base

The morphologically right atrial appendage has the shape of a blunt triangle and communicates across a broad junction with the venous component of the atrium (Fig. 5.1, left). The morphologically left appendage is long, narrow, and crenellated, and has a narrow junction with the venous component (Fig. 5.1, right). Internally, the junction of the morphologically right appendage with the smooth-walled atrium is marked by a prominent terminal crest, and the pectinate muscles encircle the entirety of the atrioventricular junction. A terminal crest is lacking within the morphologically left atrium, and the pectinate muscles are confined more or less within the tubular appendage.

Assessment of ventricular morphology is simplified by dividing the ventricles into three components. Of these components, it is the apical trabecular component that is most universally present in normal and abnormal ventricles. This trabecular component is characteristically coarse in morphologically right ventricles whether the ventricle is normally formed (Fig. 5.2, left); lacks its inlet component (Fig. 5.2, centre); or lacks both its inlet and outlet components (Fig. 5.2, right). The trabecular component of morphologically left ventricles has a much finer pattern,

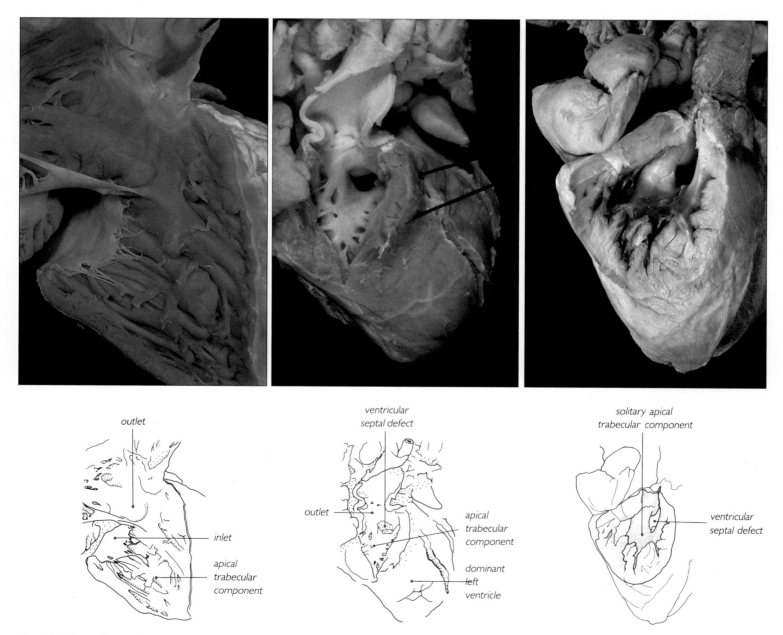

Fig. 5.2   These figures show the readily recognizable coarse apical component of the morphologically right ventricle (left) when the ventricle is normally formed; (centre) when the ventricle is incomplete and rudimentary, lacking its inlet component; and (right) when the ventricle, lacking inlet and outlet components, is represented only by the apical trabecular component.

again whether the ventricle is normally formed (Fig. 5.3, upper); lacks only its inlet (Fig. 5.3, lower left); or lacks both inlet and outlet components (Fig. 5.3, lower right). Most hearts have two ventricles, one of right and one of left morphology. Almost always, these ventricles exist together, with the inlet and outlet

components shared between the apical components in all possible combinations. Rarely, hearts are found with solitary ventricles of indeterminate morphology. The pattern of the apical portion of these ventricles is particularly coarse, more so than in a morphologically right ventricle (Fig. 5.4).

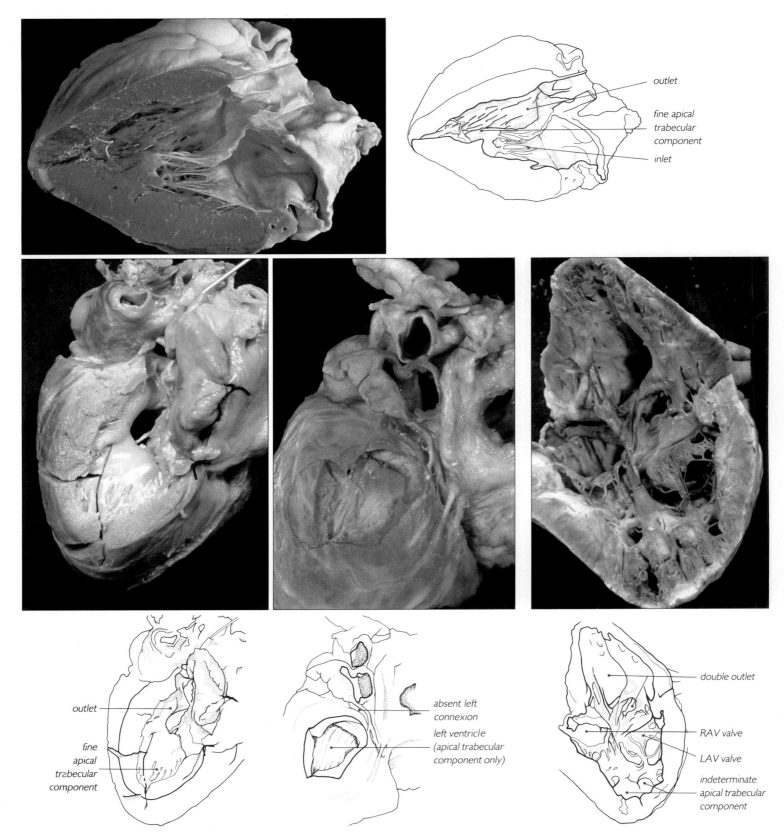

Fig. 5.3 These figures show how, in normal (upper) and abnormal (lower) morphologically left ventricles, comparable to those seen in Fig. 5.2, the fine apical trabeculations serve to identify the ventricles.

Fig. 5.4 When there is a truly solitary ventricle, its apical trabeculations are particularly coarse and are indeterminate, being of neither morphologically right nor left pattern.

When identifying arterial trunks, there is no feature unique to each of the patterns, therefore one should resort to the features most commonly present (Fig. 5.5). A normal pulmonary trunk is easily identified because its only branches are to the lungs. A normal aorta gives rise to systemic and coronary arteries. Thus, when two great arteries are present, there is little likelihood of any problem in differentiating them. On occasion, however, a single arterial trunk may leave the base of the heart. The distinction must then be made between a common arterial trunk; a solitary aortic trunk with pulmonary atresia; a solitary pulmonary trunk with aortic atresia; and a solitary arterial trunk with complete absence of the intrapericardial pulmonary arteries. The common trunk has a solitary valve and gives rise directly to systemic, pulmonary, and coronary arteries. Solitary aortic or pulmonary trunks are identified in the presence of the atretic second trunk. A solitary arterial trunk, in contrast, is a definition of exclusion, being the only logical term for description of the trunk leaving the base of the heart in the absence of a pulmonary trunk or intrapericardial pulmonary arteries.

SEQUENTIAL SEGMENTAL ANALYSIS

The first step in sequential analysis is to establish the arrangement of the atrial chambers. It could be possible to include an analysis of venoatrial connexions as the initial step, but our preference is to catalogue anomalous venous drainage in terms of associated malformations (see below). In terms of atrial arrangement, we have already established that the appendage is the best guide to atrial morphology. It has also been established that all appendages are reliably recognizable as being of either right or left morphology. There are, then, only four ways in which atrial chambers possessing either a morphologically right or a left appendage can be arranged (Fig. 5.6). Most frequently, the morphologically right appendage is right-sided, and the morphologically left appendage is to the left. This is the usual arrangement (so-called situs solitus). The mirror-image situation (inversus) is rare. A more frequent abnormality is found when either morphologically right or morphologically left appendages are found arising from both atrial chambers. Such an arrangement, known as isomerism of the appendages, occurs usually in concert with an isomeric arrangement of the thoracic organs and a jumbled up arrangement of the abdominal organs (so-called visceral heterotaxy, or the 'splenic syndromes').

At anatomical examination, it is easy to distinguish the four patterns of atrial arrangement on the basis of the morphology of the appendages. In life, other methods are often needed to determine the arrangement of the atrial chambers, although it has been shown that the appendages can be identified using transoesophageal echocardiography. More usually, nonetheless, it is necessary to infer the atrial arrangement, either from identification of bronchial morphology or by establishing the arrangement of the great vessels within the abdomen. The arrangement of the atrial chambers corresponds most closely with bronchial morphology. The morphologically left bronchus is almost twice

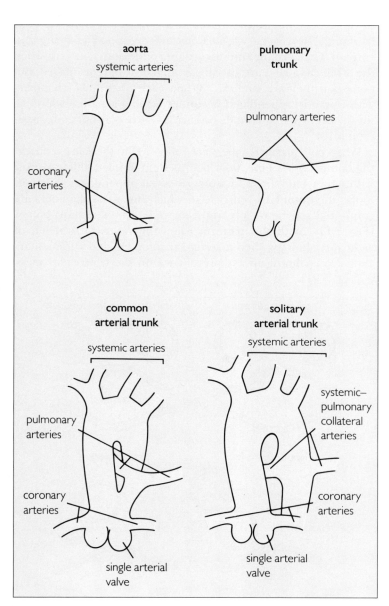

Fig. 5.5 These diagrams illustrate the patterns of branching which permit identification of arterial trunks one from the other.

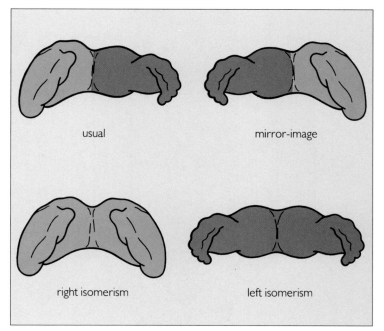

Fig. 5.6 These diagrams show the possible ways in which the atrial appendages can be combined, giving the options in terms of atrial arrangement.

as long as the morphologically right one. The morphologically left bronchus is also crossed by the left pulmonary artery before the bronchus divides, whereas the morphologically right bronchus is not. A long hyparterial bronchus on the left, therefore, is indicative of usual arrangement, whereas a long hyparterial bronchus on the right is strongly suggestive of a mirror-image arrangement. Equal bronchial length indicates isomerism, and determination of bronchial length, together with distinction of their relations to the pulmonary arteries, permits them to be diagnosed as being of right or left morphology (Fig. 5.7).

A further feature of clinical value is the arrangement of the great vessels immediately below the diaphragm. In an individual with lateralized organs, the aorta and inferior caval vein are usually on opposite sides of the spine, with the caval vein on the side of the morphologically right atrium. In patients with an isomeric arrangement, in contrast, the great vessels are usually on the same side of the spine, the caval vein being anterior to the aorta with right isomerism, and with the continuation of the inferior caval vein through the azygos system being posteriorly located in most cases with left isomerism (Fig. 5.8).

ANALYSIS OF THE ATRIOVENTRICULAR JUNCTION

Having established the atrial arrangement, the next step is to determine how the atrial chambers are connected to the ventricular mass, and to establish the morphology of the valves that guard the atrioventricular junction. In order to describe these features, it is also necessary to determine the relationships of the ventricles within the ventricular mass.

Atrioventricular connexions

In terms of the connexions between the atrial and ventricular myocardial masses, each atrium may be connected to a separate ventricle; both atrial chambers may be connected to the same ventricle; or the cavity of only one atrium may be connected with the ventricular mass. When each atrium is connected to a separate ventricle, there are three possible dispositions. The first two occur with lateralized atrial chambers (Fig. 5.9). When the morphologically right atrium is connected to the morphologically right ventricle, and the morphologically left atrium to the morphologically left ventricle, the connexions are concordant. The reverse connexions are described as being discordant. Concordant and discordant connexions can exist when the atrial chambers are usually arranged or mirror imaged, but not when they are isomeric. When each of the two chambers with isomeric appendages is connected to a separate ventricle, the atrioventricular connexions are biventricular but ambiguous (Fig. 5.10).

When both atrial chambers are connected to the same ventricle, the connexion is best described as double inlet; this can exist with either lateralized or isomeric atrial appendages. Furthermore, the dominant ventricle to which the atrial chambers are connected can be of left, right, or indeterminate morphology (Fig. 5.11). With this pattern, when the ventricle is of left or right morphology, then a second incomplete and rudimentary ventricle is almost always present within the ventricular mass,

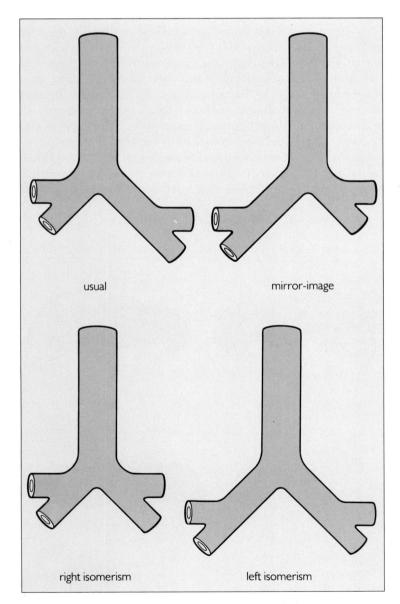

Fig. 5.7 These diagrams show the four possible bronchial arrangements, the morphologically left bronchus being significantly longer than the right.

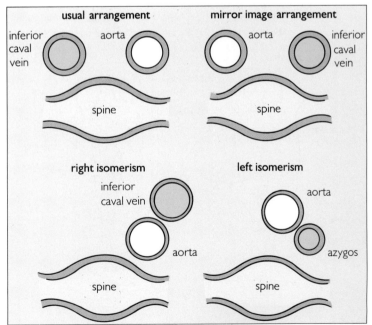

Fig. 5.8 This diagram shows the typical arrangements of the great vessels relative to the spine within the abdomen, these corresponding reasonably well with atrial arrangement.

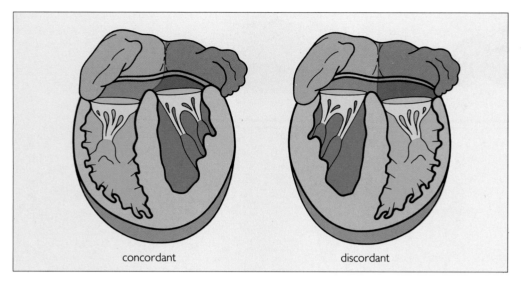

Fig. 5.9 These figures show concordant (left) or discordant (right) atrioventricular connexions. Although illustrated with usual atrial arrangement, they can also be found with mirror-image arrangement.

concordant   discordant

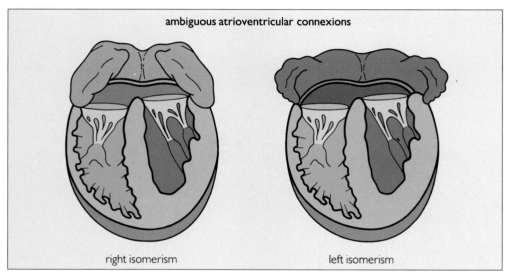

ambiguous atrioventricular connexions

right isomerism   left isomerism

Fig. 5.10 This diagram shows ambiguous and biventricular atrioventricular connexions. As seen, it can be found with right or left isomerism. It can also be found with either right hand or left hand ventricular topology (see Fig. 5.16).

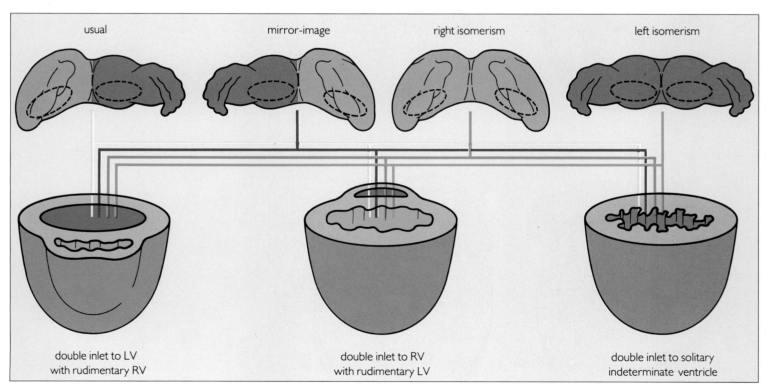

usual   mirror-image   right isomerism   left isomerism

double inlet to LV with rudimentary RV   double inlet to RV with rudimentary LV   double inlet to solitary indeterminate ventricle

Fig. 5.11 This diagram shows how a double inlet atrioventricular connexion can exist with any of the four atrial arrangements, and with the atriums connected to a dominant left, a dominant right or to a solitary and indeterminate ventricle.

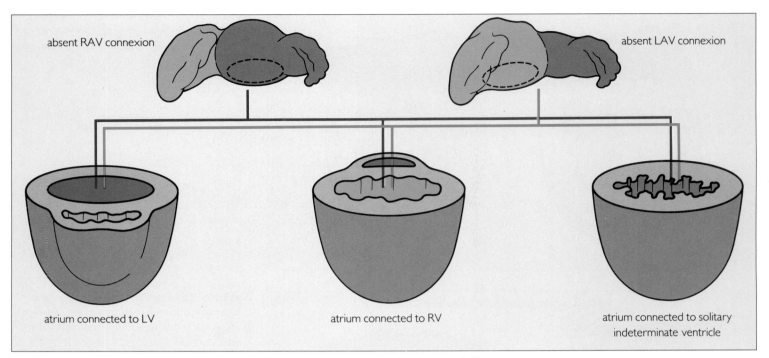

absent RAV connexion

absent LAV connexion

atrium connected to LV

atrium connected to RV

atrium connected to solitary indeterminate ventricle

Fig. 5.12 In this diagram, the combinations of ventricular morphology are shown for absence of either the right-sided or left-sided atrioventricular connexion. This can be found for any atrial arrangement, but are rare in instances other than the usual arrangement.

Fig. 5.13 This diagram shows the possible arrangements of the valves (or valve) guarding the atrioventricular junctions when both atriums are connected to the ventricular mass.

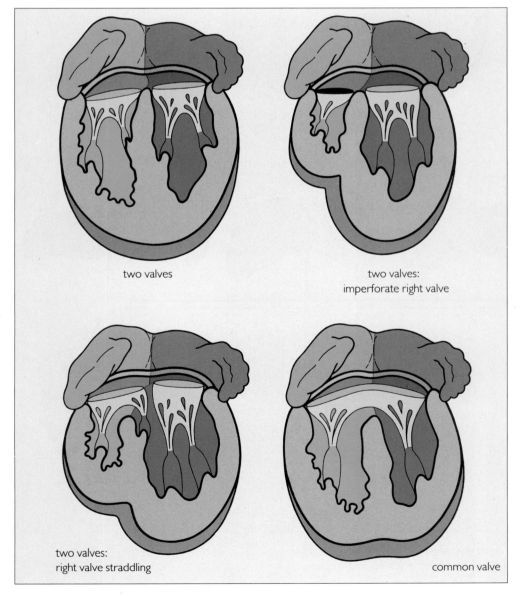

two valves

two valves:
imperforate right valve

two valves:
right valve straddling

common valve

having an apical trabecular pattern that is complementary to that of the dominant ventricle. Thus, rudimentary and incomplete right ventricles are found when there is double inlet to a left ventricle, and vice versa. When there is double inlet to a ventricle of indeterminate morphology, a second rudimentary ventricle is never found.

There is one further pattern of atrioventricular connexion. This occurs when only one atrium connects to the ventricular mass, the entirety of the other connexion being absent. Absence of one atrioventricular connexion can be found either when the atrial appendages are lateralized or when they are isomeric, although the latter is very rare. As with double inlet, the ventricle receiving the solitary atrioventricular valve may be of left, right, or indeterminate morphology (Fig. 5.12). The apical components of rudimentary ventricles, when present, are of complementary pattern to those of the dominant ventricle as in double-inlet ventricle.

Morphology of the atrioventricular valves

Describing the pattern of the atrioventricular connexion conveys no information concerning the morphology of the valves that guard the atrioventricular junction (Fig. 5.13). This feature is a further variable. There are four possibilities when both atrial chambers are connected to the ventricular mass. The first is for two valves to be present, each patent and each connecting an atrium to the ventricular mass. The second possibility is for one of the valves to be imperforate. In this respect, an imperforate valve must be distinguished from absence of an atrioventricular connexion, since each produce a variant of atrioventricular valvar atresia (Fig. 5.14). The third possibility is for a common valve to guard the junction between the two atrial chambers and the ventricular mass. The final possibility is for the tension apparatus of one valve to be attached on both sides of the ventricular septum, an arrangement described as straddling of the valve. Rarely, the tension apparatus of both valves may straddle.

When the tension apparatus of an atrioventricular valve straddles, the atrioventricular junction usually overrides the septum. There is then a spectrum between the extremes of commitment of the overriding junction to one ventricle or the other. Within this spectrum, the nomenclature of the atrioventricular connexion itself must change. Thus, when the valve is one of two valves, extreme overriding of the afflicted junction to a ventricle that is already connected to the other atrium produces a double-inlet connexion (Fig. 5.15, left). In contrast, when the overriding junction is connected for its greater part to the ventricle that is not, itself, connected to the other atrium, there will be concordant, discordant, or ambiguous connexions, the precise arrangement depending upon the morphology of the interconnected chambers (Fig. 5.15, right). There is no difficulty in diagnosing the types of connexion present at these extremes of

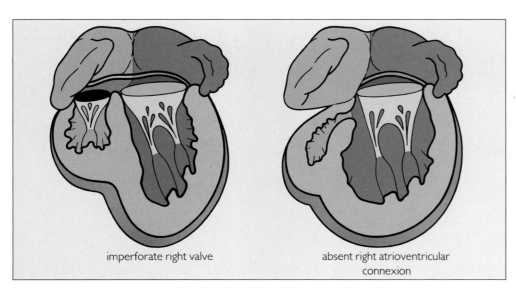

imperforate right valve

absent right atrioventricular connexion

Fig. 5.14 This diagram shows the important distinction to be made between absence of an atrioventricular connexion (right) and an imperforate atrioventricular valve (left). Both produce atrioventricular valvar atresia.

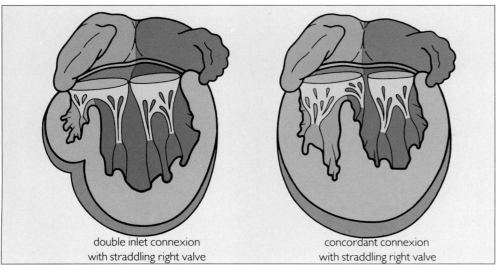

double inlet connexion with straddling right valve

concordant connexion with straddling right valve

Fig. 5.15 This diagram, illustrated in a heart with right hand pattern ventricular topology (see Fig. 5.16), shows the extremes, in terms of the atrioventricular connexion, of the spectrum of overriding of an atrioventricular junction.

the spectrum of overriding. Problems arise only when the overriding junction is committed more or less equally to the two ventricles. Our solution is then to assign the junction to the ventricle adjudged to be connected to its greater part, thus splitting the spectrum at its midpoint (the 50% rule).

The four valvar morphologies described above can exist only when each atrium is directly connected to the ventricular mass (concordant, discordant, ambiguous, or double-inlet types of connexion). When one atrioventricular connexion is absent, there is a solitary atrioventricular valve which drains only one atrium. Thus, with absence of one connexion, the different valvar morphologies are limited to either the valve (and the atrioventricular junction) straddling the septum, or the valve (and junction) being exclusively committed to one ventricle. The latter is by far the most common arrangement.

VENTRICULAR RELATIONSHIPS AND TOPOLOGY

When describing the relations of two ventricles, we describe the position of the morphologically right ventricle relative to the left in terms of right/left, anterior/posterior and, if necessary, superior/inferior co-ordinates. In most hearts, there will be one of two basic patterns of relationship, which we describe in terms of ventricular topology. The first is for the morphologically right ventricle to wrap itself around the right anterior aspect of the left ventricle, while the second is for the morphologically right ventricle to wrap around the left anterior aspect. The two basic patterns are themselves mirror images of each other, and can be designated right-hand and left-hand patterns. This is because the palmar surface of either the right or the left hand can, figuratively speaking, be placed upon the septal surface of the morphologically right ventricle in each of the two patterns (Fig. 5.16).

In general, it is possible to anticipate the pattern of topology that will be present according to the type of atrioventricular connexions. Thus, in almost all instances, concordant atrioventricular connexions will be associated with the right-hand topological pattern when the atrial chambers are usually arranged, and with the left-hand pattern in mirror-image arrangement. With few exceptions, these patterns hold true even when the ventricular relationships are not as anticipated for a given connexion, such as in the so-called criss-cross hearts or in those with ventricles arranged in superoinferior orientation. Even when exceptions do occur, the arrangement is readily clarified

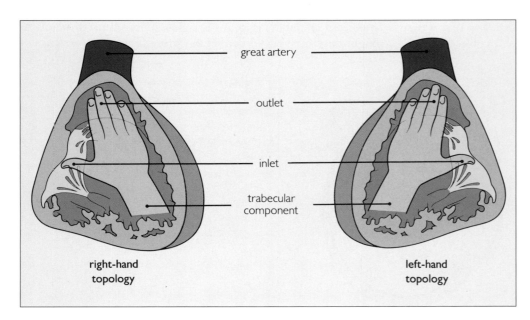

great artery

outlet

inlet

trabecular component

right-hand topology

left-hand topology

Fig. 5.16 These diagrams show how, figuratively speaking, the two isomeric arrangements of the ventricular mass can be described in terms of either the observer's right or left hand being placed upon the septal surface of the morphologically right ventricle with the thumb in the inlet and the fingers in the outlet components.

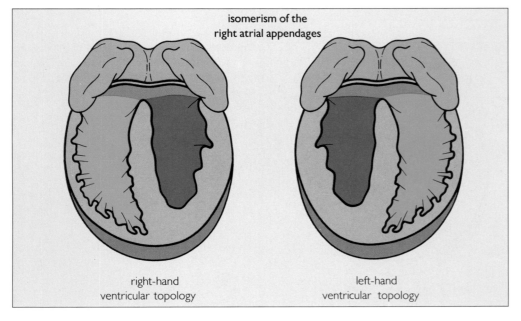

isomerism of the right atrial appendages

right-hand ventricular topology

left-hand ventricular topology

Fig. 5.17 These diagrams show the right and left hand topological arrangements as they may be found with isomerism of the right atrial appendages. They can also be found with isomerism of the left atrial appendages.

by separately describing the atrioventricular connexions, the ventricular topology, and the ventricular relationships. In one circumstance, however, it is always necessary to describe ventricular topology. This is when hearts with isomeric atrial appendages have each atrium connected to a separate ventricle. Such connexions are appropriately described as being ambiguous when, for instance, the right-sided atrium (with either a morphologically left or right appendage) is connected to a right-sided morphologically right ventricle (right-hand topology) or when it is connected to a right-sided morphologically left ventricle (left-hand topology) (Fig. 5.17). Full description of an ambiguous and biventricular connexion, therefore, requires account to be taken of both the ventricular relationships and the ventricular topology.

In hearts with rudimentary ventricles, the rudimentary ventricle is described relative to the dominant ventricle, again using right/left, anterior/posterior, and superior/inferior co-ordinates.

ANALYSIS OF THE VENTRICULO–ARTERIAL JUNCTION

As at the atrioventricular junction, it is necessary to distinguish between connexions and relationships, and to analyse separately the infundibular morphology. Each feature must be described in mutually exclusive terms. Following the approach used in the analysis of the atrioventricular junction, ventriculo–arterial connexions are described as concordant, discordant, double outlet, and single outlet. For a description of concordant and discordant connexions, it is necessary that each great arterial trunk takes origin from a separate ventricle. When one (or both) arterial valve(s) overrides the ventricular septum, it is assigned to the ventricle connected to its greater part. Concordant ventriculo–arterial connexions are present when the morphologically right ventricle (or its rudiment) is connected to the pulmonary trunk and the morphologically left ventricle (or its rudiment) to the aorta. Discordant ventriculo–arterial connexions are the reverse. A double-outlet ventriculo–arterial connexion exists when more than half of the circumference of both arterial valves are connected to the same ventricle; the ventricle may be of right, left, or indeterminate morphology. Single outlet of the heart describes the situation where the ventricular mass connects to only one arterial trunk (see Fig. 5.5). The arterial trunk may be a common trunk; an aorta when there is no connexion between a ventricle and the atretic pulmonary trunk; a pulmonary trunk where there is no connexion between a ventricle and an atretic aorta; or a solitary arterial trunk when there is no evidence of the intrapericardial pulmonary arteries (Fig. 5.18). With single outlet of the heart, it is also necessary to specify the ventricle to which the solitary trunk is predominantly connected.

Fig. 5.18 These diagrams show the four possible arrangements with a solitary arterial trunk leaving the base of the heart (see also Fig. 5.5).

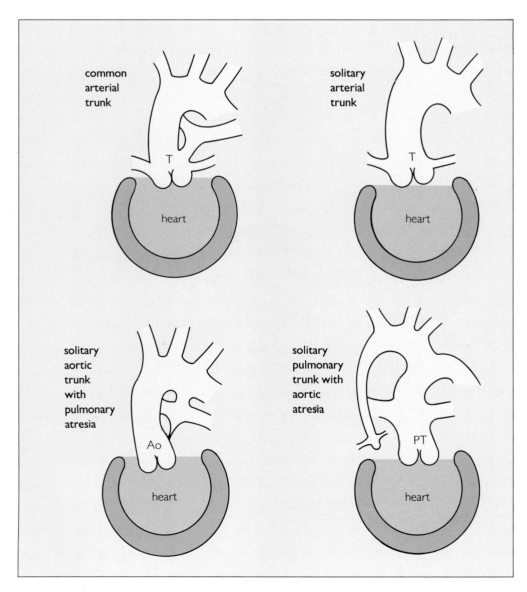

The arrangement of the valves at the ventriculo–arterial junction is limited, since an arterial valve has no tension apparatus. Both valves may be perforate or one valve can be imperforate. One or both valves may override the ventricular septum. A common truncal valve can be exclusively committed to one ventricle or, more usually, be overriding. When one valve is perforate, and the other imperforate, but its ventricular origin can be defined, the connexion is described as concordant, discordant, or double outlet complicated by an imperforate valve. It is not coded as single outlet of the heart.

When accounting for infundibular morphology, we are concerned with the arrangement of the ventricular myocardium supporting the arterial valves. The most usual arrangement is for the arterial valve of the right ventricle to be supported by a complete muscular infundibulum, but with fibrous continuity to be present between the leaflets of the arterial and atrioventricular valves within the left ventricle. Alternatively, there may be a complete muscular infundibulum supporting the leaflets of both arterial valves completely, or there may be continuity bilaterally between the leaflets of both arterial valves and the atrioventricular valves. When describing the components of these infundibular regions (Fig. 5.19), the structure separating the two arterial valves and their supporting ventricular outflow portions is known as the outlet septum. Any muscular structure separating the leaflets of an arterial from those of an atrioventricular valve is the ventriculo–infundibular fold. The extensive trabeculation reinforcing the septal surface of the morphologically right ventricle is not an infundibular structure; it is described as the septomarginal trabeculation.

Arterial relationships are categorized by considering the location of the aortic valve relative to the pulmonary valve in terms of right/left and anterior/posterior co-ordinates (Fig. 5.20).

CARDIAC POSITION

When describing the position of the heart within the chest, it is necessary to account for both the basic position of the heart as well as the orientation of the cardiac apex. The heart itself may be predominantly within the left chest, the right chest, or midline. The cardiac apex may point to the left, middle, or right. Any direction of the apex can be found with any cardiac position, although usually a left-sided heart has an apex pointing to the left and so on.

ADDITIONAL CARDIAC MALFORMATIONS

Additional cardiac malformations are catalogues that must be considered within the framework established from sequential segmental analysis. The individual malformations are described in subsequent chapters of the section on congenital malformations, together with certain sequential arrangements that are sufficiently constant to constitute recognized malformations. These associated lesions can exist in all parts of the heart and, to continue a logical sequence, they are described by progressing from the venous to arterial poles of the heart. Analysis of congenital malformations of the cardiac subsystems conclude the section.

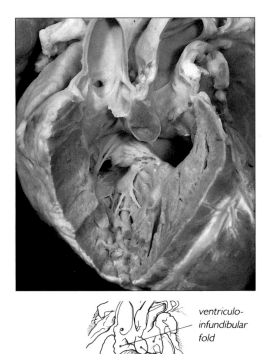

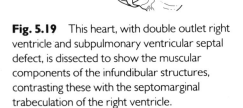

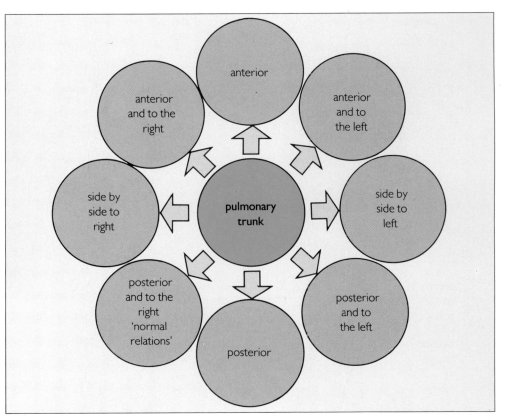

Fig. 5.19 This heart, with double outlet right ventricle and subpulmonary ventricular septal defect, is dissected to show the muscular components of the infundibular structures, contrasting these with the septomarginal trabeculation of the right ventricle.

Fig. 5.20 This diagram shows how the location of the aortic valve can be related to the pulmonary valve in terms of right/left and anterior/posterior coordinates.

MALFORMATIONS OF THE ATRIAL CHAMBERS

In this, the first of the sections devoted to associated lesions, malformations of the atrial chambers are discussed, in particular, abnormal connexions of the systemic and pulmonary veins; lesions of the atrial septum and its surrounds which produce the potential for interatrial communications; and various miscellaneous lesions such as divisions of an atrium in its various forms (cor triatriatum) and juxtaposition of the atrial appendages. This section begins, however, with a consideration of the abnormal arrangement of the organs of the thorax and abdomen, concentrating on the forms in which so many of these atrial lesions are seen and usually recognized, namely hearts that have an isomeric arrangement of the atrial appendages.

Anomalies of atrial arrangement

By far, the greatest majority of patients with congenital cardiac malformations have the atrial chambers arranged in their expected positions and, in keeping with this, a normal arrangement of the organs of the thorax and abdomen, so-called 'situs solitus' (Fig. 6.1). Very rarely, patients with congenital heart disease are encountered with the atrial chambers and the organs of the thorax and abdomen arranged in mirror-image fashion (Fig. 6.1, right). In some instances, the heart can be entirely normal with such mirror-image arrangement (Fig. 6.2). More usually, a lesion is present which is the mirror image of the better-known pattern found in patients with usual arrangement; for example, in the patient with complete transposition in the mirror-image

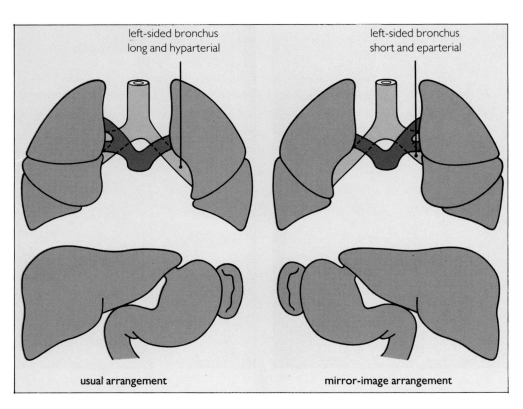

left-sided bronchus
long and hyparterial

left-sided bronchus
short and eparterial

usual arrangement

mirror-image arrangement

Fig. 6.1 These diagrams show the typical positions of the thoracic and abdominal organs with (left) usual and (right) mirror-imaged lateralized arrangements.

Fig. 6.2 This heart is normally structured, but is arranged in mirror-image fashion.

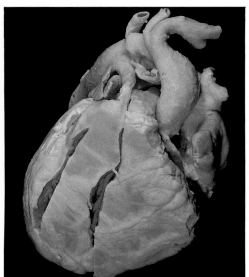

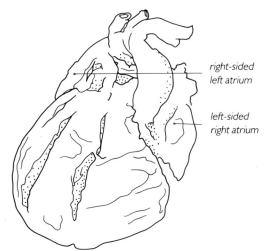

right-sided
left atrium

left-sided
right atrium

arrangement, the aorta, which is connected to the left-sided morphologically right ventricle, is usually anterior and to the left of the pulmonary trunk, while the heart is almost always found in the right chest with its apex pointing to the right (Fig. 6.3). Any congenital cardiac lesion must be anticipated to exist in the mirror-image arrangement, although some, such as congenitally corrected transposition, are found more frequently in the mirror-image arrangement than would be anticipated from their known frequency in patients with usual atrial arrangement.

Other well-recognized syndromes of cardiac malformation exist with some frequency in patients who have neither a usual nor a mirror-imaged arrangement of their organs. These are the patients with so-called 'visceral heterotaxy'. The essence of the usual arrangement and its mirror-image variant is lateralization of the morphologically distinct organs of the thorax and abdomen, including the atrial appendages. The key to understanding 'visceral heterotaxy' (or the so-called 'splenic syndromes') is that the organs of the thorax, again including the atrial appendages, are isomeric rather than lateralized. These anomalies are readily interpreted in terms of the existence on both sides of the body of organs found normally only on the right side of the body (morphologically right organs), or of organs normally found only on the left side of the body (morphologically left organs). When approached in this way, there is nothing ambiguous about these patients with heterotaxy, particularly when attention is concentrated within the thorax. The patient with right isomerism has bilateral trilobed lungs

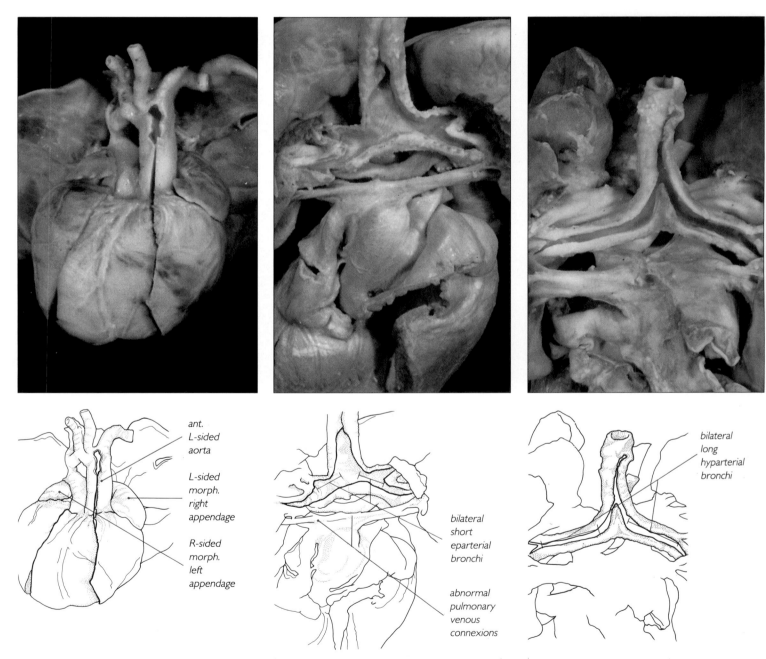

ant.
L-sided
aorta

L-sided
morph.
right
appendage

R-sided
morph.
left
appendage

bilateral
short
eparterial
bronchi

abnormal
pulmonary
venous
connexions

bilateral
long
hyparterial
bronchi

Fig. 6.3   In this heart, which has the segmental combination producing complete transposition, all the structures are mirror-imaged in comparison to typical examples of this lesion.

Fig. 6.4   This posterior view of the bronchial tree shows the arrangement of right isomerism. Note the abnormal connexions of the pulmonary veins to the atrial roof.

Fig. 6.5   In this specimen, seen from behind, there is left isomerism of the bronchial tree.

with bilaterally short bronchi that branch before being crossed by the pulmonary artery supplying the segments of the lower lobe (Fig. 6.4). In contrast, the patient with left isomerism has bilateral bilobed lungs with bilaterally long bronchi that do not branch until already crossed by the artery to the lower lobe (Fig. 6.5). Almost always, the patient with right isomerism has absence of the spleen (asplenia) while the patient with left isomerism has multiple spleens (polysplenia; Fig. 6.6).

The beauty of classifying the heterotaxic syndromes on the nature of readily identifiable structures (such as the bronchi and the appendages) is enhanced by the fact that the arrangement of the spleen does not always correspond to the anticipated isomeric arrangement. Thus, cases with all the features of right isomerism can be found when the spleen is formed normally. Similarly,

cases with all the evidence of left isomerism do not always have multiple spleens, while patients with multiple spleens can be found to have normally structured hearts. Almost always, however, there is correspondence between the arrangement of the bronchi and the appendages, although disharmonious cases have been reported.

From the standpoint of the heart, hearts with isomeric appendages are well recognized as harbouring complex intra-cardiac malformations. Again, this emphasizes the importance of having a system of classification that concentrates upon the heart. There is nothing ambiguous about the morphology of the atrial appendages in such cases. As might be expected, both are of right morphology in cases with right isomerism (Figs 6.7 and 6.8) while, in left isomerism, both appendages have left morpho-

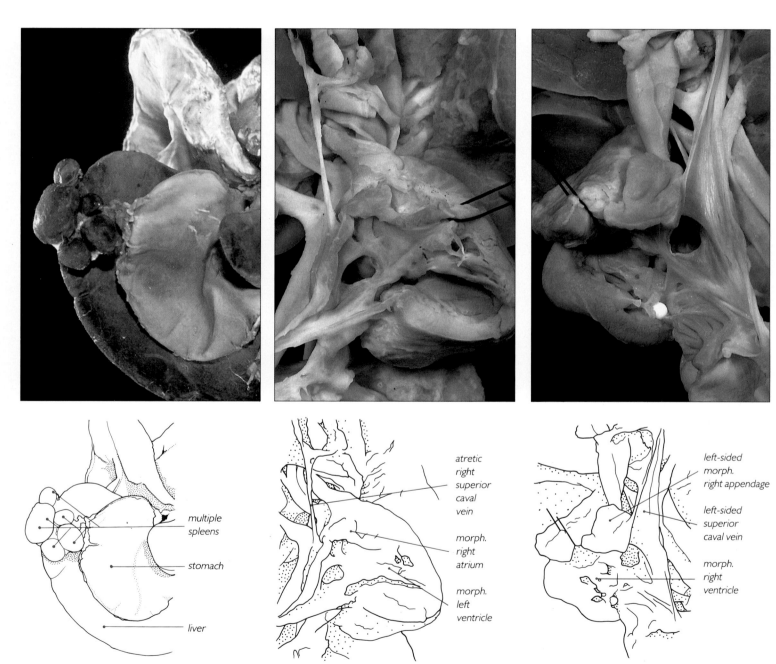

Fig. 6.6 This view of the abdominal organs from behind shows the multiple spleens typically found in the presence of left isomerism.

Fig. 6.7 This heart, with an atretic superior caval vein, has a right-sided appendage of right morphology. The right-sided atrium is connected to a morphologically left ventricle (left hand topology).

Fig. 6.8 This is the left side of the heart shown in Fig. 6.7. The left-sided appendage is also of right morphology (right isomerism). Note the left-sided superior caval vein connecting to the atrial roof.

logy (Figs 6.9 and 6.10). This holds true not only for their external shape, but particularly for their internal anatomy. Cases with right isomerism having bilateral terminal crests, have broad openings to both appendages, and pectinate muscles encircling the atrioventricular junction on both sides (Fig. 6.11). Those with left isomerism, in contrast, lack a terminal crest, have a narrow opening to the appendage, and the extent of the pectinate muscles is much more limited. This morphology also determines the site of the sinus node, right isomerism being associated

with bilateral sinus nodes while the node is abnormally located and usually hypoplastic with left isomerism.

It should not be construed from the above descriptions that, simply because the appendages are bilaterally isomeric, the entire atrial chambers are duplicated. Thus, hearts with left isomerism do not have eight pulmonary veins. Only the appendages are mirror images of each other and, hence, isomeric. The veno-atrial connexions are abnormal to various extents, and all such abnormalities must be described. In over 50% of all cases, there

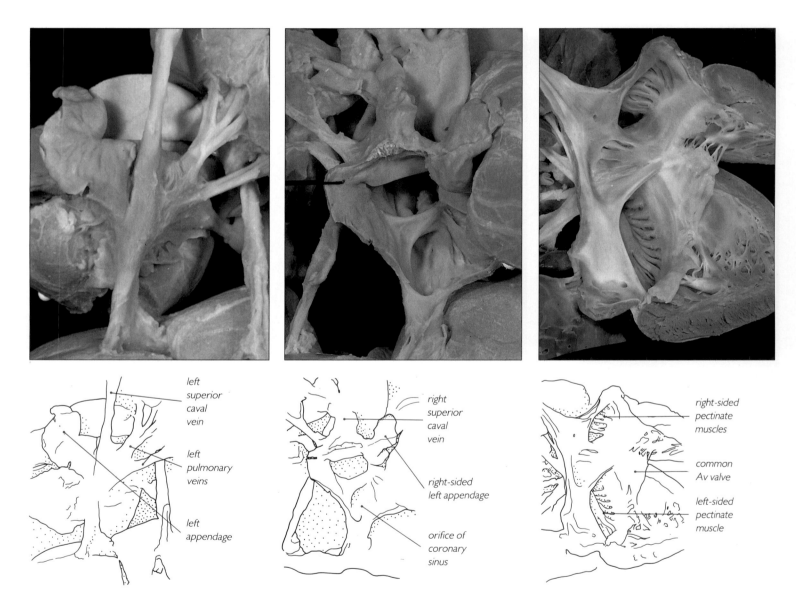

left superior caval vein

left pulmonary veins

left appendage

right superior caval vein

right-sided left appendage

orifice of coronary sinus

right-sided pectinate muscles

common Av valve

left-sided pectinate muscle

Fig. 6.9 This shows a typical left-sided morphologically left atrial appendage, with a left superior caval vein between the appendage and the pulmonary veins.

Fig. 6.10 The right side of the heart shown in Fig. 6.9 reveals another appendage of left morphology (left isomerism) and shows the enlarged orifice of the coronary sinus, into which drains the left superior caval vein. There is also a right superior caval vein.

Fig. 6.11 This view of the common atrial chamber in a heart with isomerism of the right appendages shows the pectinate muscles encircling the atrioventricular junction on both sides.

are superior caval veins bilaterally, which usually drain to the atrial roof, in association with absence of the coronary sinus when there is right isomerism. Totally anomalous pulmonary venous connexion is also the rule in right isomerism. Even when the pulmonary veins drain to the atrial roof, their connexions are abnormal and, hence, anomalous (see Fig. 6.4). Very rarely, the pulmonary veins may all drain to one atrium and the systemic veins to the other, both atrial chambers having morphologically right appendages (Figs 6.12, 6.13). The site of pulmonary venous drainage, nonetheless, is usually to an extracardiac site. The

anatomy is then as found in hearts in which anomalous pulmonary venous connexions are an isolated lesion (see below).

In left isomerism, the pulmonary venous drainage may be to one or other atrial chamber; frequently, however, the veins drain bilaterally to the right-sided and left-sided chambers, each with a morphologically left appendage. Interruption of the inferior caval vein, with return through the azygos venous system, is the most frequent systemic venous anomaly associated with isomerism of the left appendages (Fig. 6.14).

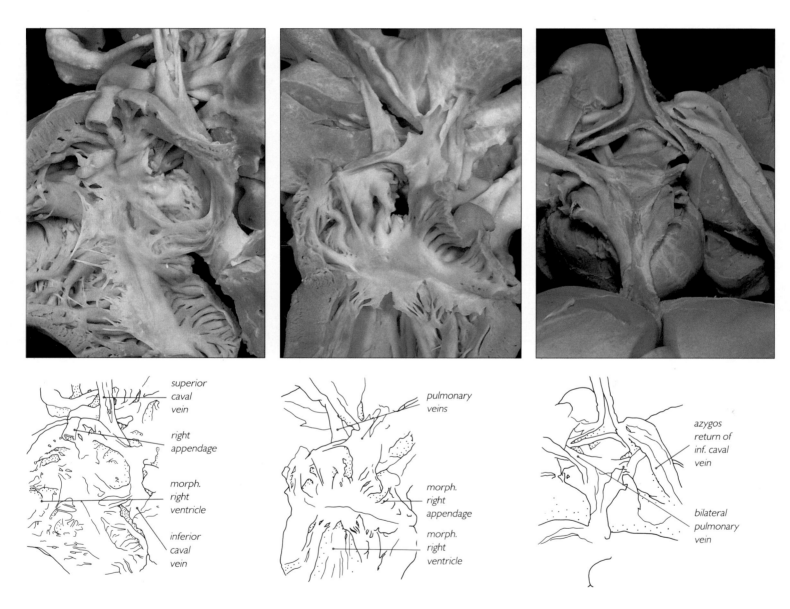

Fig. 6.12 This view of left-sided chambers shows an atrium with a right appendage connecting with a morphologically right ventricle (apparently a concordant connexion).

Fig. 6.13 The right-sided chambers of the heart seen in Fig. 6.12 are shown to be another atrium with a morphologically right appendage (note the terminal crest and the pectinate muscles) which receives the pulmonary veins and connects with the morphologically left ventricle. The connexions are biventricular and ambiguous with left hand ventricular topology.

Fig. 6.14 This posterior view of a heart with isomerism of the left appendages shows continuation of the inferior caval vein through the azygos venous system and bilateral connexions of the pulmonary veins. There is a confluent channel draining the hepatic venous return to the atrium.

Deficient atrial septation is the rule, particularly in right isomerism where the atrial septum is frequently reduced to a single strand crossing a common chamber (Fig. 6.15). The atrial septum is usually better formed in left isomerism and may even be intact, as may rarely be the case in right isomerism. When taken overall, however, the haemodynamic arrangement at atrial level is such that there is marked mixing of systemic and pulmonary venous returns so that it is rare to find cases with 'quasi-usual' or 'quasi-mirror-image' patterns (see Figs 6.12 and 6.13).

In terms of the atrioventricular junction, the greater majority of cases with isomeric appendages will have either an ambiguous and biventricular atrioventricular connexion or double-inlet ventricle. When there is an ambiguous and biventricular atrioventricular connexion, it is also necessary to account for the ventricular topology, which can be of right-hand or left-hand pattern. When there is double inlet, then, as with any heart with double-inlet connexions, this can be to a left, right, or morphologically indeterminate ventricle. Irrespective of the connexion, there is usually a common valve guarding the atrioventricular junctions (see Fig. 6.10) but two perforate valves may be present. Very rarely, cases may be found with absence of one atrioventricular connexion, the left connexion usually being the one that is lacking.

It is the ventricular topology which determines the disposition of the atrioventricular conduction tissues, irrespective of whether there is isomerism of the right or left appendages. A normal atrioventricular node is the rule with right-hand topology, whereas either an anomalous anterior node or a sling of conduction tissue is usually found with left-hand topology.

Variability at the ventriculo–arterial junction is as great as is permitted by the ventricular morphology. When considered as a whole, concordant ventriculo–arterial connexions with normally related great arteries are more frequent with left isomerism, while pulmonary atresia or double-outlet right ventricle with bilateral infundibulum is more common with right isomerism; in any individual case, however, any connexion is possible.

Taken overall, therefore, isomerism of the right appendages is almost universally associated with complex cardiac malformations, dominated by anomalous pulmonary venous connexions, a common atrioventricular valve, double-inlet ventricle, and pulmonary atresia. Left isomerism, on the other hand, may show a wider range in the severity of lesions. In general, it is associated with more normal connexions, although a common atrioventricular valve and interruption with azygos continuation of the inferior caval vein should always be anticipated.

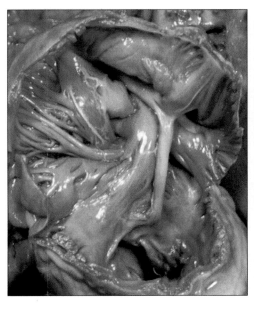
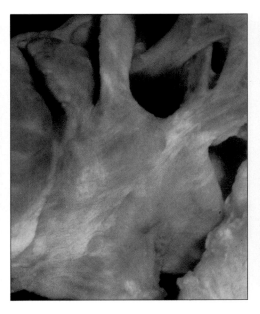
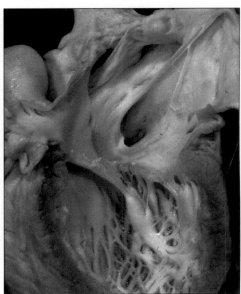

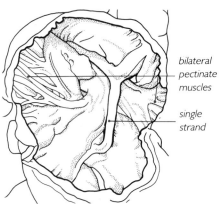
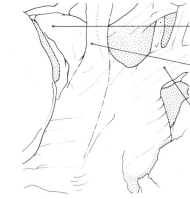
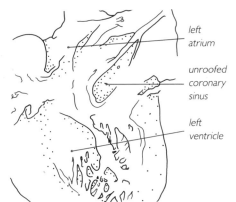

Fig. 6.15 This view of the common atrial chamber in a heart with isomerism of the right appendages shows the typical strand which is all that remains of the atrial septum.

Fig. 6.16 In this heart with usual atrial arrangement, a persistent left superior caval vein passes into the left atrioventricular groove between the pulmonary veins and the left appendage.

Fig. 6.17 This view of the opened left atrium shows unroofing of the course of the coronary sinus along the left atrioventricular groove. It drains to the right atrium through the enlarged orifice of the coronary sinus (see Fig. 6.18).

Anomalous systemic venous connexions

In the presence of lateralized atrial chambers, as opposed to those with isomeric appendages, anomalous systemic venous drainage is rarely of haemodynamic significance. The most common malformation type (presuming usual arrangement) is persistence of the left superior caval vein (Fig. 6.16). The persistent channel usually drains to the right atrium via the enlarged but normally positioned orifice of the coronary sinus. When there is mirror-image arrangement, it is the right superior caval vein which persists to drain in anomalous fashion. Most frequently, the persisting vein is present in addition to the normally connected venous channel but, on occasion, the normal vein (the right one with usual arrangement) is atretic or even absent. A variant is found when the venous channel connects directly to the roof of the morphologically left atrium emptying between the appendage and the left pulmonary veins (Fig. 6.17). This is the site at which the persistent left superior caval vein should have crossed the left atrial wall. In this variant, therefore, the left-sided systemic venous return enters into the pulmonary venous atrium as opposed to the more usual form of anomalous drainage where the deoxygenated blood continues to reach the systemic venous atrium. The constellation of termination of the left superior caval vein in the roof of the left atrium, together with an interatrial communication at the site of the coronary sinus, can be considered as unroofing of the coronary sinus. The enlarged orifice of the coronary sinus will then act as an interatrial communication (Fig. 6.18). The lesion is the extreme form

of fenestration between the coronary sinus and the left atrium. So-called levoatrial cardinal vein is a similar anomaly in which a vein from the roof of the left atrium carries the pulmonary venous return to a systemic venous channel.

Anomalous connexion of the inferior caval vein is a rarer malformation. Direct connexion to the morphologically left atrium is described, albeit rarely, but we have never encountered the lesion. We have seen the orifice of the inferior caval vein straddling the atrial septum so as to drain predominantly to the left atrium. This latter arrangement is accentuated by undue prominence of the valve of the vein (the Eustachian valve). The most common anomaly of the inferior caval vein is interruption of its abdominal course with continuation via the azygos or hemiazygos system of veins to the superior caval vein. The anomaly can be found in the presence of usual or mirror-image atrial arrangement but is more frequent when there is isomerism of the left appendages.

Although rare, and of limited clinical significance, obstruction of the coronary sinus can be produced by a stenotic orifice. Even more rarely, obstruction of the venous return to the heart can be produced by hypertrophy of valves, particularly those in the great cardiac vein (valve of Vieussens). Another strange malformation of the coronary sinus is gross dilatation of its floor, with herniation as a diverticulum into the diaphragmatic wall of the right ventricle (Fig. 6.19). Such dilatations are accompanied by anomalous pathways of conduction, and have been discovered in patients dying suddenly.

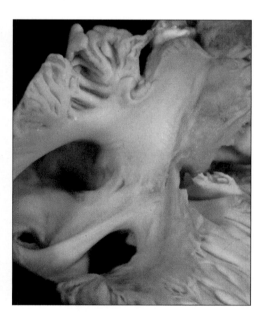

Fig. 6.18 This view of the right atrium of the heart seen in Fig. 6.17 shows the enlarged orifice of the coronary sinus which functions as an interatrial communication.

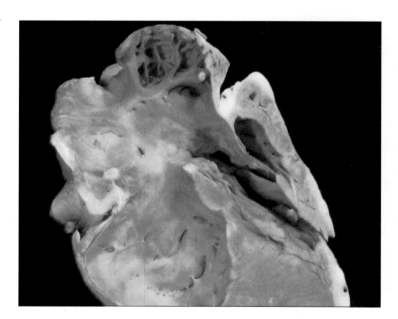

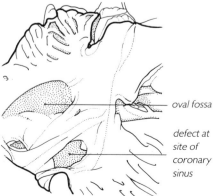

oval fossa

defect at site of coronary sinus

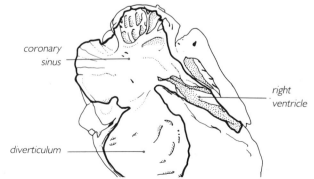

coronary sinus

right ventricle

diverticulum

Fig. 6.19 In this heart, an extensive diverticulum from the floor of the coronary sinus excavates into the diaphragmatic surface of the right ventricle.

Anomalous pulmonary venous connexions

All the pulmonary veins normally drain to the morphologically left atrium, usually with two veins draining each of the lungs so that four veins enter the atrium posteriorly at its corners. Anomalous connexion is present when one or more of these veins drain to a site other than to the left atrium. Classification depends upon the amount of lung draining anomalously together with the site of drainage.

Traditionally, the anomalous connexion has been classed as 'total', when both lungs are abnormally connected, 'hemianomalous' when one lung is affected, and 'partial anomalous drainage'

when only part of one lung is concerned. There is much to commend the system that advocates treating each lung as an entity. It is then easy to describe totally anomalous connexion when both lungs are abnormally connected. Unilateral anomalous connexion is defined as the situation in which only one lung drains anomalously (either right or left). This may be complete or partial. Partially anomalous connexion (Fig. 6.20) can then be said to be unilateral or bilateral according to whether part of one or both lungs is affected.

Whether the anomalous connexion is bilateral, unilateral, or partial, the potential sites of drainage are the same. The usual

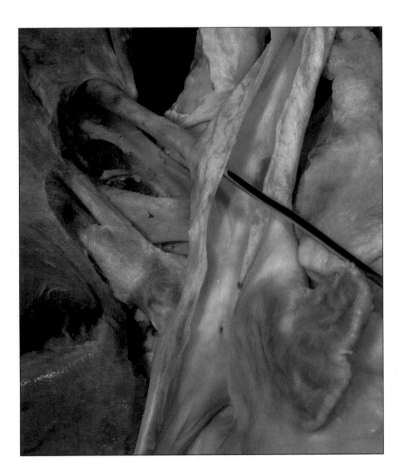

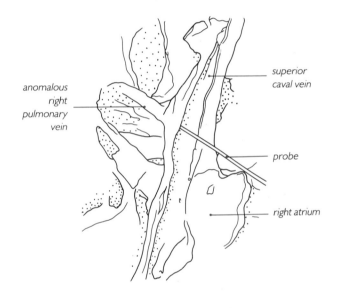

Fig. 6.20 The probe is placed into one of the pulmonary veins which connects anomalously into the superior caval vein.

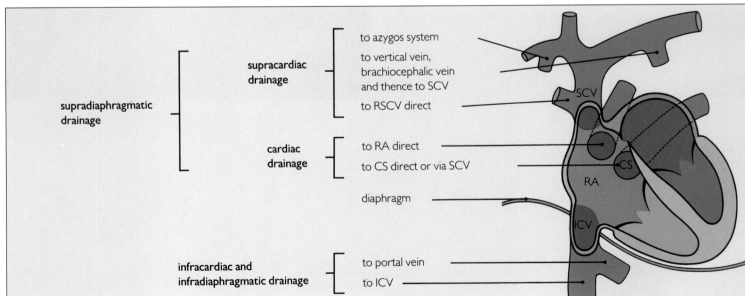

Fig. 6.21 This diagram shows the potential sites for anomalous connexion of the pulmonary veins.

convention when dividing sites of connexion (Fig. 6.21) is first to distinguish drainage to an abdominal site (infradiaphragmatic or infracardiac connexion). Drainage within the thorax can then be divided into the form occurring to one or more of the systemic veins (supracardiac connexion) or drainage to the heart itself (cardiac connexion).

Supradiaphragmatic connexion is more frequent than infradiaphragmatic. The most typical arrangement is for the four pulmonary veins to join into a confluence. A vertical vein then ascends from the confluence to join the left brachiocephalic vein and thence to reach the right atrium via the superior caval vein (Fig. 6.22). It is this circular course of the abnormal venous channel which produces the upper part of the 'snowman' silhouette so characteristic of the chest radiograph of this form of anomalous connexion. Less frequently, totally anomalous connexion can be to the superior caval vein via a channel that does not take the 'snowman' course, crossing instead beneath the heart to ascend on the right side of the spine and terminate in the azygos vein (Fig. 6.23). Cardiac connexion can be directly to the cavity of the right atrium, as occurs most frequently in right isomerism (see Fig. 6.12), but is usually to the coronary sinus (Fig. 6.24).

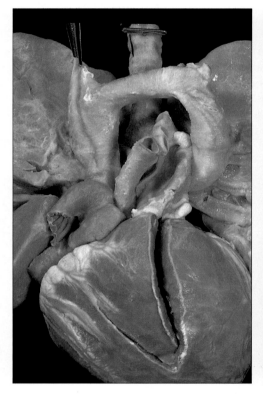
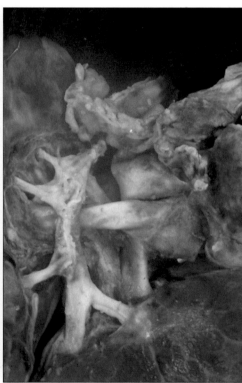
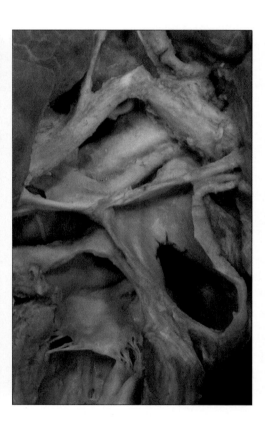

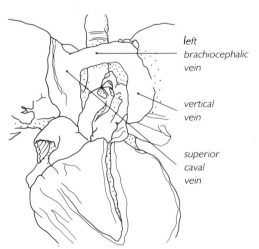

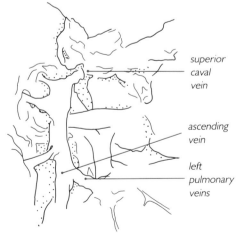

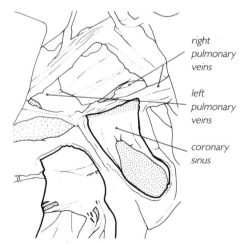

Fig. 6.22 In this heart, seen from the front, the pulmonary veins join a confluence which then drains in snowman-fashion to the superior caval vein.

Fig. 6.23 In this heart with totally anomalous pulmonary venous connexion to the superior caval vein, the anomalous vein passes beneath the heart and ascends to the right of the spine.

Fig. 6.24 This posterior view shows all four pulmonary veins connecting anomalously to the coronary sinus.

In infradiaphragmatic connexion, the confluence of veins turns downwards and passes through the diaphragm along with the oesophagus and drains usually to the venous duct or the portal venous system (Fig. 6.25). Occasionally, it may connect directly to the inferior caval vein. Unilateral anomalous drainage, or partial drainage, can be to any of these sites. A further important variant occurs when the different lungs, or different parts of the lungs, drain to different sites; this is known as mixed anomalous connexion, any combination being possible.

Obstructed drainage is another significant complication. This is found most frequently with the infradiaphragmatic variety, when the obstruction is within the hepatic portal venous plexuses. Obstruction can also occur with supracardiac connexion, the site then usually being found where the vertical vein crosses the bronchial tree, or where the venous channel becomes trapped in a vascular 'vice' (Fig. 6.26). Anomalous pulmonary venous connexion is an important anomaly in its own right, but also has important associations. Totally anomalous connexion is the rule in right isomerism (see above). A unilateral and partially anomalous connexion is also the rule with an interatrial communication of the sinus venous type (see below), while another unusual form of partially anomalous connexion is found in the Scimitar syndrome. In this malformation, the right lung is either hypoplastic or part of it is sequestrated, having its own anomalous systemic arterial supply. All or part of its veins connect anomalously through a common channel to the inferior caval vein.

Interatrial communications

Although there are several types of defects that produce an interatrial communication, all but one are outside the confines of the normal atrial septum. The normal septum is composed mostly of the flap-valve of the oval fossa. It is only the immediate circumference of the fossa and its floor which is a muscular interatrial structure (see Chapter 1). The remainder of the anterosuperior rim is an interatrial fold, while the inferior rim is, for its greater part, an atrioventricular septal structure. Categorization of interatrial communications, therefore, must be viewed in the light of this normal septal morphology.

Traditionally, such defects are divided into the secundum type (to be distinguished from a patent foramen ovale) and the primum, sinus venosus, and coronary sinus variants (Fig. 6.27). The so-called secundum defect is the only true defect of the atrial septum. It is due to deficiency (or perforation) of the flap-valve of the oval fossa and, hence, is more accurately termed an oval fossa defect. It can be a small hole when the flap-valve is marginally deficient (Fig. 6.28, upper); larger when the valve is deficient and fenestrated (Fig. 6.28, lower); or of considerable size when the flap-valve is totally lacking. A small defect should be distinguished from patency of the oval foramen. In this lesion, the flap-valve is not adherent to the left side of the rim. There is then no atrial shunting as long as the left atrial pressure is higher than that of the right, but this arrangement can produce

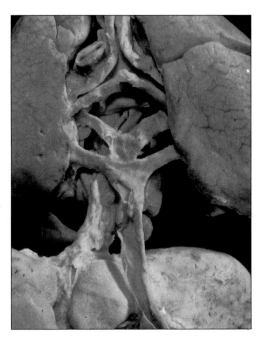

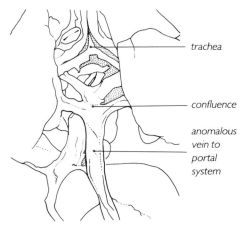

Fig. 6.25 In this case, again viewed from behind, the four pulmonary veins join a confluence which then connects infradiaphragmatically via a descending channel with the portal venous system.

trachea

confluence

anomalous vein to portal system

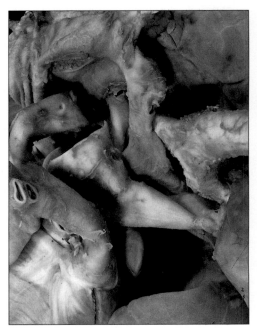

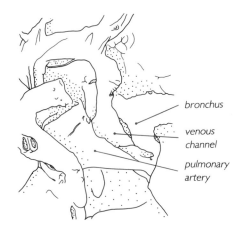

Fig. 6.26 This view of the left side of the bronchial tree shows an anomalous pulmonary venous channel caught in a vice between bronchus and pulmonary artery.

bronchus

venous channel

pulmonary artery

problems in deep-sea divers, or can be a source of paradoxical embolism. Occasionally, however, when there is marked atrial dilatation, such as in hearts with longstanding mitral insufficiency, the flap-valve may be stretched to the extent that a small defect is produced. Patency of the oval foramen is an incidental finding in approximately 25% of all normal hearts. The so-called ostium primum defect is due to absence of the atrioventricular septal structures. It is an atrioventricular septal defect rather than an atrial defect, and its morphology is described below.

The essence of the sinus venosus defects is that they, too, are outside the confines of the oval fossa. Thus, while unequivocally permitting an interatrial communication, they are not strictly atrial septal defects. The sinus venosus defect is usually located in the mouth of the superior caval vein, which overrides the left atrial cavity. The anomaly is associated either with anomalous connexion of the upper and middle-right pulmonary veins, or anomalous attachment of these veins to the overriding parts of the caval vein (Fig. 6.29). Sinus venosus defects can, much more rarely, be found in the mouth of the inferior caval vein, again almost always in association with anomalous connexion or attachment of the right pulmonary veins, in this case, the lower ones.

The final defect that provides the potential for interatrial communication is also outside the confines of the true atrial septum. This is the defect at the site of the orifice of the coronary sinus which permits interatrial shunting when a left superior caval vein drains directly to the left atrium and its intracardiac course is unroofed (see Figs 6.17 and 6.18).

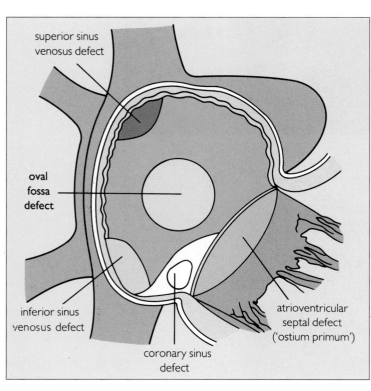

superior sinus venosus defect

oval fossa defect

inferior sinus venosus defect

coronary sinus defect

atrioventricular septal defect ('ostium primum')

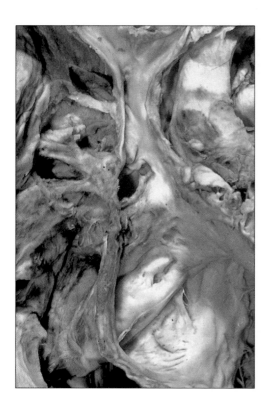

Fig. 6.27 This diagram shows the sites of interatrial communication. Only the holes within the oval fossa are truly atrial septal defects.

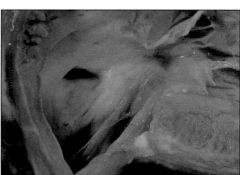

Fig. 6.28 These views show small (upper) and large (lower) holes within the oval fossa – true deficiencies of the atrial septum.

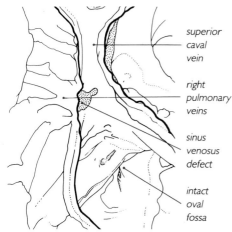

superior caval vein

right pulmonary veins

sinus venosus defect

intact oval fossa

Fig. 6.29 This view of a so-called superior sinus venosus defect shows how the hole is outside the confines of the oval fossa with overriding of the orifice of the superior caval vein. Note the anomalous connexions of the right pulmonary veins.

Miscellaneous atrial malformations

Discussion of the malformations of the atrial chambers is concluded by considering their division, so-called cor triatriatum, together with malformations of the atrial appendages.

Either atrium can be divided but, when unspecified, the term 'cor triatriatum' is usually used in the context of a divided left atrium. There are several variants of this lesion. In the most frequent form, the pulmonary veins drain to a proximal chamber that is separated by an oblique muscular partition from the vestibule of the atrium (Fig. 6.30). The distal chamber contains the left atrial appendage, and usually the flap-valve of the oval fossa, and it communicates with the left ventricle. The variants of this classical form depend upon the site of communication of the oval fossa and the association with anomalous pulmonary venous connexion.

Division of the right atrium is almost always the consequence of undue prominence of the valves of the venous sinus (Eustachian and Thebesian valves). Usually prominent in fetal life when they divert the richly oxygenated inferior caval venous blood to the left atrium, these valves tend to regress during infancy. They may persist as prominent structures in tricuspid atresia, when there is no egress blood from the right atrium other than across the atrial septum, but are rare in the otherwise normally structured heart. Their presence can then lead to obstruction of the right atrial outflow and, on occasion, a valve may herniate through the orifice of the tricuspid valve like a spinnaker sail (Fig. 6.31), even extending as far as the pulmonary valve. An anomaly also related to persistence of the valves of the venous sinus is the Chiari network. This is the filigreed remnant that extends across the cavity of the atrial chamber, but is usually of no clinical significance.

The most obvious anomaly of the appendages is their juxta-position. With this malformation, it is usually the right appendage that is abnormally located within the transverse sinus so that it lies alongside the left, an arrangement known as left juxtaposition (Fig. 6.32). More rarely, the left appendage can extend through the transverse sinus to lie alongside the right, producing right

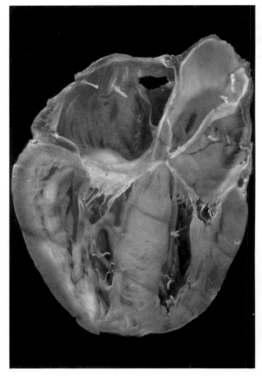

Fig. 6.30 This four chamber section shows the typical anatomy of a divided left atrium.

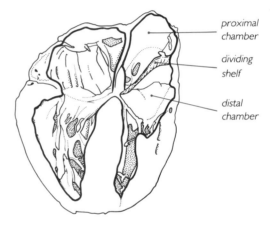

proximal chamber

dividing shelf

distal chamber

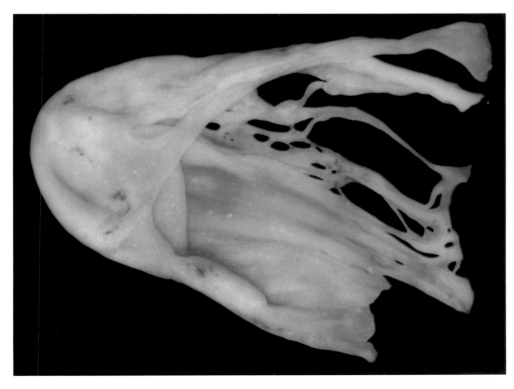

Fig. 6.31 This fibrous structure, removed at surgery, was herniated from the valve guarding the entrance of the inferior caval vein to the right atrium (the Eustachian valve) and was producing tricuspid stenosis.

juxtaposition. Left juxtaposition almost invariably is an accompaniment of complex intracardiac lesions such as tricuspid atresia or complete transposition. In some of the hearts with right juxtaposition, in contrast, there are relatively minor lesions such as atrial septal defects. In the others, right juxtaposition is a harbinger of complex malformations.

Another significant, but rare, anomaly of the appendages is giant aneurysm of the left appendage, usually found in association with a pericardial defect.

ANOMALIES OF THE ATRIOVENTRICULAR JUNCTION

This section concentrates on malformations that distort and malform the atrioventricular junction. Firstly, complete absence of the atrioventricular septal structures, a lesion that produces a characteristic defect often referred to in the past as an 'endocardial cushion defect' or an 'atrioventricular canal malformation', is considered. This is followed by discussion of two abnormal connexions, the discordant ones and double-inlet ventricle, and

description of the other lesions that so frequently accompany them. Finally, the various lesions that affect either the right-sided or left-sided atrioventricular junctions, including so-called valvar atresia, are grouped together. In these latter sections, lesions are described together when they affect the right-sided or left-sided junctions, irrespective of whether it is the morphologically mitral or the morphologically tricuspid valve that is involved.

Atrioventricular septal defects

Atrioventricular septal defects comprise a group of anomalies unified by the characteristically abnormal structure of both the atrioventricular junction and the ventricular mass. When compared with the normal heart (see Fig. 1.61), the primary lesion occupies the site normally filled by the membranous and muscular parts of the septum (Fig. 6.33). Hence, the most appropriate, and anatomically correct, name for the group is atrioventricular septal defects.

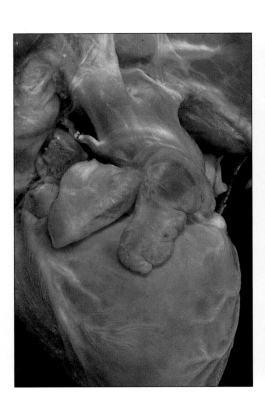

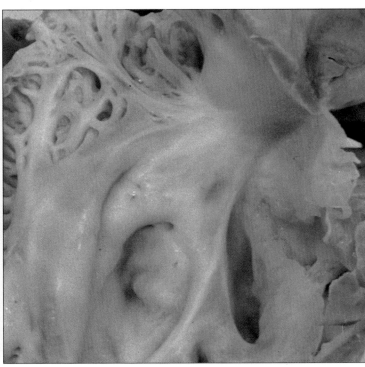

Fig. 6.33 This view of a so-called ostium primum defect shows how the hole occupies the site normally filled by the atrioventricular septal structures. Note that the atrial septum itself is virtually normal.

intact atrial septum

septal defect

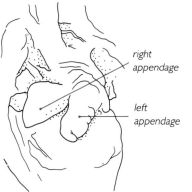

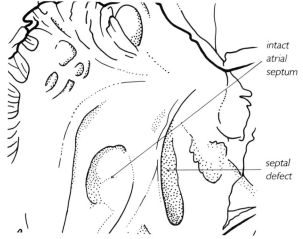

right appendage

left appendage

Fig. 6.32 This anterior view of the heart shows left juxtaposition of the atrial appendages.

Comparison with the normal heart (see Fig. 1.16) also shows that, in addition to the lack of normal atrioventricular septal structures, atrioventricular septal defects have a common atrioventricular junction (Fig. 6.34) rather than separate right and left junctions guarded by the mitral and tricuspid valves. Due to this, the leaflets of the atrioventricular valve that guard the common orifice differ markedly from the normal, particularly those guarding the left-sided aspect of the junction (Fig. 6.35). Furthermore, the aortic valve is no longer 'wedged' between the left atrioventricular valve and the septum. Instead, in hearts with deficient atrioventricular septation, the outflow tract from the left ventricle is directly anterior to the left-sided component of the common atrioventricular valve. Taken together, the leaflets of the valve guarding the common junction in all atrioventricular septal defects are arranged in five components (Fig. 6.36). Two of the leaflets are contained entirely within the right ventricle (the anterosuperior and inferior leaflets) and are comparable with these leaflets in the normal tricuspid valve. The other leaflets have no counterpart in the normal heart. In the normal mitral valve, the mural leaflet guards at least two-thirds of the junction and is tethered by papillary muscles in anterolateral and posteromedial positions (Fig. 6.36, left). In atrioventricular septal defects, irrespective of their type (see below), the mural leaflet is a much less significant structure (Fig. 6.36, centre and left), tethered before and after between paired paired papillary muscles (see Fig. 6.35). The other two of the

five leaflets are tethered to papillary muscles in both the right and left ventricles, that is, they are bridging leaflets. They are located superiorly and inferiorly, and have left ventricular and right ventricular components (Fig. 6.36).

Thus far, our discussion has been confined to atrioventricular septal defects in general. It is usual, however, to divide hearts grouped under this heading into those with a common valvar orifice (often called complete defects) and those with separate right and left valvar orifices (known as partial, or ostium primum defects). In terms of the overall arrangement of the atrioventricular junction, nonetheless, the two patterns are comparable. The major difference is that, in the so-called primum or partial defect, a tongue of valvar tissue connects the facing edges of the bridging leaflets along the crest of the ventricular septum (Fig. 6.37). In those with a common orifice, in contrast, the bridging leaflets are discrete and separate structures (Fig. 6.38). Indeed, if the leaflets are stripped away completely from an atrioventricular septal defect, there is no way of knowing whether, initially, it had a common valvar orifice or separate right and left orifices (Fig. 6.39). Two other aspects are common to all atrioventricular septal defects: the first feature is the 'scooped-out' appearance of the septal crest, the scoop being greater in the presence of a common orifice; and the second feature is the gross disproportion between the inlet and outlet dimensions of the septal surface, the ratio being the same for all defects.

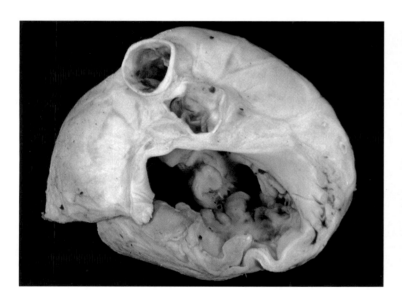

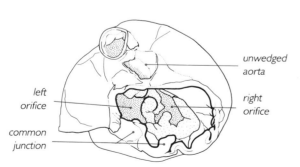

Fig. 6.34 This superior view of a heart with deficient atrioventricular septation, with the atrial chambers removed, shows the typical common atrioventricular junction (compare with Fig. 1.16).

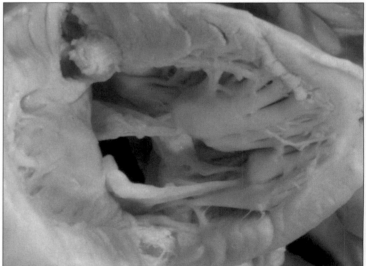

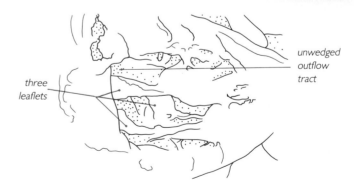

Fig. 6.35 This view of the left ventricle of a heart with deficient atrioventricular septation shows the typical trifoliate arrangement of the left atrioventricular valve, and demonstrates how the outflow tract is not, as in the normal heart, interposed between the valve and the septum (compare with Fig. 1.53).

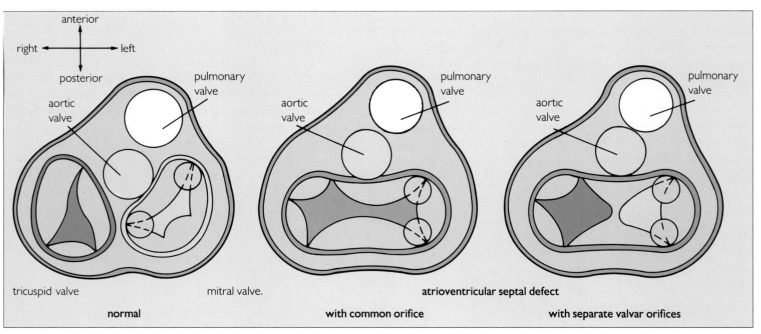

Fig. 6.36 This diagram compares the arrangement of the atrioventricular junction in (left) the normal heart, (centre) atrioventricular septal defect with common valvar orifice and (right) atrioventricular septal defect with separate right and left atrioventricular valves. The short axis sections are viewed from beneath.

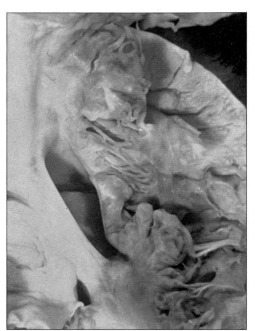

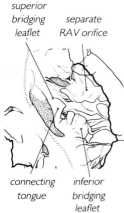

Fig. 6.37 This view shows an atrioventricular septal defect with separate right and left atrioventricular valves.

superior bridging leaflet

separate RAV orifice

connecting tongue

inferior bridging leaflet

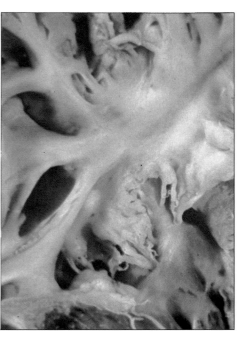

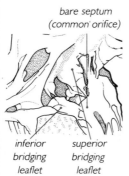

Fig. 6.38 This view from behind, taken in similar orientation to Fig. 6.37, with the right atrioventricular junction opened, shows an atrioventricular septal defect with common atrioventricular valve.

bare septum (common orifice)

inferior bridging leaflet

superior bridging leaflet

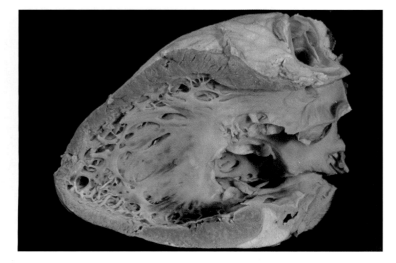

Fig. 6.39 In this heart with an atrioventricular septal defect, the valvar leaflets have been removed from the ventricular mass to show its typical configuration.

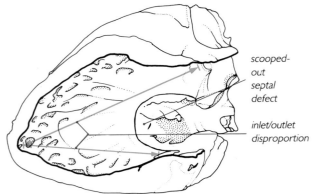

scooped-out septal defect

inlet/outlet disproportion

Atrioventricular septal defects, therefore, although constituting a discrete entity, are generally categorized according to whether they have a common atrioventricular valvar orifice or separate right and left valvar orifices. They are then further divided according to the potential for shunting across the septal defect, this depending on the relationship between the bridging leaflets and the leading edges of the atrial and ventricular septal structures (Fig. 6.40). Almost always, when there are separate right and left valvar orifices, the bridging leaflets are firmly attached to the scooped-out crest of the ventricular septum. Shunting of blood through the defect can then occur only at atrial level (Fig. 6.40, left). In this particular setting, the leading edge of the atrial septum often extends down almost to the atrioventricular junction, with a crescentic bow towards the atria, but most of the interatrial shunting occurs below the level of the junction. When there is a common valvar orifice, in contrast, it is very rare to find the bridging leaflets fused to the scooped-out crest of the ventricular septum. Shunting, therefore, can occur on both the atrial and ventricular aspects of the bridging leaflets. There is also the potential to shunt between the facing surfaces of the bridging leaflets (Fig. 6.40, centre). There is then one further variation, albeit much rarer, in terms of the potential for

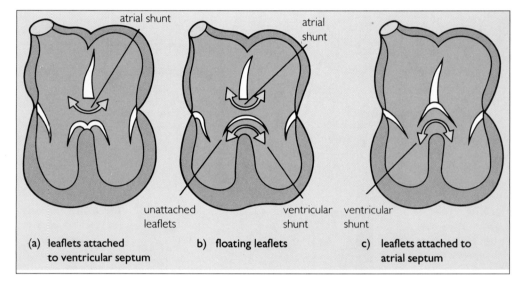

Fig. 6.40 In this diagram, it is shown how shunting through an atrioventricular septal defect is dependant upon the relationships of the bridging leaflets and the septal structures.

(a) leaflets attached to ventricular septum

b) floating leaflets

c) leaflets attached to atrial septum

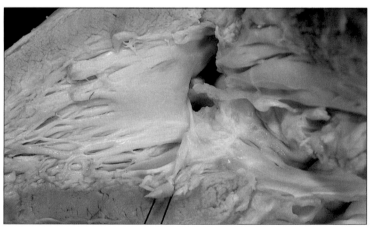

Fig. 6.41 This view of the left ventricle shows an atrioventricular septal defect in which fusion of the bridging leaflets to the underside of the atrial septum confines the potential for shunting at ventricular level.

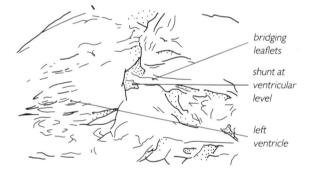

Fig. 6.42 This four chamber section shows an atrioventricular septal defect in which there is a balanced arrangement of the chambers.

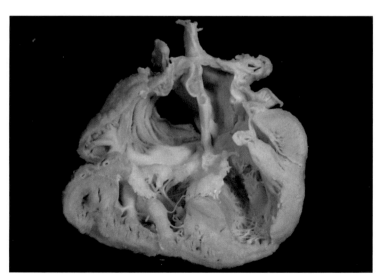

shunting through an atrioventricular septal defect. This occurs when the bridging leaflets are fixed to the underside of the atrial septum (Fig. 6.40, right). This arrangement permits shunting only at ventricular level. Although rare, it can occur both with a common valvar orifice and with separate right and left atrioventricular orifices (Fig. 6.41).

Another important feature of hearts with deficient atrioventricular septation is the mode of sharing of the atrioventricular junction between the atrial chambers and ventricles. Usually, the junction is shared more or less equally, giving the so-called balanced arrangement (Fig. 6.42). In contrast, the junction may be arranged so as to favour one or the other side of the heart – so-called right or left ventricular dominance (Fig. 6.43). It is also possible for the junction to be equally shared between the ventricles but to be attached almost exclusively to one atrium, either the right (Fig. 6.44) or the left. These lesions, unequivocally examples of atrioventricular septal defect, are sometimes described as 'double-outlet atrium'. The other exemplar of a double-outlet atrium is when a heart with absence of one atrioventricular connexion co-exists with straddling and overriding of its solitary atrioventricular valve.

Another significant feature is the anomalous disposition of the conduction tissues. The cardinal feature in this respect is posterior displacement of the atrioventricular node into a nodal triangle at the crux of the heart (Fig. 6.45). Having penetrated the fibrous atrioventricular junction, a long nonbranching bundle extends down the crest of the scooped-out ventricular septum beneath the inferior bridging leaflet. The subaortic outflow tract, unlike in the normal heart (see Fig. 1.94), is no longer related to the ventricular conduction tissues.

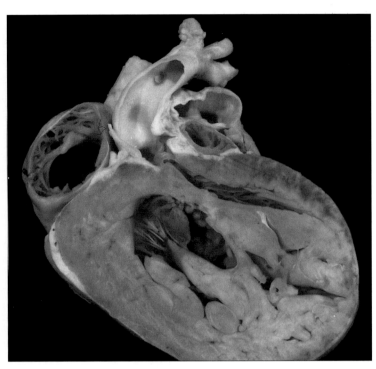

Fig. 6.43 In this atrioventricular septal defect, there is dominance of the right-sided chambers at the expense of the left.

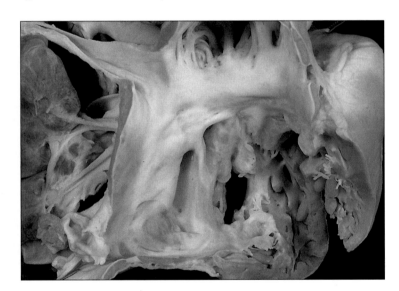

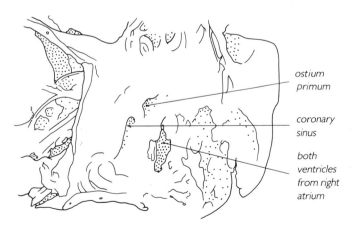

ostium primum

coronary sinus

both ventricles from right atrium

Fig. 6.44 In this atrioventricular septal defect, both ventricles drain from the right atrium, the ostium primum defect being the only exit for the left atrium. Note the enlarged mouth of the coronary sinus which drains a persistent left superior caval vein.

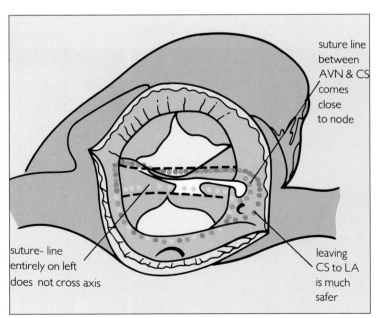

suture line between AVN & CS comes close to node

suture-line entirely on left does not cross axis

leaving CS to LA is much safer

Fig. 6.45 This diagram shows the course of the atrioventricular conduction tissues in a typical atrioventricular septal defect with separate right and left atrioventricular orifices.

Discordant atrioventricular connexions

Discordant connexions constitute one specific arrangement of the atrioventricular junction, the morphologically right atrium being connected to the morphologically left ventricle (Fig. 6.46) and the morphologically left atruim to the morphologically right ventricle (Fig. 6.47). Such discordant connexions can exist with the atrial chambers arranged in the usual fashion, or in the mirror-image variant, but not when there is isomerism of the appendages. In the setting of isomerism, the resulting biventricular connexions would, by definition, be ambiguous.

Discordant atrioventricular connexions can exist with any type of ventriculo–arterial connexions but, most frequently, they are found with discordant ones (Fig. 6.48). The segmental combination thus produced is termed congenitally corrected

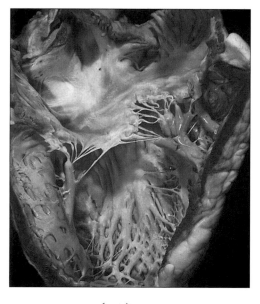

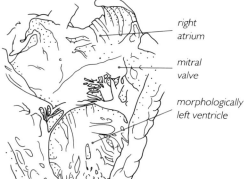

Fig. 6.46 This view of the right-sided chambers in a heart with congenitally corrected transposition shows the right atrium connected to the morphologically left ventricle through a mitral valve.

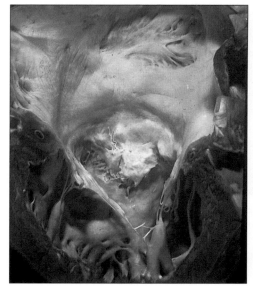

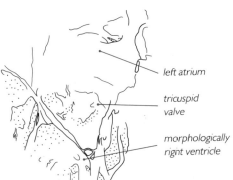

Fig. 6.47 This, the other side of the heart shown in Fig. 6.46, shows the left atrium connected to the morphologically right ventricle through a tricuspid valve.

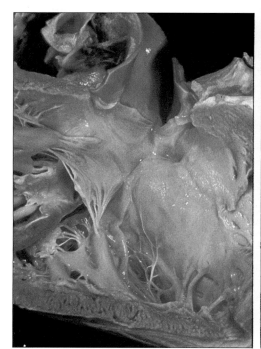

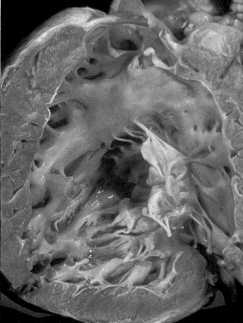

Fig. 6.48 These views of the right and left sides of a heart with congenitally corrected transposition show (left) the pulmonary trunk arising from the morphologically left ventricle and (right) the aorta arising from the morphologically right ventricle.

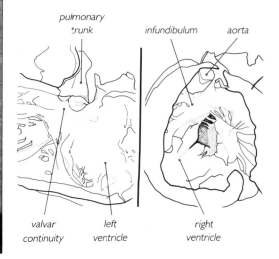

transposition. When this combination exists with usual atrial arrangement, the morphologically left ventricle is usually right-sided relative to the morphologically right ventricle, while the aorta tends to be to the left of the pulmonary trunk (Fig. 6.49). An important variant is found, however, when, because of rotation of the ventricular mass, the morphologically left ventricle is predominantly left-sided despite the discordant atrioventricular connexions. The aorta is then usually to the right of the pulmonary trunk. This arrangement, in which the ventricular and arterial relationships are not as anticipated for the connexions present, is known as a 'criss-cross' heart. When congenitally corrected transposition is found in its mirror-image variant, then the morphologically left ventricle is usually left-sided while the aorta is right-sided (Figs 6.50, 6.51).

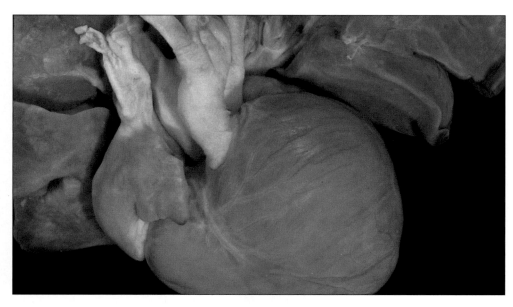

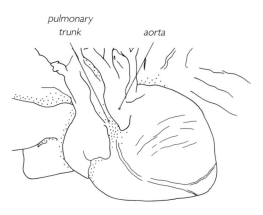

Fig. 6.49 This anterior view shows the typical left-sided location of the aorta in a heart with congenitally corrected transposition.

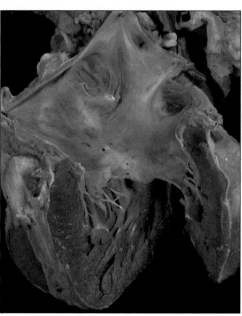

Fig. 6.50 This view of the right-sided chambers in a heart with mirror-image arrangement and congenitally corrected transposition shows the right-sided morphologically left atrium connected to the morphologically right ventricle.

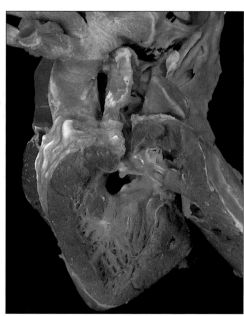

Fig. 6.51 This view of the left-sided chambers of the heart shown in Fig. 6.50 reveals the pulmonary|trunk arising from the left-sided morphologically left ventricle. Note the right-sided location of the aorta.

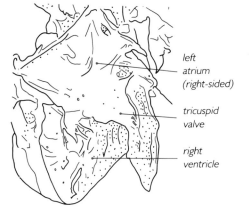

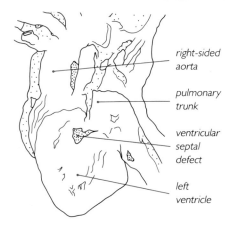

Since the discordant connexions are existing in series, the circulation in congenitally connected transposition is basically 'corrected'. The usual presence of associated anomalies, none theless, tends to 'uncorrect' the arrangement. It is rare to find cases with intact atrial and ventricular septal structures and no other lesions (Fig. 6.52). Three of the associated lesions are so frequent as to be considered almost part of the anomaly. They are, firstly, a ventricular septal defect; secondly, pulmonary stenosis; and, thirdly, Ebstein's malformation of the morphologically tricuspid valve. The ventricular septal defect is usually subpulmonary and perimembranous, extending to open between the ventricular inlets (Fig. 6.53). It can also extend to open between the outlets (doubly committed and juxta-arterial), or be encased in the muscular septum. Pulmonary stenosis can be due

to any of the lesions that produce obstruction of the morphologically left ventricular outflow tract (see below), obstruction due to tags derived from fibrous tissue being of particular significance. The tags herniate either from a partially formed membranous septum (Fig. 6.54) or from adjacent valvar tissues. When Ebstein's malformation is present (Fig. 6.55), it is unusual to find thinning and dilatation of the 'atrialized' inlet portion as occurs with concordant atrioventricular connexions, although it can occur.

The discordant atrioventricular connexions are often accompanied by conduction abnormalities. These relate to the grossly abnormal disposition of the atrioventricular conduction tissues. The hallmark of the discordant atrioventricular connexions when the atrial chambers are usually arranged is malalignment

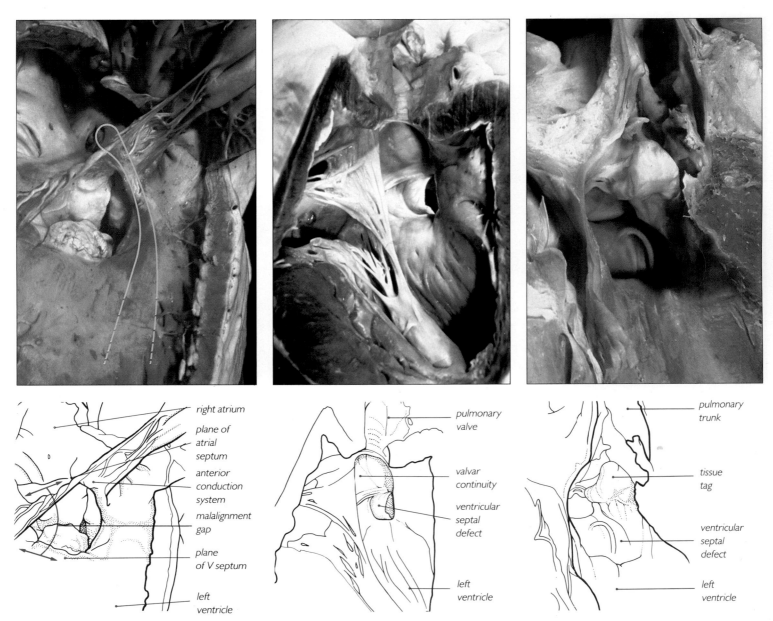

Fig. 6.52 This view of the right-sided morphologically left ventricle in a case of congenitally corrected transposition with intact septal structures shows the malalignment of the atrial and ventricular septal structures which underscores the abnormal location of the conduction tissues (superimposed on the photograph).

Fig. 6.53 This view through the morphologically left ventricle shows the typical perimembranous ventricular septal defect as found in congenitally corrected transposition.

Fig. 6.54 In this heart with congenitally corrected transposition, a tissue tag is obstructing the subpulmonary outflow tract from the morphologically left ventricle.

of the atrial relative to the ventricular septal structures, the subpulmonary outflow tract being wedged into the gap between them (see Fig. 6.52). Due to this, an atrioventricular node occupying its normal position at the apex of the triangle of Koch would be unable to make contact with the conduction tissues carried on the ventricular septum. Instead, an anomalous anterior node takes over the function of atrioventricular conduction, giving rise to a long nonbranching bundle that runs anteriorly relative to the pulmonary outflow tract (Fig. 6.56). The bundle descends anterocephalad relative to a perimembranous ventricular septal defect, if such a defect is present. It is fibrosis within the abnormally long nonbranching bundle which underscores the frequent finding of progressive disturbances of conduction in congenitally corrected transposition. When congenitally corrected transposition is found with mirror-image atrial arrangement,

there is much better alignment between the septal structures. Consequently, a normally positioned atrioventricular node and bundle are more frequently found.

Other associated lesions are much less frequent but do occur in congenitally corrected transposition. Of particular surgical significance is straddling of the right or left atrioventricular valves (see below). Various ventriculo–arterial connexions also co-exist with discordant atrioventricular connexions. Double outlet from the morphologically right ventricle and single outlet with pulmonary atresia are the most frequent. They, together with double-outlet left ventricle, are 'close cousins' of congenitally corrected transposition. Concordant ventriculo–arterial connexions are less frequent but are significant because, when combined with the discordant atrioventricular connexions, they present clinically as complete transposition.

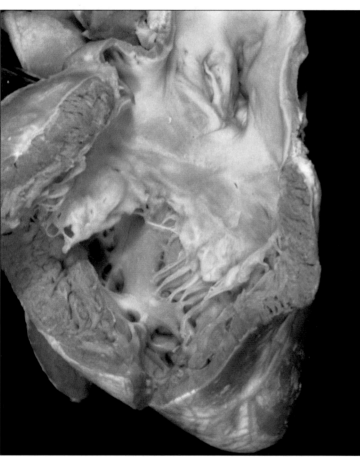

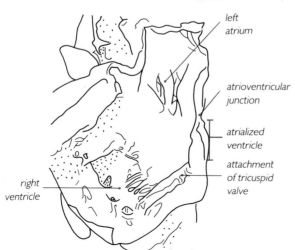

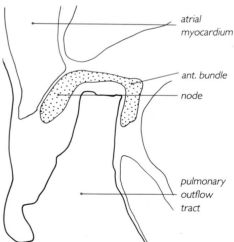

Fig. 6.55 This view of the left-sided chambers in a heart with congenitally corrected transposition shows Ebstein's malformation of the morphologically tricuspid valve.

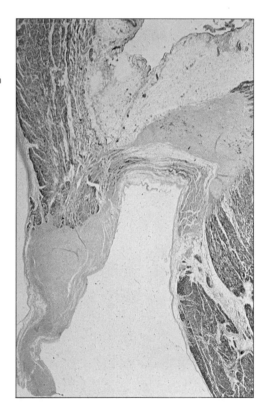

Fig. 6.56 This histological section through the subpulmonary outflow tract of a heart with congenitally corrected transposition shows the abnormal anterior location of the atrioventricular node and conduction tissues.

Double-inlet ventricle

Hearts that are unified by a double-inlet atrioventricular connexion have, in the past, tended to be described as 'single ventricle'. This makes little sense, since most of the hearts have two ventricles. They can more accurately, and simply, be described in terms of double-inlet ventricle. Similar ventricular morphologies also exist when either the right or left atrioventricular connexion is absent (see below).

Double-inlet left ventricle

By far the most common type of double inlet is when both atrial chambers connect to a dominant left ventricle, either through two separate valves (Fig. 6.57) or through a common atrioventricular valve (Fig. 6.58). An anterior septum, which never extends to the crux, separates the left ventricle from the anterior rudimentary and incomplete right ventricle, which usually gives rise to at least one arterial trunk (Fig. 6.59). The rudimentary right

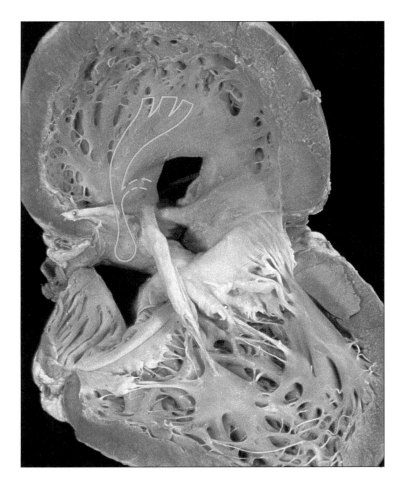

Fig. 6.57 This heart, opened like a clamshell, shows double inlet to a dominant left ventricle. Note the origin of the pulmonary trunk from the dominant ventricle and the ventricular septal defect which feeds the rudimentary and incomplete right ventricle (shown in Fig. 6.59).

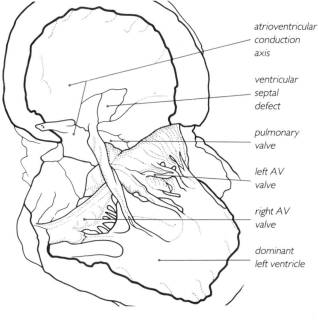

Fig. 6.58 In this heart, opened through the right atrioventricular junction, there is double inlet to a dominant left ventricle through a common atrioventricular valve.

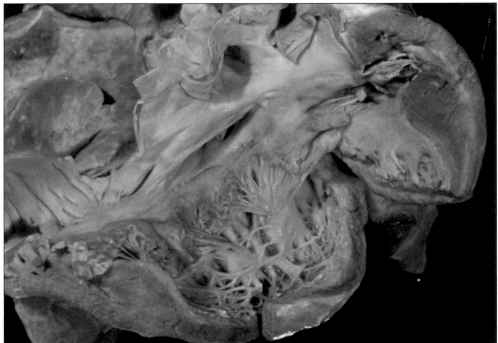

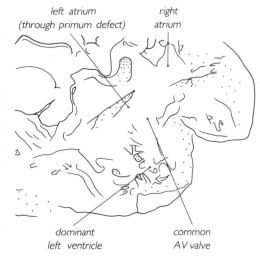

ventricle is incomplete since it lacks its inlet component. One, or even both of the atrioventricular valves, nonetheless, can straddle and override the ventricular septum as long as most of the overriding valve is connected to the dominant ventricle (Fig. 6.60). A common valve can also override and straddle. Other abnormalities of the atrioventricular valves are frequent in addition to straddling, stenosis being common. One atrioventricular valve, either the left or the right, can also be imperforate (Fig.

6.61). The rudimentary right ventricle can be positioned directly anterior, but, more usually, is positioned to one or other side of the dominant left ventricle. Nonetheless, the rudimentary ventricle is always anterosuperior, and is left-sided more frequently than right-sided.

Most frequently, the ventriculo–arterial connexions are discordant (see Fig. 6.59). Concordant ventriculo–arterial

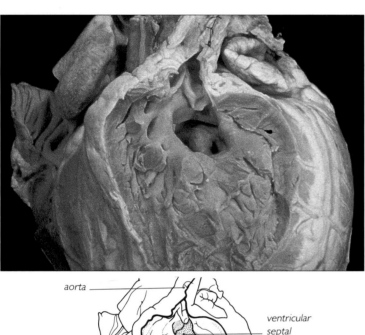

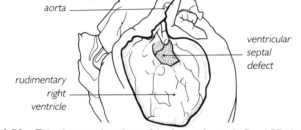

Fig. 6.59 This, the anterior view of the heart shown in Fig. 6.57, shows the incomplete and rudimentary right ventricle giving rise to the aorta.

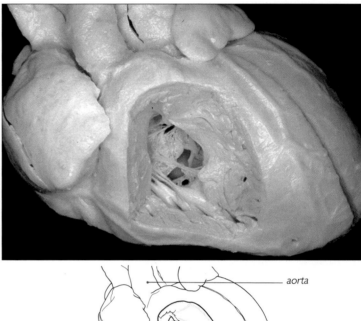

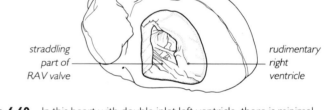

Fig. 6.60 In this heart with double inlet left ventricle, there is minimal straddling and overriding of the right atrioventricular valve into the rudimentary right ventricle. Photographed and reproduced by kind permission of Dr L.H.S. Van Mierop, University of Florida.

Fig. 6.61 In this heart with double inlet left ventricle and discordant ventriculo–arterial connexions, there is an imperforate left atrioventricular valve.

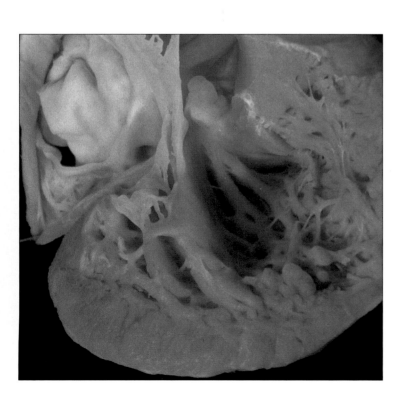

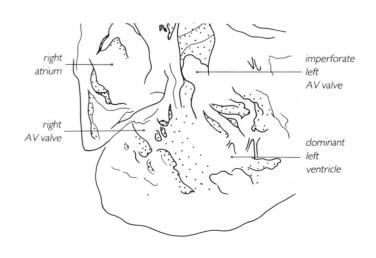

connexions can also exist, and then the rudimentary and in-complete right ventricle (Fig. 6.62) is virtually indistinguishable from the right ventricle seen in classical tricuspid atresia (see Fig. 6.72). Double outlet can also, rarely, be found from the rudimentary right ventricle and, more frequently, from the dominant left ventricle. When both arterial trunks are connected to the dominant left ventricle, the incomplete right ventricle is represented only by its apical trabecular component (Fig. 5.3).

Single outlet of the heart via a common arterial trunk is exceedingly rare, as is a solitary pulmonary trunk with aortic atresia. Solitary aortic trunk with pulmonary atresia is more frequent and, almost always, the solitary trunk is connected to the rudimentary right ventricle. Irrespective of the precise connexions, subarterial stenosis is a frequent finding, usually below the level of the arterial valves. It affects more frequently the subpulmonary infundibulum. Obstruction of the subaortic outlet, however, is frequent with discordant ventriculo–arterial connexions, usually due to narrowing of the ventricular septal defect. Coarctation, usually severe, tends to accompany subaortic obstruction.

By virtue of the abnormal orientation of the ventricular septum, the disposition of the conduction tissues is also grossly abnormal. An anomalous atrioventricular node is situated in the anterolateral quadrant of the right atrioventricular orifice. This gives rise to a long nonbranching bundle, which then runs anterosuperiorly before dividing to form the bundle branches astride the ventricular septum. When the rudimentary right ventricle is left-sided and there are discordant ventriculo–arterial connexions, this long bundle passes anterosuperiorly relative to the orifice of the pulmonary valve (Fig. 6.63 lower). When the

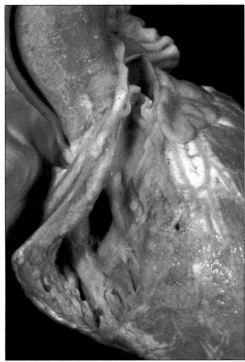

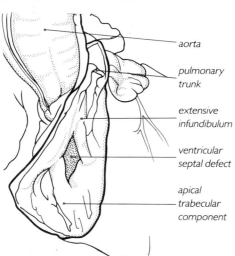

aorta

pulmonary trunk

extensive infundibulum

ventricular septal defect

apical trabecular component

Fig. 6.62 This heart with double inlet left ventricle has concordant ventriculo–arterial connexions. Note the similarity of the rudimentary right ventricle (shown) to the anterior chamber seen in hearts with tricuspid atresia (see Fig. 6.72).

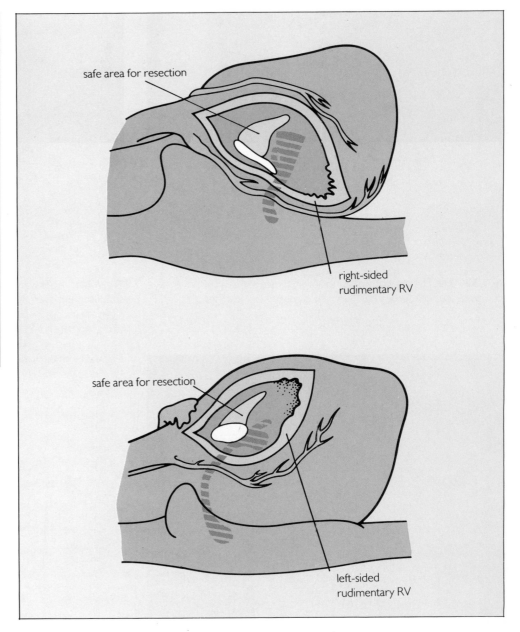

safe area for resection

right-sided rudimentary RV

safe area for resection

left-sided rudimentary RV

Fig. 6.63 This diagram shows the course of the axis of atrioventricular conduction tissue in hearts with double inlet left ventricle when the rudimentary right ventricle is (lower) left-sided and (upper) right-sided.

rudimentary right ventricle is right-sided, in contrast, the bundle descends directly to the muscular septum without running round the subpulmonary outflow tract (Fig. 6.63 upper). The abnormal location of the septum also influences the disposition of the coronary arteries. There is no prominent artery at the crux. Instead, prominent arteries arise from both right- and left-sided coronary arteries and descend anteriorly to delimit the position of the incomplete right ventricle.

Double-inlet right ventricle

The essence of the lesion, double-inlet right ventricle, is that both atrial chambers are connected to a dominant right ventricle (Fig. 6.64) in the presence of a posteroinferior rudimentary and incomplete left ventricle that is usually left-sided (Fig. 6.65). The connexion can be through two atrioventricular valves (see Fig.

6.64) or a common valve (Fig. 6.66). Occasionally, the rudimentary left ventricle can be posterior and right-sided. As with double-inlet left ventricle, the coronary arteries delimit the position of the incomplete ventricle, and either of the atrioventricular valves (or a common valve) can straddle and override the ventricular septum (see Fig. 6.65). Imperforate valves must also be anticipated. The ventriculo–arterial connexions are usually either double outlet from the right ventricle (see Fig. 6.64), concordant (Fig. 6.66), or single outlet with either pulmonary or aortic atresia, the solitary trunk then arising from the right ventricle. Since the ventricular septum extends to the crux, there is usually a regularly positioned conduction system. When the rudimentary ventricle is right-sided, however, the ventricular topology is of left-handed pattern and the atrioventricular conduction tissues have an abnormal disposition, comparable to those seen in congenitally corrected transposition.

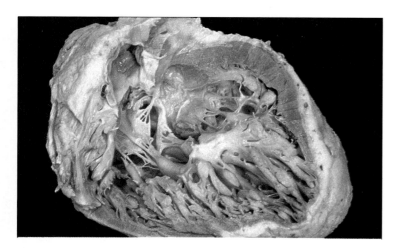

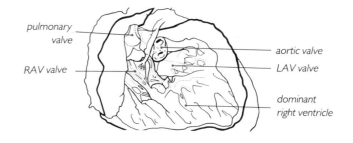

Fig. 6.64 This heart, dissected by removing the anterior wall of the ventricular mass, has double inlet to and double outlet from the dominant right ventricle.

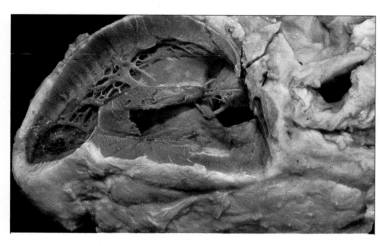

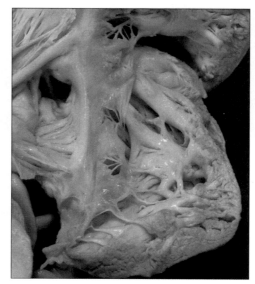

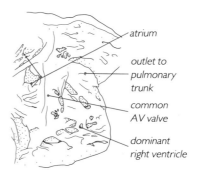

Fig. 6.66 This heart has double inlet to the dominant right ventricle through a common atrioventricular valve. There are concordant ventriculo–arterial connexions.

Fig. 6.65 This is the posterior aspect of the heart shown in Fig. 6.64. It shows the rudimentary and incomplete left ventricle with minimal straddling of the left atrioventricular valve (one papillary muscle remains in the left ventricle).

Double-inlet solitary and indeterminate ventricle

Double-inlet solitary and indeterminate ventricle is the rarest type of double-inlet ventricle. It is characterized by presence of a solitary ventricle with neither right nor left ventricular trabeculations (Fig. 5.4). Instead, the trabeculations are coarser than those of the right ventricle, and the ventricular apex is frequently crossed by larger free-standing trabeculations that often extend either into the ventricular outlet or to the atrioventricular junction. These trabeculations can give rise to tension apparatus of the atrioventricular valves, which may be two in number or a common structure. The trabeculations may also carry the axis of atrioventricular conduction tissue, which takes the form of a solitary bundle, descending from an anomalous anterolateral node. Often, there is a well-formed posterior ridge between the two atrioventricular connexions, which peters out when traced towards the ventricular apex. The trabeculations are then equally coarse to either side of the ridge (Fig. 6.67), which does not carry the axis of atrioventricular conduction tissue. This arrangement of double inlet to a solitary and indeterminate ventricle

must be distinguished from hearts in which a remnant of the ventricular septum separates apical trabecular components of unmistakably right and left ventricular pattern (Fig. 6.68). The latter anomaly is best considered in terms of a huge ventricular septal defect rather than double-inlet ventricle. With double-inlet to a solitary and indeterminate ventricle, the ventriculo–arterial connexions are, of necessity, either double-outlet or single outlet from the heart. There are no prominent descending coronary arteries when there is double-inlet to a solitary and indeterminate ventricle, reflecting the fact that the only ventricular septal structure present is the outlet septum.

Anomalies of the right atrioventricular junction

The greater majority of hearts encountered with abnormal right atrioventricular junctions will have usually arranged atrial chambers, so the affected junction will compromise the morphologically right atrium, most often guarded by a morphologically tricuspid valve. It must be remembered, nonetheless, that in hearts with discordant atrioventricular connexions (see above),

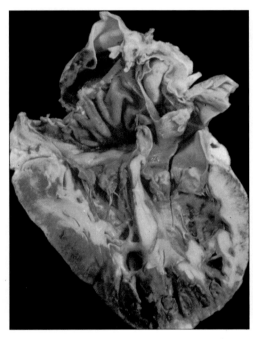
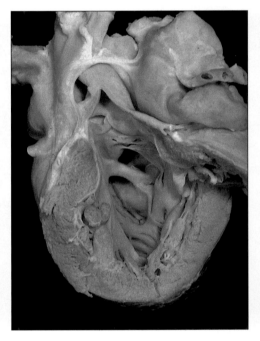
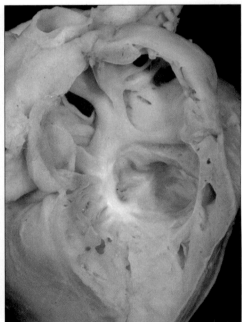

Fig. 6.67 This four chamber section through a solitary and indeterminate ventricle (see Fig. 5.4) shows a prominent posterior ridge between the atrioventricular valves. Note, however, that the apical trabeculations are uniformly coarse to both sides of the ridge.

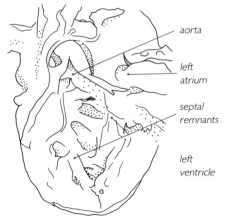

Fig. 6.68 This view shows the left ventricle in a heart with a huge ventricular septal defect. The remnants of the septum are clearly seen.

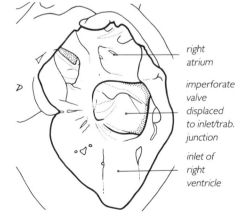

Fig. 6.69 This heart, seen from behind, has concordant atrioventricular connexions with an imperforate right atrioventricular valve which shows Ebstein's malformation.

this right-sided junction is guarded by the morphologically mitral valve. Similarly, in those with mirror-image arrangement, the right-sided atrium will also be of left morphology and its valve will again be a mitral valve. In hearts with isomeric appendages, the right-sided atrium may have an appendage of either morphologically right or left type. The right-sided valve will be of tricuspid or mitral morphology, nonetheless, depending on the ventricular rather than the atrial topology. These abnormal arrangements are rare in comparison to the frequency of anomalies of the right-sided morphologically tricuspid valve in hearts with usual atrial arrangement. Unless otherwise indicated, therefore, lesions of the morphologically tricuspid valve are described, starting with a consideration of its most extreme pathology, total absence, or, as more usually expressed, valvar atresia.

Atresia of the right atrioventricular valve

There is a significant difference between an imperforate valve (Fig. 6.69) and absence of the atrioventricular connexion (Fig. 6.70) as the cause of atrioventricular valvar atresia. When found in the right atrium, both usually produce tricuspid atresia. The imperforate variant, however, is rare and usually also exhibits Ebstein's malformation (see Fig. 6.69). Tricuspid atresia is much more frequently due to complete absence of the right atrioventricular connexion. The right atrium then has a completely muscular floor (Fig. 6.70) that is separated in its entirety from the ventricular mass by the fibrofatty tissues of the atrioventricular groove (Fig. 6.71). A dimple, if present, overlies the atrioventricular component of the central fibrous body, so that the right atrium is in potential communication with the morphologically left rather than the right ventricle.

Irrespective of the substrate for the atresia in these settings, all right atrial blood must traverse an atrial septal defect in tricuspid atresia and then pass from the left atrium to the left ventricle. When the connexion is absent then, as in double-inlet left ventricle (see Fig. 6.62), the right ventricle is incomplete and rudimentary, lacking its inlet portion (Fig. 6.72). The rudimentary ventricle is again delimited by prominent downgoing coronary arteries, and there is no prominent coronary artery at

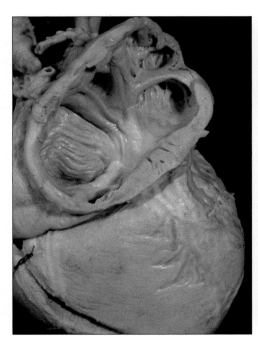

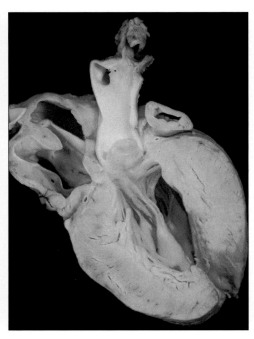

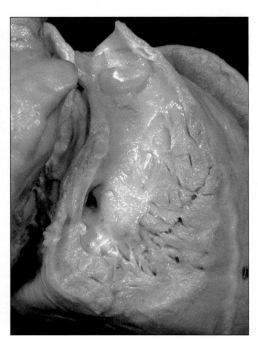

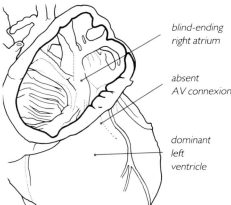

blind-ending
right atrium

absent
AV connexion

dominant
left
ventricle

Fig. 6.70 In this heart, with classical tricuspid atresia, there is complete absence of the right atrioventricular connexion and the right atrium has a muscular floor (compare with Fig. 6.69).

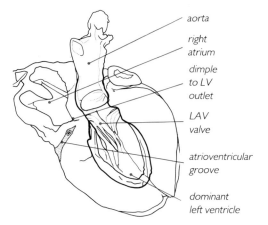

aorta

right
atrium

dimple
to LV
outlet

LAV
valve

atrioventricular
groove

dominant
left ventricle

Fig. 6.71 This "four chamber" section through a heart with classical tricuspid atresia shows absence of the right atrioventricular connexion and reveals how the dimple overlies the atrioventricular component of the membranous septum, pointing to the left ventricular outflow tract.

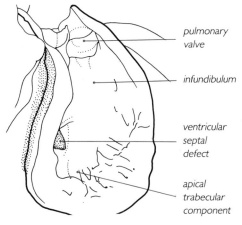

pulmonary
valve

infundibulum

ventricular
septal
defect

apical
trabecular
component

Fig. 6.72 This view, from the front, shows the incomplete and rudimentary right ventricle in a heart with classical tricuspid atresia and concordant ventriculo–arterial connexions. Compare with the heart shown in Fig. 6.62.

the crux (Fig. 6.73). Usually, the ventriculo–arterial connexions are concordant, and pulmonary stenosis, a common finding, is then due to stenosis at the ventricular septal defect. Pulmonary atresia may also be found, and then the right ventricle is usually grossly hypoplastic in addition to being incomplete. In a minority of cases, the ventriculo–arterial connexions may be discordant, with the aorta arising from the rudimentary right ventricle. Other connexions, such as double outlet or single outlet via a common arterial trunk, can occur from either dominant or rudimentary ventricles but are rare. The atrioventricular node is found in the floor of the right atrium, overlapping the dimple. The ventricular conduction tissues branch on the apical trabecular septum, the branching bundle being on the left ventricular aspect beneath the septal crest.

Although tricuspid atresia is almost always found in the variants described above, other patterns do exist. An imperforate right valve can, for example, be found with double-inlet ventricle. Absence of the right atrioventricular connexion can also be seen when the left atrium is connected to a dominant right ventricle. This variant is usually seen with a right-sided rudimentary left ventricle, and with straddling and overriding of the left atrioventricular valve (Fig. 6.74). It is fair to presume that, had the right atrioventricular valve been formed in this setting, it would have been of mitral morphology. Some, therefore, might prefer to describe this rare variant as mitral atresia, even though it is the right atrium that is blind-ending.

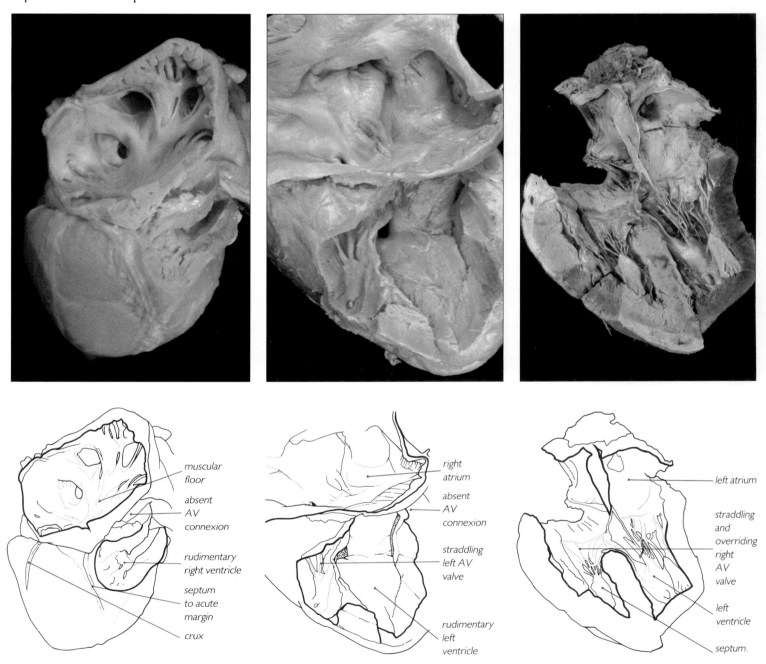

Fig. 6.73 This dissection of a heart with classical tricuspid atresia shows how the septum between dominant left and incomplete and rudimentary right ventricles comes to the acute margin of the ventricular mass and not to the crux.

Fig. 6.74 In this heart with absence of the right atrioventricular connexion (compare with Fig. 6.70), the left atrium is connected to a dominant right ventricle, with straddling of the left atrioventricular valve into the right-sided incomplete and rudimentary left ventricle.

Fig. 6.75 This four chamber section shows straddling and overriding of the tricuspid valve in a heart with basically concordant atrioventricular connexions.

Straddling right atrioventricular valve

Straddling of the right atrioventricular valve is found most frequently when there is right-hand ventricular topology. A series of anomalies are then found which vary according to the degree of override of the straddling valve. The extremes of the spectrum are concordant atrioventricular connexions (Fig. 6.75) and double-inlet left ventricle (Fig. 6.76). The essence of straddling tricuspid valve, whether the atrioventricular connexions are concordant or double inlet, is malalignment between the atrial and ventricular septal structures (Fig. 6.77). Due to this, the regular atrioventricular node within the triangle of Koch is

unable to make contact with the ventricular conduction tissues carried astride the ventricular septum. Instead, an anomalous node is formed posteriorly and laterally in the overriding junction at the point of origin of the ventricular septum.

Straddling of the right atrioventricular valve can also be found with left-hand ventricular topology. The straddling valve is then of mitral morphology (Fig. 6.78). According to the precise connexion of the overriding junction, the connexions will then either by discordant or double-inlet right ventricle with right-sided rudimentary left ventricle. There is an abnormal disposition of the atrioventricular conduction tissues because of the left-handed ventricular topology.

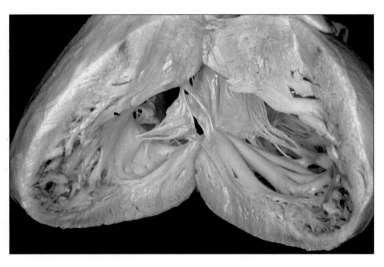

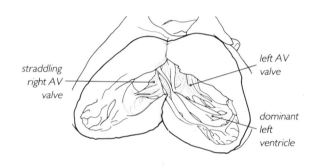

Fig. 6.76 This view of the left ventricle of the heart shown in Fig. 6.60 reveals overriding and straddling of the right atrioventricular valve in a basically double inlet connexion. Photographed and reproduced by kind permission of Dr L.H.S. Van Mierop, University of Florida.

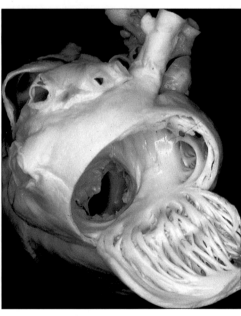

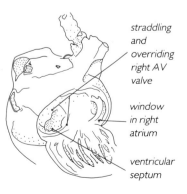

Fig. 6.77 This heart with straddling and overriding of the tricuspid valve is revealed by a window in the right atrium. Note the anomalous location of the ventricular septum.

Photographed and reproduced by kind permission of Dr L.H.S. Van Mierop, University of Florida.

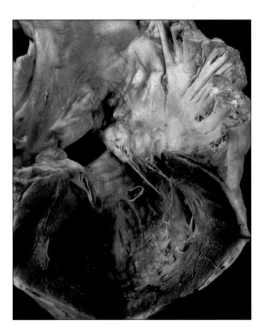

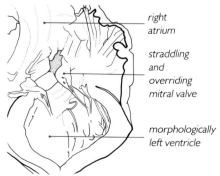

Fig. 6.78 This view of the right atrioventricular junction in a heart with congenitally corrected transposition shows straddling and overriding of the mitral valve with basically discordant atrioventricular connexions.

Ebstein's malformation

The essence of Ebstein's malformation is displacement of the hinge point of some of the leaflets of the tricuspid valve from the atrioventricular junction into the cavity of the right ventricle, the leaflets themselves often being dysplastic. It is the septal and mural leaflets which are usually affected (Fig. 6.79). The extent of the displacement varies, but it is never further than the junction of the inlet and apical trabecular components of the ventricle. In its severest form, the attachment of the leaflets is displaced down to the junction of these components, and is often heaped onto a prominent muscular shelf. The annular attachment of the anterosuperior leaflet is almost never displaced. It is the distal attachments of this leaflet which show important variation. They may be focally attached, in which case the blood is able to reach the subpulmonary outlet across the leading edge of the leaflet (Fig. 6.80). Alternatively, there may be an abnormal linear attachment (Fig. 6.81). The only communication with the ventricular outlet component is then through the commissure between the deformed septal and inferior leaf-

lets, or through perforations in the malformed anterosuperior leaflet itself. In this severe form, the inlet component of the ventricle is usually dilated and thinned, so-called atrialization. Such atrialization, nonetheless, can also be found with focal attachment. In rare circumstances, the commissures between the valve leaflets may be closed, producing an imperforate variant of Ebstein's malformation (see Fig. 6.69).

Other malformations of the tricuspid valve

While dysplasia of the leaflets of the morphologically tricuspid valve is most universally associated with Ebstein's malformation, it can exist as an isolated lesion without any downwards displacement of the hinge points of the leaflets (Fig. 6.82). Such isolated dysplasia can occur in a valve of normal dimensions but, more usually, it is seen in pulmonary atresia with intact septum, either in combination with Ebstein's malformation or alone. Congenital anomalies producing stenosis or incompetence of the morphologically tricuspid valve other than Ebstein's malformation or isolated dysplasia are exceedingly rare. One rare lesion of

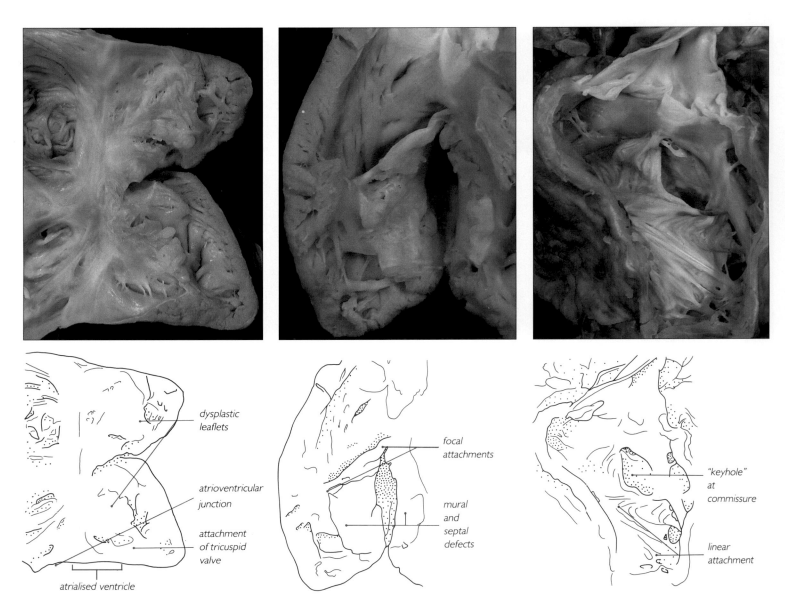

Fig. 6.79 This heart has been opened through the right atrioventricular juncton to show the typical features of Ebstein's malformation.

Fig. 6.80 In this heart with Ebstein's malformation, there is a focal attachment of the tension apparatus supporting the antero-superior leaflet of the tricuspid valve.

Fig. 6.81 In this example of Ebstein's malformation, the antero-superior leaflet is tethered in linear fashion.

significance is congenitally unguarding of the tricuspid orifice. In this lesion, which is again usually found with pulmonary atresia where the ventricular septum is intact, there is either total absence of the leaflets of the valve, or they are grossly deficient and plastered down onto the ventricular walls.

Anomalies of the left atrioventricular junction

As with the previous section, the greater part of the discussion here is devoted to the left atrioventricular junction in hearts with usual atrial arrangement and concordant atrioventricular connexions. We are, therefore, concerned with malformations of the morphologically mitral valve. It should be remembered, nonetheless, that, in the heart with mirror-image arrangement and concordant atrioventricular connexions, the left-sided junction is guarded by the morphologically tricuspid valve. This can be afflicted by all the lesions discussed above, which are specific for the morphologically tricuspid valve. Equally, in the patient with usual atrial arrangement and discordant atrioventricular connexions, the left-sided junction is again guarded by a

morphologically tricuspid valve. This valve can also be affected by lesions specific to the tricuspid valve, such as Ebstein's malformation (Fig. 6.54). These lesions and anomalies of the left-sided valve in hearts with isomeric appendages, are not discussed. Straddling of the left-sided valve, in contrast, will be described irrespective of its morphology, and atresia of the left-sided valve will be considered in the setting of various segmental combinations.

Atresia of the left atrioventricular valve

As with the right atrioventricular junction, it is essential to distinguish between an imperforate left atrioventricular valve (Fig. 6.83) and absence of the atrioventricular connexion (Fig. 6.84) as the substrate for atresia of the left atrioventricular valve. In hearts with mitral atresia, the morphologically right atrium is almost always connected to a morphologically right ventricle (Fig. 6.84). When the left atrioventricular connexion is absent, however, the left ventricle is rudimentary and incomplete as well as hypoplastic, lacking its inlet portion. The size of the left

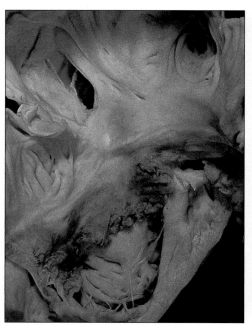

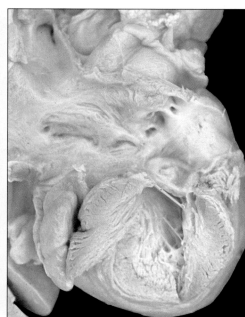

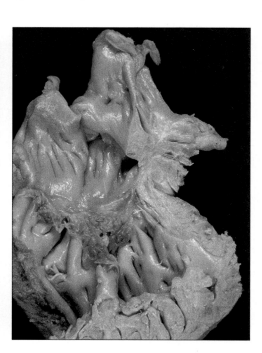

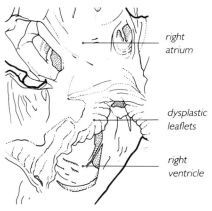

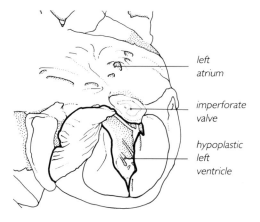

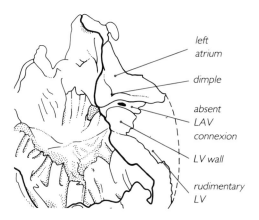

right atrium

dysplastic leaflets

right ventricle

left atrium

imperforate valve

hypoplastic left ventricle

left atrium

dimple

absent LAV connexion

LV wall

rudimentary LV

Fig. 6.82 This tricuspid valve has normal junctional attachments but gross dysplastic changes in all its leaflets.

Fig. 6.83 This heart has an imperforate mitral valve blocking a concordant atrioventricular connexion.

Fig. 6.84 In this heart, mitral atresia is produced by absence of the left atrioventricular connexion. The right atrium is connected to a dominant right ventricle.

ventricle, nonetheless, whether there is an imperforate valvar membrane or absent atrioventricular connexion, usually relates to the state of the aortic outflow tract. When there is coexisting aortic atresia, the left ventricle is almost always grossly hypoplastic (Fig. 6.84). When there is a patent aortic root, the left ventricle can be considerably larger; this is usually because there is a co-existing ventricular septal defect, either with concordant ventriculo–arterial connexions (Fig. 6.85), or double-outlet right ventricle. Any of these combinations with a patent aortic root may be found either with an imperforate valvar membrane or with absence of the atrioventricular connexion.

Another common variant of left atrioventricular valvar atresia is seen when the right atrium is connected to a dominant morphologically left ventricle. The left atrioventricular connexion is usually absent (Fig. 6.86) and there is an anterior left-sided rudimentary and incomplete right ventricle, usually with discordant ventriculo–arterial connexions. If the left valve is formed in these circumstances, it would almost certainly be of tricuspid morphology. It is customary, therefore, to categorize this combination as tricuspid atresia.

Anatomic lesions of the morphologically mitral valve

The congenital lesions that produce mitral stenosis or incompetence are more common than those that affect the morphologically tricuspid valve. Overall, miniaturization and dysplasia of the valve (Fig. 6.87) are usually found with co-existing aortic atresia and mitral stenosis. Miniaturization of the valve, sufficient to produce stenosis, can be found without dysplasia, while dysplasia can occur in isolation or in other lesions such as clefts. A cleft in the aortic leaflet of the normally constructed mitral valve (Fig. 6.88) points directly to the subaortic outflow tract. It is this feature that distinguishes the true cleft in an aortic leaflet from the septal commissure between the left ventricular components of the bridging leaflets in atrioventricular septal defect, often referred to erroneously as a 'cleft mitral valve'. A more common cause of mitral incompetence than the isolated cleft is prolapse of individual scallops of the mural leaflet of the valve. Most severe in diseases such as Marfan's syndrome (Fig. 6.89), prolapse may occur in a variety of conditions, particularly with the so-called floppy valve. From the morphological standpoint, there is

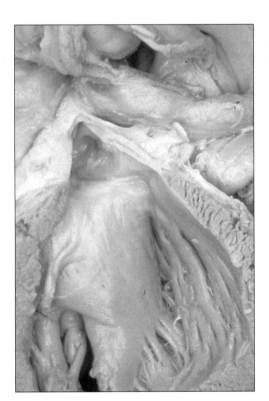

Fig. 6.85 This heart with mitral atresia due to an imperforate valve has a patent aortic root and a ventricular septal defect.

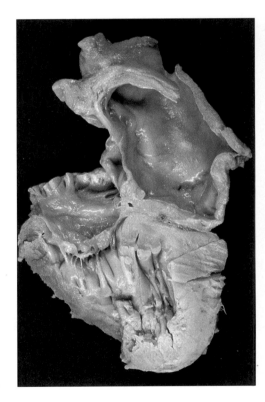

Fig. 6.86 In this heart with absence of the left atrioventricular connexion, the right atrium is connected to a dominant left ventricle. Photographed and reproduced by kind permission of Prof. Gaetano Thiene, University of Padova.

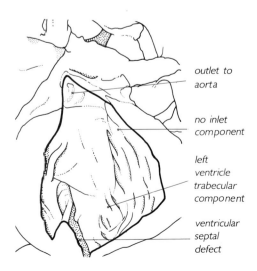

outlet to aorta

no inlet component

left ventricle trabecular component

ventricular septal defect

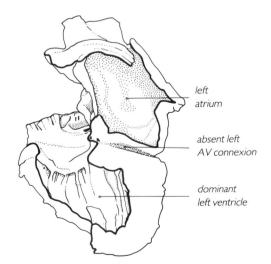

left atrium

absent left AV connexion

dominant left ventricle

evidence·that prolapse and its related lesion of valvar hooding, results from lack of cordal support to the affected segment of the leaflet.

Several congenital lesions produce mitral stenosis over and above the miniaturization discussed above. The most frequently described is the so-called 'parachute' deformity. The lesion that most closely resembles a parachute occurs when one of the paired papillary muscles is either grossly hypoplastic or absent

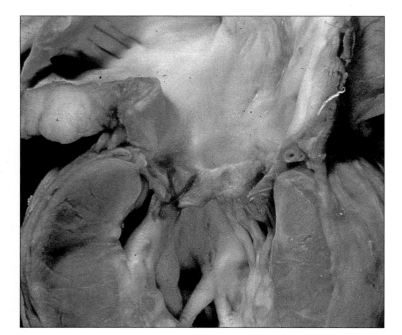

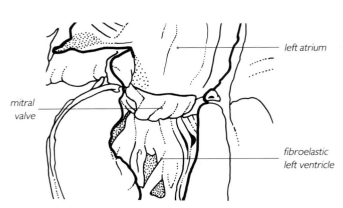

Fig. 6.87 This heart, opened through the left atrioventricular junction, has mitral stenosis, fibroelastosis of the left ventricle and aortic atresia (the hypoplastic left heart syndrome).

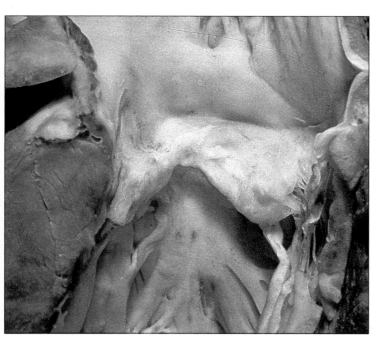

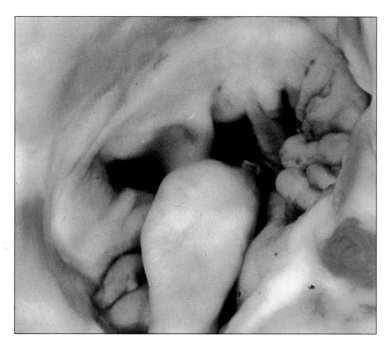

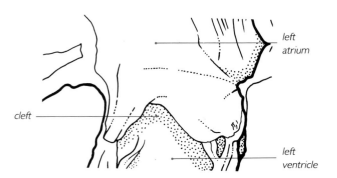

Fig. 6.88 This heart has a cleft in the aortic leaflet of the mitral valve. It "points" to the subaortic outlet.

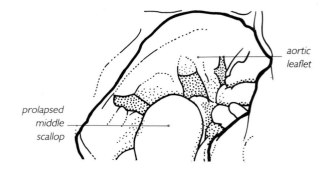

Fig. 6.89 This heart is viewed from the left atrium and shows prolapse of the middle scallop of the mural leaflet of the mitral valve in a patient with Marfan's syndrome.

(Fig. 6.90). The leaflets then insert directly into the ventricular wall and all the tendinous cords stream to the solitary papillary muscle. A parachute arrangement can also be produced when the two papillary muscles are fused together.

A rarer form of congenital mitral stenosis is produced by the arcade lesion. In this anomaly, the cords are muscularized from the papillary muscles to the leaflets so that the muscles fuse to form an arcade along the edge of the leaflet (Fig. 6.91).

Another lesion that may produce congenital stenosis occurs when the valve has a double orifice; this is found in two forms. In one, there is a tongue of tissue between the aortic leaflet and one of the scallops of the mural leaflet (Fig. 6.92), the valve itself having normal papillary muscles. This variant is often found in the left valve of atrioventricular septal defects. In the other form, there are two discrete orifices within the valve, with each orifice supported by a separate tension apparatus (Fig. 6.93).

Although Ebstein's malformation usually affects the tricuspid valve, a similar lesion can rarely affect the mitral valve. It is the mural leaflet that is affected, with the hinge point displaced into the ventricular inlet portion (Fig. 6.94).

Straddling left atrioventricular valve

A straddling left atrioventricular valve is found most frequently with usual atrial arrangement and right-hand ventricular topology. The valve is then connected in part to the right ventricle and in part to the normally positioned left ventricle. When the valve is connected mostly to the left ventricle, there are concordant atrioventricular connexions (see Fig. 6.93). This variant is seen most frequently with either complete transposition or double-outlet right ventricle. In contrast, if the straddling valve is connected mostly to the right ventricle, there would be double-inlet atrioventricular connexion.

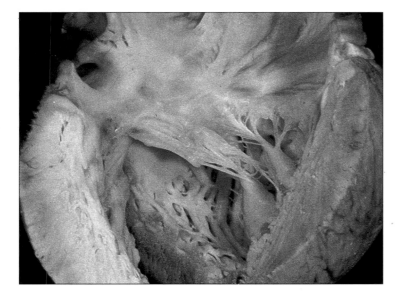

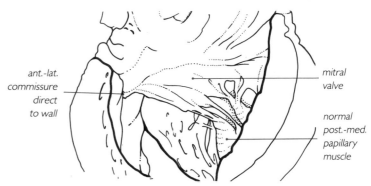

Fig. 6.90 In this heart with tricuspid atresia, there is a parachute arrangement of the left atrioventricular valve by virtue of absence of one of the papillary muscles.

Fig. 6.91 This heart, viewed from the left ventricle, has an arcade lesion of the mitral valve, the musculature of the papillary muscles meeting on the leading edge of the aortic leaflet of the valve.

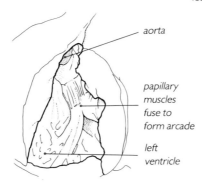

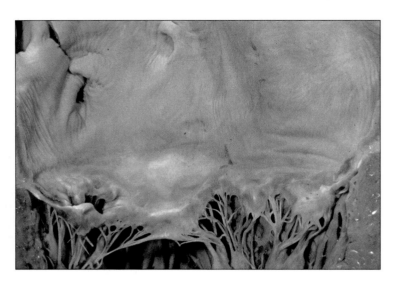

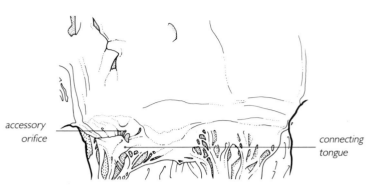

Fig. 6.92 This otherwise normal heart has a dual orifice within the mitral valve produced by a tongue of tissue running from the aortic to the mural leaflet.

accessory orifice

connecting tongue

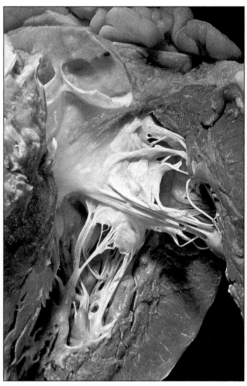

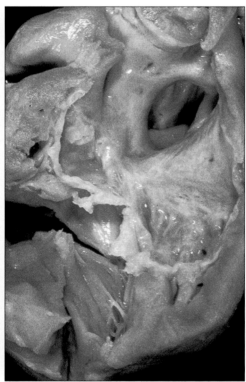

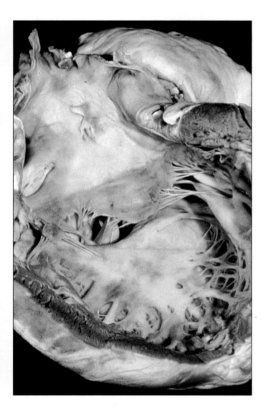

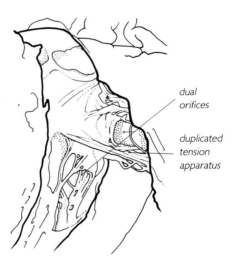

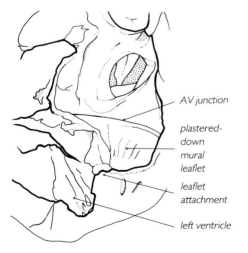

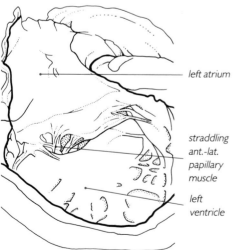

dual orifices

duplicated tension apparatus

AV junction

plastered-down mural leaflet

leaflet attachment

left ventricle

left atrium

straddling ant.-lat. papillary muscle

left ventricle

Fig. 6.93 In this mitral valve with dual orifices, seen from the left ventricle, each orifice is supported by its own set of tension apparatus.

Fig. 6.94 This heart, seen from the left side, has Ebstein's malformation of the mitral valve.

Fig. 6.95 This heart, seen from the left ventricle, has minimal straddling of the mitral valve in the setting of basically concordant atrioventricular connexions.

The other variant of straddling left valve is found with usual atrial arrangement and left-hand ventricular topology. The straddling valve is then connected partly to the right-sided morphologically left ventricle, and partly to the left-sided morphologically right ventricle. When connected mostly to the morphologically right ventricle, the combination is that of congenitally corrected transposition with straddling tricuspid valve (Fig. 6.96). An anomalous conduction system is found as in corrected transposition. When the straddling valve connects mostly to the morphologically left ventricle, there is a double inlet with a left-sided rudimentary right ventricle. The arrangement of the conduction tissue is comparable with that found in typical double-inlet left ventricle.

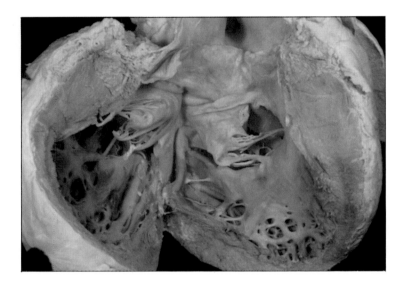

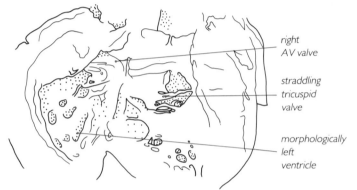

Fig. 6.96 In this heart, seen from the morphologically left ventricle, there is minimal straddling and overriding of the left-sided tricuspid valve with basically discordant atrioventricular connexions.

In Chapter 6, malformations of the atrioventricular junction have been discussed, including numerous anomalies that affect the inlet portions of the ventricles. In this chapter, we discuss defects of the ventricular septum along with malformations of the ventricular outlets in hearts with both normal and abnormal ventriculo—arterial connexions. Also included are miscellaneous lesions such as divided ventricles, supernumerary ventricles, and Uhl's malformation.

ANOMALIES OF THE VENTRICLES

Ventricular septal defects

It is well recognized that defects can be found at various sites between the ventricles. Our approach to categorization is based upon the premise that the septum itself has membranous and muscular components (Fig. 7.1). In this respect, it should also be

Fig. 7.1 In this septum removed from a normal heart, the membranous component has been isolated, together with parts of the muscular septum corresponding to the inlet, apical trabecular and outlet components of the right ventricle.

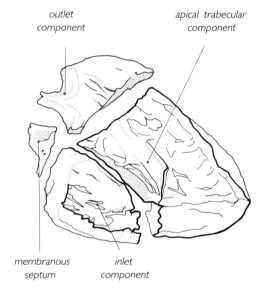

outlet component   apical trabecular component

membranous septum   inlet component

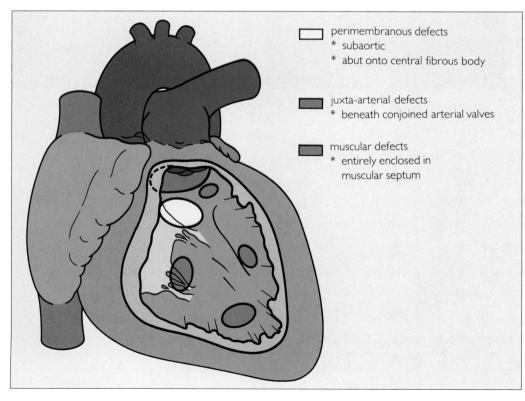

perimembranous defects
* subaortic
* abut onto central fibrous body

juxta-arterial defects
* beneath conjoined arterial valves

muscular defects
* entirely enclosed in muscular septum

Fig. 7.2 This diagram shows the basic system used for categorization of ventricular septal defects.

remembered that the attachment of the tricuspid valve to the right side of the septum is more towards the ventricular apex than is the attachment of the mitral valve. Due to this, part of the muscular septum, together with part of the membranous septum, are atrioventricular in position (see Figs 1.62 and 1.63). It is absence of these components which produce the atrioventricular septal defects that were discussed in Chapter 6. Defects of the ventricular septum, in contrast, are all found below the level of junctional attachment of the leaflets of the tricuspid valve.

Three discrete anatomic types can be distinguished according to the nature of their borders as seen from the right ventricle (Fig. 7.2). The majority are found adjacent to the area of the membranous septum. Although frequently termed 'membranous', the defects almost invariably occupy an area of septum far greater than that normally filled by the interventricular component of the membranous septum (see Fig. 7.1). When viewed from the left ventricle (Fig. 7.3), their distinguishing feature is that they abut directly on the central fibrous body,

of which the atrioventricular component of the membranous septum is an integral part. Moreover, part (or all) of the inter-ventricular component of the membranous septum is often still present, hanging as a fibrous fold in the posterior margin of the defect. The defects, therefore, are perimembranous rather than membranous. They can be further divided according to the way in which they open into the right ventricle.

Occasionally, defects are large and open towards both inlet and outlet components. These are called confluent defects (Fig. 7.4). More usually, however, the defects open either towards the inlet or the outlet. When viewed from the right ventricle, the usual view obtained by the surgeon, a defect opening towards the inlet is mostly shielded by the septal leaflet of the tricuspid valve. The medial papillary muscle is then in superocephalad position (Fig. 7.5). Reflection of the valvar leaflet shows that the roof of the defect is an extensive area of fibrous continuity between the leaflets of the aortic, mitral, and tricuspid valves.

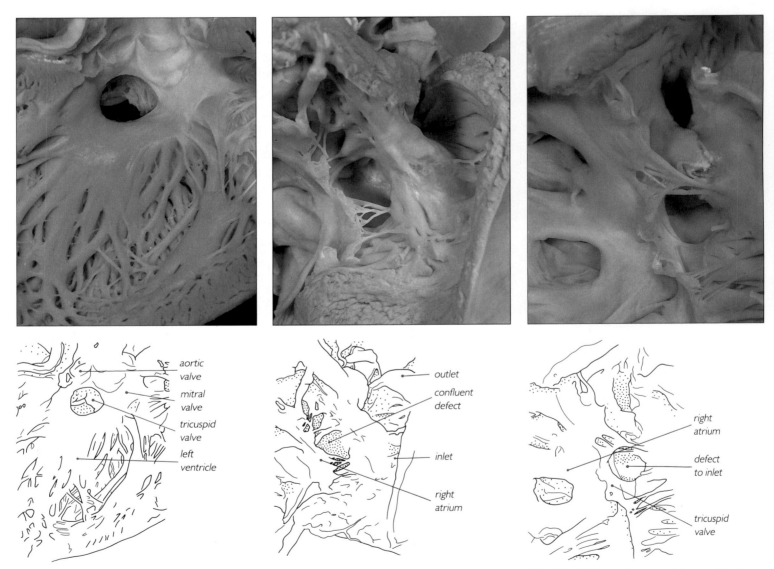

Fig. 7.3 This view from the left ventricle shows how perimembranous defects are directly related to the area of fibrous continuity between the leaflets of the aortic, mitral and tricuspid valves.

Fig. 7.4 In this heart, seen from the right ventricle, a perimembranous defect opens from the inlet to the outlet – a so-called confluent defect.

Fig. 7.5 This view from the right ventricle shows the appearance of a perimembranous defect opening to the inlet.

Perimembranous defects opening towards the infundibulum of the right ventricle have the medial papillary muscle beneath and behind them (Fig. 7.6). Such defects are frequently associated with malalignment of the outlet septum, either into the right ventricle as in tetralogy of Fallot, or into the left ventricle (Fig. 7.7). Posterior deviation of the outlet septum into the left ventricle produces obstruction of its outflow tract and is usually associated with coarctation or interruption of the aortic arch. All perimembranous defects (when the ventriculo–arterial connexions are concordant) are directly related to and beneath the aortic orifice. Furthermore, the axis of atrioventricular conduction tissue is always positioned posteroinferiorly to a perimembranous defect, except when there is straddling and overriding of the tricuspid valve (see Fig. 6.77).

The second anatomic type of ventricular septal defect is that which, when viewed from the right ventricle, is completely surrounded by the musculature of the septum, the so-called

muscular defect. As with perimembranous defects, muscular defects can be divided according to whether they open into the inlet, trabecular, or outlet components of the right ventricle. Inlet muscular defects, like perimembranous defects opening to the right ventricular inlet, are covered by the septal leaflet of the tricuspid valve (Fig. 7.8). They are distinguished from perimembranous defects because of the bar of muscular tissue that intervenes between the edge of the defect and the central fibrous body. The muscle bar is important since it carries the axis of atrioventricular conduction tissue above the defect. Apical muscular defects are found within the confines of the apical trabecular septum; they can be large and single, or multiple. Multiple defects can take two forms: there may be two or three large defects, usually situated to either side of the septomarginal trabeculation, or many small defects may percolate through the septum. The latter arrangement is known as a 'Swiss cheese

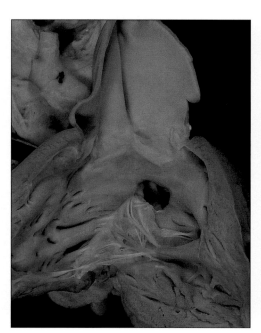
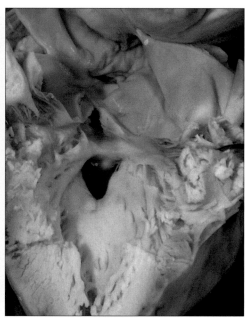
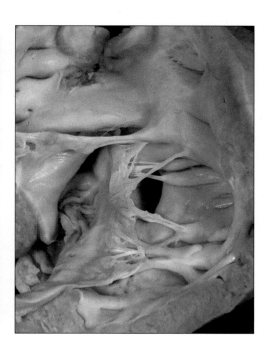

Fig. 7.6 This view, again from the right ventricle, shows the features of a perimembranous defect opening to the outlet.

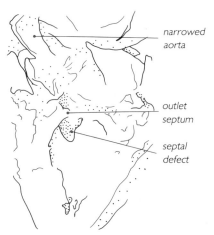

narrowed aorta

outlet septum

septal defect

Fig. 7.7 This view from the left ventricle shows posterior deviation of the outlet septum in a heart with interruption of the aortic arch.

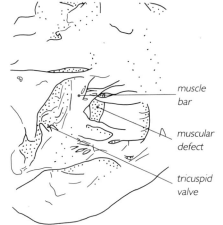

muscle bar

muscular defect

tricuspid valve

Fig. 7.8 This heart has a muscular defect opening to the inlet of the right ventricle.

septum'. The third type of muscular defect is that opening directly to the subpulmonary infundibulum. These outlet defects are usually relatively small (Fig. 7.9).

The third anatomic pattern for a ventricular septal defect is produced when there is complete absence of the outlet component of the septum, together with the posterior aspect of the subpulmonary infundibulum. With this arrangement, the defect opens beneath both the aortic and pulmonary valves which form an area of fibrous continuity in the roof of the defect. Such defects are accurately described as being doubly committed and juxtaarterial (Fig. 7.10). Most frequently in such defects, a muscle bar formed by the fusion of the septomarginal trabeculation and the ventriculo–arterial fold separates the edge from the central fibrous body and protects the conduction tissues. Occasionally, however, when the muscle bar is attenuated, a doubly committed

defect can extend to become perimembranous. The axis of atrioventricular conduction tissue is then much closer to the edge of the defect, but is still usually carried on the left ventricular aspect of the septum. Due to the absence of the outlet septum, the leaflets of the aortic valve are relatively unsupported, and prolapse of the right coronary leaflet is frequent. Such prolapse can also occur with perimembranous defects. We have also seen prolapse in a muscular defect when the outlet septum was particularly hypoplastic (Fig. 7.11).

Many ventricular septal defects close spontaneously and, while it is not possible from autopsy material determine how many defects close, insight can be gained into the mechanics of closure. Muscular defects, when small, can close simply by overgrowth of the muscular septum. Perimembranous defects close either by the plastering of the leaflets of the tricuspid valve across the

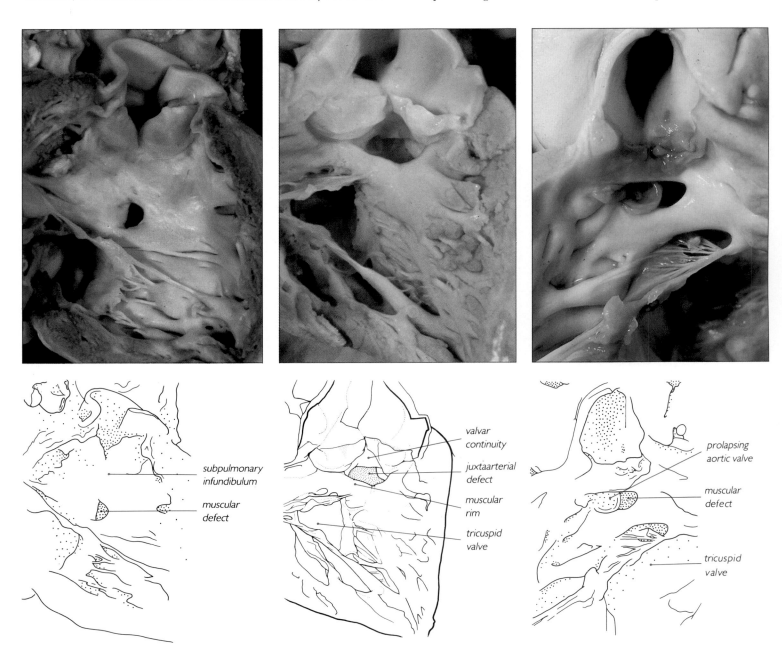

subpulmonary infundibulum

muscular defect

valvar continuity

juxtaarterial defect

muscular rim

tricuspid valve

prolapsing aortic valve

muscular defect

tricuspid valve

Fig. 7.9 This muscular defect opens to the outlet of the right ventricle.

Fig. 7.10 In this heart, a ventricular septal defect, opening between the outlets is roofed by fibrous continuity between the leaflets of the arterial valves – the criterion for a doubly committed and juxtaarterial defect. Note the muscular postero-inferior rim.

Fig. 7.11 In this heart with a muscular outlet defect, prolapse of one leaflet of the aortic valve has partially closed the hole.

defect (Fig. 7.12) or by herniation of tissue tags derived from the underside of the valvar leaflets (so-called aneurysm of the membranous septum). Defects characterized by malalignment of septal components are unlikely to close spontaneously, as are doubly committed and juxtaarterial defects, although the latter may regress in size due to herniation of a leaflet of the aortic valve (see Fig. 7.11).

Discussion thus far has been confined to ventricular septal defects in hearts with concordant atrioventricular and ventriculo–arterial connexions. The categorization into perimembranous, muscular, and doubly committed and juxtaarterial is equally valid in hearts with abnormal connexions of the chambers, such as complete or corrected transposition or double-outlet ventricles. We will also see that, in hearts with complete transposition, posterior deviation of the outlet septum into the left ventricle again produces stenosis but, because of the abnormal ventriculo–arterial connexions, it is subpulmonary rather than subaortic.

Miscellaneous right ventricular anomalies

There are several malformations of the ventricles which, although dissimilar themselves, fall into none of the categories discussed thus far or in subsequent sections. Uhl's malformation afflicts the entirety of the right ventricular myocardium. The heart originally described was characterized by total absence of the right ventricular myocardium, the remainder of the heart being normal. The essence of the lesion, therefore, is that the parietal right ventricular wall is composed only of apposed layers of epicardium and endocardium. The myocardium of the septo-marginal trabeculation and its ramifications, in contrast, are normal (Fig. 7.13). Care must be taken to distinguish between Uhl's malformation and lipomatous infiltration of the myocardium (Fig. 7.14). The latter lesion has recently become of importance because of its implication as the cause of arrhythmogenesis in the right ventricle (see Section 5). Since the arrhythmogenic

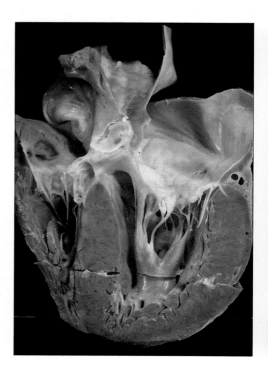

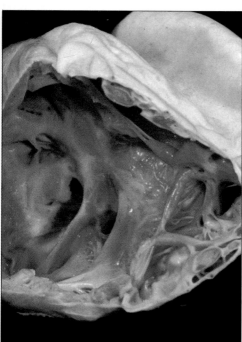

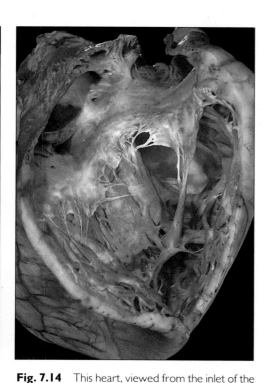

Fig. 7.14 This heart, viewed from the inlet of the right ventricle, is transilluminated to show the thinning of the outlet produced by fatty infiltration.

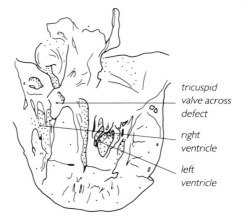

tricuspid valve across defect

right ventricle

left ventricle

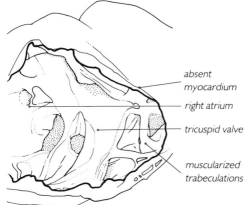

absent myocardium

right atrium

tricuspid valve

muscularized trabeculations

Fig. 7.12 This four chamber section shows how a perimembranous defect has been closed by plastering of the septal leaflet of the tricuspid valve across the defect.

Fig. 7.13 This heart has complete absence of the myocardium in the parietal wall of the right ventricle – Uhl's malformation.

ventricle can be a familial disease, and the substrate for sudden death, it is all the more important to distinguish fatty infiltration from Uhl's malformation.

Division of the ventricles into two parts is described as two-chambered ventricle, and occurs most frequently in the morphologically right ventricle, although several varieties of division can rarely be found in the left ventricle. An anomalous muscle bundle is often considered as the least severe form of divided right ventricle. This does not really produce two separate chambers, but simply crosses the ventricular cavity (Fig. 7.15).

Such a simple anomalous muscle bundle rarely produces problems. The ventricular division is much more obvious, and obstruction much more severe, when it is the apical portion of the septomarginal trabeculation that is hypertrophied to produce a shelf dividing the right ventricle into discrete inlet and outlet components (Fig. 7.16). This is the most common form of two-chambered right ventricle. Although it can exist in isolation, it usually co-exists with either an isolated ventricular septal defect or with tetralogy of Fallot. The right ventricle can also be divided by overgrowth of the septomarginal trabeculation in association

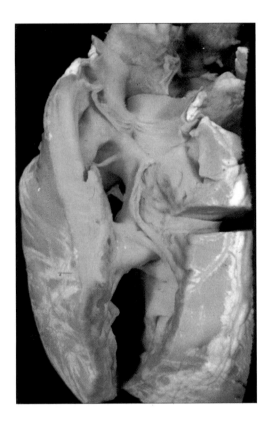

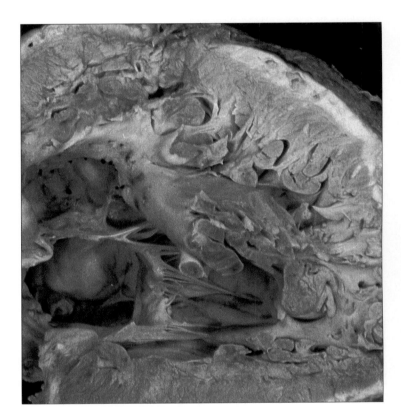

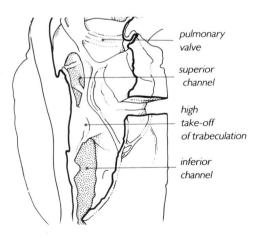

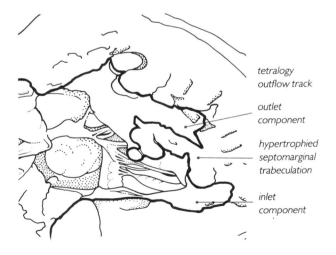

Fig. 7.15 This heart, seen from the infundibular aspect, has an anomalous muscle bundle crossing the cavity of the right ventricle.

Fig. 7.16 In this heart, the apical trabecular component of the right ventricle is divided by hypertrophy of the apical part of the septomarginal trabeculation.

with a ventricular septal defect communicating with the outlet component. If the dividing shelf becomes excessively large, the outlet component can then effectively be incorporated as part of the morphologically left ventricle. Such anomalies can pose problems for clinical diagnosis because of the impression that it is the left rather than the right ventricle that is divided.

Division of the right ventricle can also occur when one of its anatomical components is sequestrated, either partially or completely, from the rest of the chamber. A stenotic ring between the body of the right ventricle and the subpulmonary infundibulum produces the typical arrangement often found in tetralogy of Fallot. A stenotic muscular ring between the trabecular and outlet components is also a common cause of subpulmonary obstruction when rudimentary and incomplete right ventricles give rise to the pulmonary trunk in tricuspid atresa or double-inlet left ventricle. The inlet component can also be completely separated from the remainder of the right ventricle by a thick muscular shelf. In this lesion, the leaflets of the right atrioventricular valve are usually absent so that the heart presents as a bizarre variant of tricuspid atresia (Fig. 7.17, left). The remainder of the right ventricle persists as a rudimentary chamber supplied from the left ventricle through a ventricular septal defect (Fig. 7.17, right).

ANOMALIES OF THE VENTRICULAR OUTFLOW TRACTS

This section is concerned with lesions that affect the outflow tracts of the morphologically right and left ventricles. The same lesions which then produce subaortic obstruction in the heart with concordant connexions produce subpulmonary obstruction in the hearts with discordant ventriculo–arterial connexions and vice versa. We describe, therefore, the basic anatomy of the obstructive lesions, irrespective of the ventriculo–arterial connexions. In addition, atresia of the outflow tracts is discussed, including cases that can appropriately be designated as single outlet of the heart.

Tetralogy of Fallot

The combination of four morphological features that make up the anomaly called tetralogy of Fallot was recognized long before Arthur Etienne-Louis Fallot implicated it as the most common cause of 'la maladie bleu'. It was also described by Stensen, John Hunter, and Peacock, but it was Fallot who recognized its clinical significance.

The classical features are a ventricular septal defect, overriding of the aorta, infundibular pulmonary stenosis, and right ventricular hypertrophy (Fig. 7.18). The most important anatomical

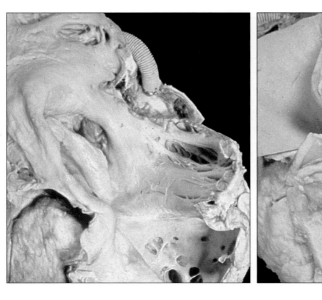
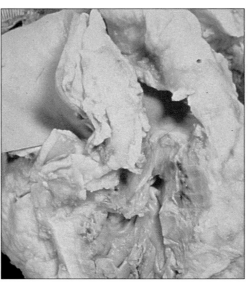
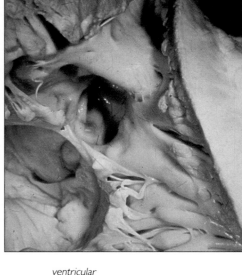
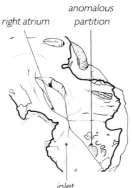
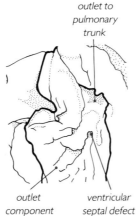
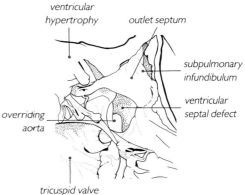

right atrium — anomalous partition

outlet to pulmonary trunk

ventricular hypertrophy — outlet septum

subpulmonary infundibulum

overriding aorta

ventricular septal defect

inlet

outlet component — ventricular septal defect

tricuspid valve

Fig. 7.17 These views of a heart with tricuspid atresia show, to the left, complete unguarding of the right atrioventricular junction and, to the right, a complete muscular partition separating the apical and outlet parts of the right ventricle from its inlet component. The ventricular septal defect leads to the left ventricle.

Fig. 7.18 This view from the apex of the right ventricle shows the four cardinal features of tetralogy of Fallot.

feature, however, is anterocephalad insertion of the outlet septum relative to the limbs of the septomarginal trabeculation. This anomalous insertion produces malalignment of the outlet septum with the rest of the septum and, hence, a ventricular septal defect. Due to its right ventricular location, the aorta, of necessity, has a biventricular connexion and, at the same time, there is a narrowing of the subpulmonary infundibulum. The right ventricular hypertrophy can be considered as a haemodynamic consequence of these anatomic abnormalities.

Although all cases of tetralogy have this same basic arrangement, there is important variability in detailed morphology of the anatomical components. The ventricular septal defect is perimembranous in the majority of cases (Fig. 7.18) but, in approximately 20% of cases, it has a muscular posterior rim (Fig. 7.19). Either type of defect may extend to become doubly committed and juxtaarterial, although this is rare (Fig. 7.20). When found, because of the absence of the outlet septum, such hearts are not strictly examples of tetralogy of Fallot. The typical ventricular septal defect extends into the infundibular region, but it may also excavate to open between the inlets in association with a common atrioventricular orifice (Fig. 7.21). On rare occasions, hearts with the unequivocal anatomy of tetralogy of

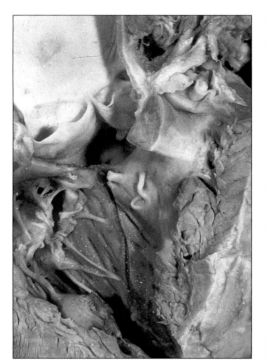

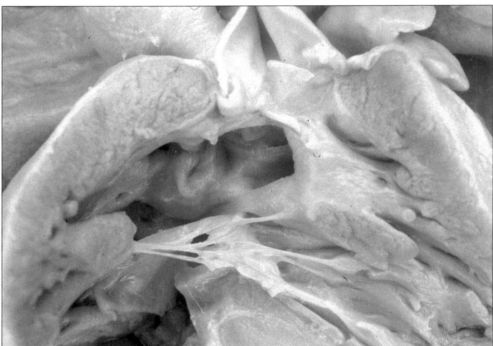

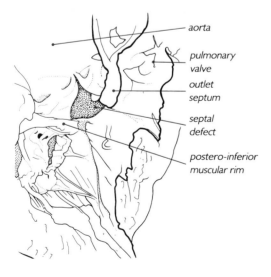

aorta

pulmonary valve

outlet septum

septal defect

postero-inferior muscular rim

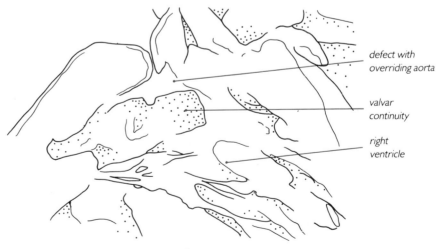

defect with overriding aorta

valvar continuity

right ventricle

Fig. 7.19 In this heart with tetralogy of Fallot, a muscle bar separates the leaflets of the tricuspid and aortic valves in the postero-inferior margin of the ventricular septal defect.

Fig. 7.20 In this heart with overriding aorta and pulmonary stenosis, the ventricular septal defect is doubly committed and juxtaarterial due to complete absence of the outlet septum.

Fallot can also exist with an obstructed ventricular septal defect, either because of reduplication of leaflets of the tricuspid valve around the defect or because of an anomaly of the mitral valve.

As with isolated ventricular septal defects, the perimembranous or muscular nature of a defect changes its relationship to the axis of atrioventricular conduction tissue. When perimembranous, the axis usually penetrates through the area of aortic–mitral–tricuspid valvar continuity and, in this area, may be overlaid by a remnant of the interventricular membranous septum. The branching segment of the axis then tends to be carried just below the septal crest on the left ventricular aspect, where it is

safe from surgical trauma. On occasion, nonetheless, the bundle may be disposed directly astride the septum. It is then vulnerable to stitches placed through the septal crest (Fig. 7.22).

The ventricular septal defect is sited so that the aorta takes its origin from both ventricles. Thus, it overrides the ventricular septum, being connected to the right ventricle to a greater or lesser extent. The extent of this connexion determines the ventriculo–arterial connexions, which can be concordant or double outlet from the right ventricle.

The subpulmonary stenosis is primarily due to the antero-cephalad insertion of the outlet septum (Fig. 7.18). This is usually

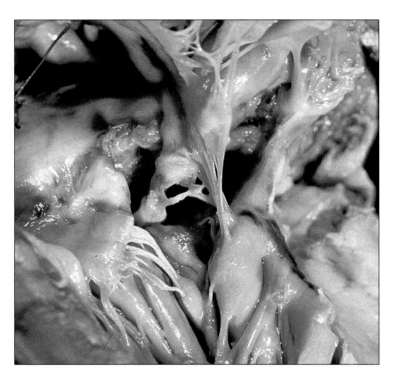

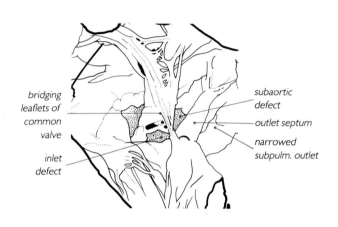

Fig. 7.21 This example of tetralogy of Fallot also has an atrioventricular septal defect with a common atrioventricular valve.

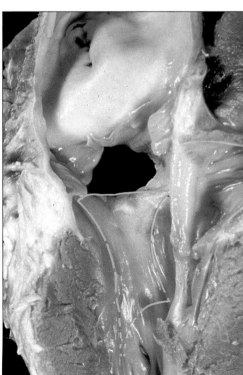

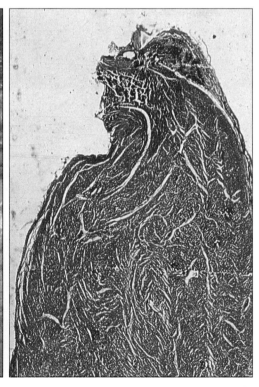

Fig. 7.22 In this heart with tetralogy of Fallot, stitches for repair were passed through the crest of the ventricular septum (left). As shown by the section (right), the conduction axis was directly astride the septum and, hence, was destroyed by the stitches.

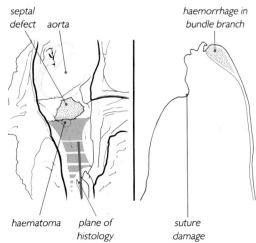

exacerbated by hypertrophy of septoparietal trabeculations (see Fig. 7.23). Obstructive lesions of the pulmonary valve are also frequent, the valve itself often having only two leaflets. On occasion, the leaflets of the pulmonary valve may be absent, in the sense that only a rim of dysplastic valvar tissue is present. The pulmonary trunk is dilated in these instances (Fig. 7.24), with dilatation of its branches often producing bronchial compression. Other than in these cases, the pulmonary arteries are usually smaller than normal, often with peripheral stenosis.

Pulmonary atresia

Pulmonary atresia describes the situation in which the pulmonary circulation has no patent communication with the ventricular mass. This can either be because the leaflets of the pulmonary valve are formed but imperforate (Fig. 7.25), or because the pulmonary trunk narrows down and ends blindly at its sinuses (Fig. 7.26). In the latter instance, there is a myocardium interposing between the ventricular and arterial cavities. A further

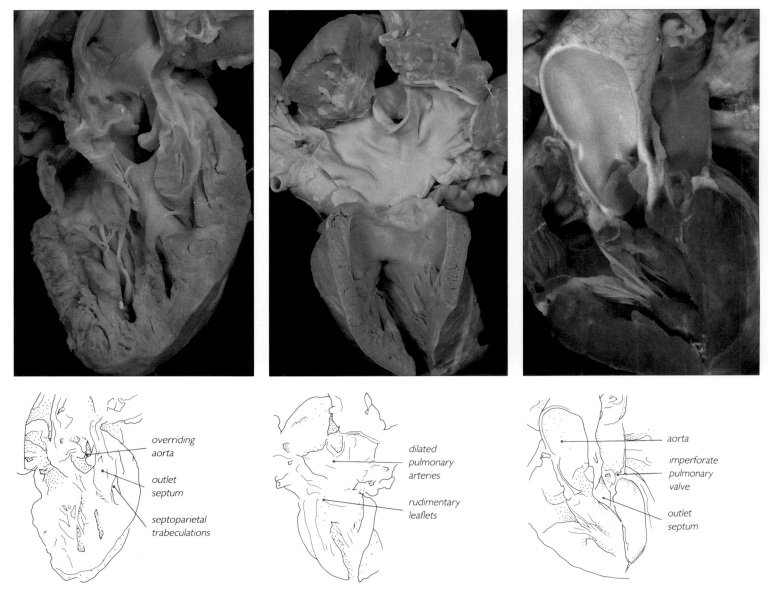

Fig. 7.23 This section along the long axis of the right ventricle shows how subpulmonary stenosis in tetralogy of Fallot is produced by the deviated outlet septum and the hypertrophied septoparietal trabeculations.

Fig. 7.24 In this heart with tetralogy of Fallot, the leaflets of the pulmonary valve are rudimentary ("absent valve syndrome") and the pulmonary arteries are grossly dilated.

Fig. 7.25 In this heart with tetralogy of Fallot, there is pulmonary atresia due to an imperforate pulmonary valve.

variation is seen when the entire pulmonary trunk, or even the entire intrapericardial pulmonary arteries, are absent (Fig. 7.27). In this latter instance, it is more correct to describe a solitary arterial trunk, since it is impossible to know whether, if the pulmonary arteries had been present, they would have connected to the arterial trunk or to the ventricular mass.

Pulmonary atresia in its different variants is essentially a malformation of the ventriculo–arterial junction, and can, therefore, occur with any possible combination of atrioventricular and ventriculo–arterial connexions. This section is concerned with the most common variant, namely, pulmonary atresia in the setting of usual atrial arrangement, concordant atrioventricular connexions, and essentially concordant ventriculo–arterial connexions. This arrangement itself can then occur in two further basic varieties, those with an intact ventricular septum and those with a ventricular septal defect. The rarer variants can be understood in terms of the anatomy described for these two variants existing in the settings of, for example, complete transposition, congenitally corrected transposition, double-inlet ventricle, and so on.

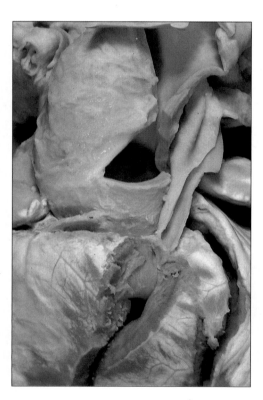

Fig. 7.26 In this example of tetralogy with pulmonary atresia, the subpulmonary outlet is muscular and blind-ending, the pulmonary trunk starting immediately above the sinuses with no evidence of valvar tissue.

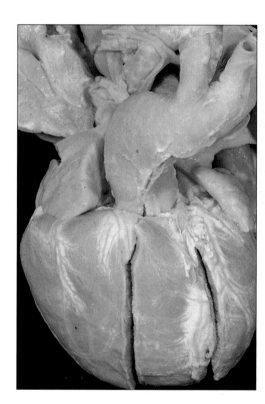

Fig. 7.27 This heart has complete absence of the intrapericardial arteries – the vessel leaving the base of the heart is best described as a solitary arterial trunk.

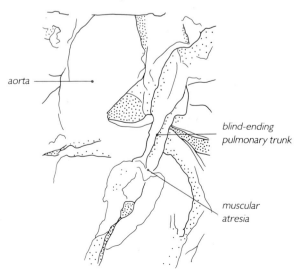

aorta

blind-ending pulmonary trunk

muscular atresia

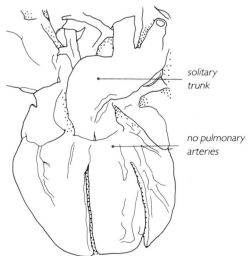

solitary trunk

no pulmonary arteries

Pulmonary atresia with intact septum

The most obvious feature of the variant with an intact ventricular septum is the degree of hypoplasia of the right ventricle. There is a spectrum of size, ranging from the cavity being tiny, through normal dimensions, to, rarely, some cavities being dilated and paper thin. The size of the cavity is related to the degree of obliteration of its various components by hypertrophy of the ventricular wall. In those that are smallest, the cavity is composed effectively of only the ventricular inlet. Hypertrophy of the wall obliterates both the apical trabecular component and the infundibulum (Fig. 7.28). The obliteration of the outlet produces the muscular form of pulmonary atresia and, consequently, there is no evidence of leaflets at the base of the pulmonary trunk. The trunk, therefore, commences blindly above the radiating and fused arterial sinuses (Fig. 7.29).

In cases in which the cavity is larger, the apical trabecular component again tends to be obliterated by mural hypertrophy (Fig. 7.30). The outlet portion, in contrast, is patent. It extends to the undersurface of an imperforate valvar membrane, which separates the cavity of the right ventricle from that of the pulmonary trunk (Fig. 7.31). In the cases with right ventricular cavities of more-or-less normal size, there is less hypertrophy of the wall and all components of the cavity are well represented, the atresia again being the consequence of an imperforate valve. Whatever the size of the right ventricular cavity, the tricuspid valve tends to be abnormal, exhibiting dysplasia with short and thick cords and, occasionally, the features of Ebstein's malformation. Almost always, cases that have dilated right ventricles have Ebstein's malformation or a congenitally unguarded orifice. The ventricular cavity is then enlarged by gross dilatation, and the muscular wall is thinned and attenuated. These hearts

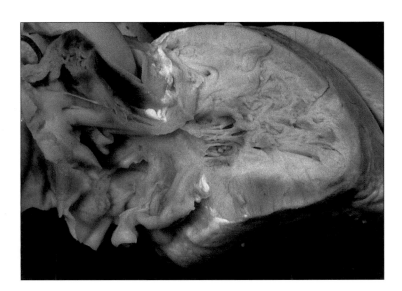

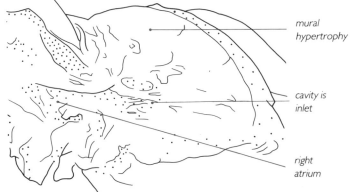

Fig. 7.28 In this heart with pulmonary atresia and intact ventricular septum, the cavity of the right ventricle is represented only by the inlet component, the other parts being virtually obliterated by hypertrophy of the ventricular walls.

mural hypertrophy

cavity is inlet

right atrium

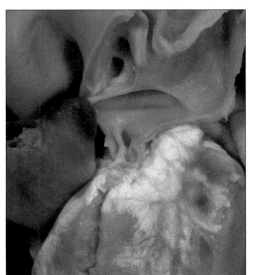

Fig. 7.29 This shows the typical arrangement of the pulmonary trunk in atresia with an intact ventricular septum when the outlet component is obliterated by muscular hypertrophy. There is no evidence of the leaflets of the pulmonary valve.

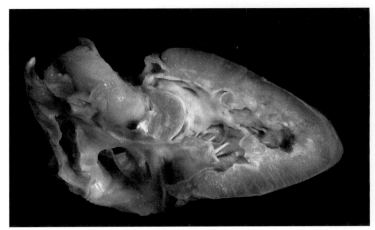

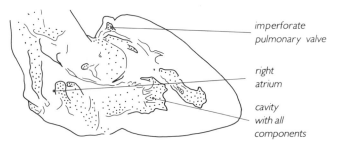

imperforate pulmonary valve

right atrium

cavity with all components

Fig. 7.30 In this example of pulmonary atresia with intact ventricular septum, there is less hypertrophy than in the heart shown in Fig. 7.28. The cavity is represented by all of its components and the pulmonary valve is imperforate.

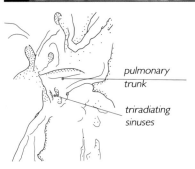

pulmonary trunk

triradiating sinuses

should be distinguished from Uhl's malformation, in which the pulmonary and tricuspid valves are normal and the parietal myocardium of the right ventricle is congenitally absent (see Fig. 7.13).

Of considerable significance in pulmonary atresia with an intact ventricular septum is the presence of fistulous communications from the ventricular cavity through the hypertrophied myocardium to the coronary arteries. These can, in some cases, become grossly dilated. Usually, they are associated with interruptions along the coronary arteries (Fig. 7.32). Although hypoplasia of the right ventricular cavity is the rule in pulmonary atresia with an intact ventricular septum, the pulmonary arteries are usually of good size and, almost always, are fed through a patent arterial duct.

Pulmonary atresia with ventricular septal defect

When pulmonary atresia with ventricular septal defect is found in the setting of concordant atrioventricular and ventriculo–arterial connexions, the ventricular morphology is almost always that of extreme tetralogy of Fallot in which the outlet septum is deviated sufficiently far anteriorly to produce muscular pulmonary atresia rather than stenosis (Fig. 7.33). In some cases, nonetheless, there may be valvar atresia, probably acquired (see Fig. 7.25). The ventricular septal defect is usually perimembranous (Fig. 7.33) and only rarely has a muscular inferior rim. Occasionally, examples will be found without any evidence of a subpulmonary infundibulum, but these are very much the exceptions. Cases can also rarely be encountered in which the

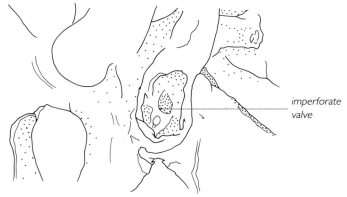

Fig. 7.31 This shows the pulmonary aspect of an imperforate valve in pulmonary atresia with intact ventricular septum but with a patent outlet component.

imperforate valve

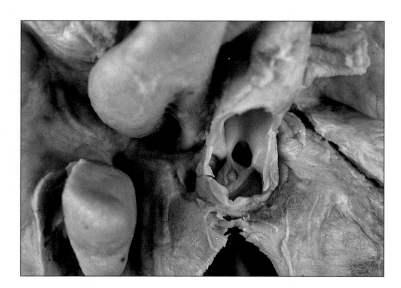

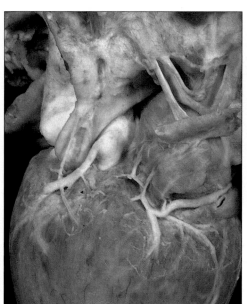

Fig. 7.32 This view of the left side of the ventricular mass in a heart with pulmonary atresia and intact ventricular septum shows distortion of the coronary arteries, which communicate via fistulous tracts with the cavity of the right ventricle.

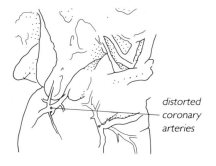

distorted coronary arteries

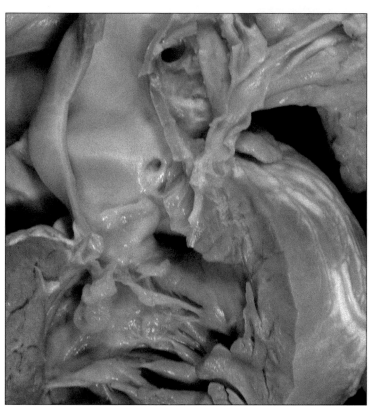

Fig. 7.33 This view of the right ventricle shows the typical arrangement of the outflow tract when tetralogy of Fallot is associated with pulmonary atresia rather than stenosis. The confluent pulmonary arteries are fed by the arterial duct.

ventricular septal defect is closed secondarily, thus presenting as pulmonary atresia with intact septum.

Most variation is found in the morphology and source of the pulmonary blood supply. In this respect, the pulmonary circulation must be assessed in its entirety, since it is the potential to reconnect this circulation back to the heart which determines the options for surgical repair. The simplest form is when the intrapulmonary arteries from all segments of both lungs are themselves connected by confluent right and left pulmonary arteries. This produces the arrangement termed unifocal supply, almost always fed through an arterial duct (Fig. 7.33). More rarely, unifocal supply may come from other sources, such as an aortopulmonary window or a fifth aortic arch.

More complicated patterns are found when the arterial duct is absent. Different compartments of intrapulmonary arterial circulation are then supplied from different sources, giving a multifocal supply. Multifocal supply usually comes from major aortopulmonary collateral arteries, which arise most frequently from the descending aorta (Fig. 7.34). The collateral arteries

may also take origin from branches of the aorta, such as the brachiocephalic or coronary arteries. Major collateral arteries tend to vary in number from two to five, and each collateral artery tends to supply a different part of the intrapulmonary arterial circulation. When collateral arteries are present, the duct is usually absent, but this does not imply that a pulmonary arterial confluence is lacking. Indeed, it is possible, rarely, to have unifocal supply of the lungs via a collateral artery feeding the central pulmonary arteries. More frequently, when central pulmonary arteries co-exist with collateral arteries, the central arteries do not supply the entire intrapulmonary circulation. It is important then to determine the number of broncho-pulmonary segments fed exclusively by collateral arteries, and to distinguish these from segments fed through central pulmonary arteries, the blood reaching the central arteries themselves via anastomoses with collateral arteries (Fig. 7.35). In some instances, bronchopulmonary segments can be supplied both from collateral arteries directly, and from central pulmonary arteries fed themselves via collateral vessels (Fig. 7.36).

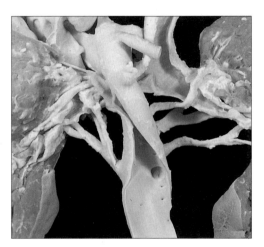

Fig. 7.34 In this patient with tetralogy of Fallot and pulmonary atresia, in which the heart and lungs are seen from behind, pulmonary arterial supply was derived through four systemic-to-pulmonary collateral arteries.

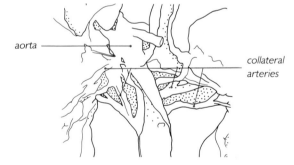

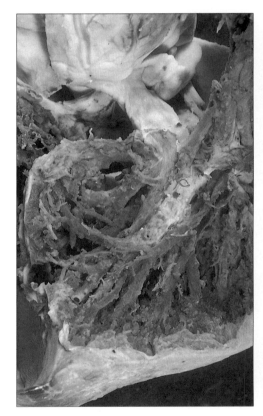

Fig. 7.36 In this segment of a lung from a patient with tetralogy and pulmonary atresia, dissection has been made of branches from the intraperi-cardial pulmonary arteries (coloured red) and a systemic-to-pulmonary collateral artery (blue). They supply the same segment.

Fig. 7.35 In this patient with tetralogy and pulmonary atresia, again seen from behind, a large systemic-to-pulmonary collateral artery is seen passing behind the oesophagus and anastomosing with the left pulmonary artery at the hilum.

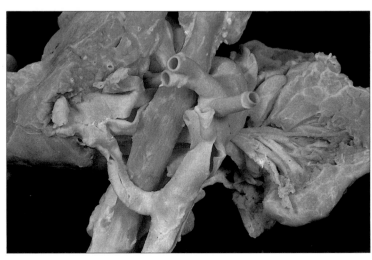

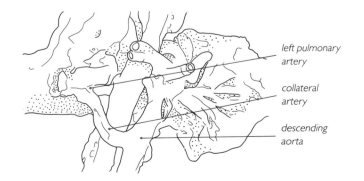

Aortic atresia

As with pulmonary atresia, the aortic outflow tract can be rendered atretic by either an imperforate aortic valve or by fibromuscular tissue interposing between the ventricular outlet and the blind and hypoplastic aortic trunk. The latter lesion is more common (Fig. 7.37). In both of these types, it is usually possible to determine the ventricular origin of the atretic aorta, and this most frequently is concordantly connected. It can, nonetheless, rarely be found with discordant ventriculo–arterial connexions or with double outlet ventricle. As might be expected, the atretic ventriculo–arterial connexion can also be found with any of the atrioventricular connexions, such as discordant ones producing congenitally corrected transposition with aortic atresia (Fig. 7.38).

The further variability in aortic atresia, as in cases with pulmonary atresia, is found according to the integrity of the ventricular septum. Most cases have an intact ventricular septum, and the ventricle supporting the atretic aorta is then grossly hypoplastic. This produces the so-called hypoplastic left heart syndrome. The left ventricle is slit-like when there is co-existing mitral atresia, which itself may be due to either absent left connexion (Fig. 7.39) or an imperforate mitral valve. The ventricle can be somewhat larger, although still grossly hypoplastic, when there is a patent but stenotic mitral valve. When the mitral valve is patent, the hypoplastic ventricle is always lined by a thick, pearly layer of fibroelastosis (see Fig. 6.87). These cases with gross hypoplasia of the left ventricle, if left untreated, have an exceedingly poor prognosis. Of late, none-

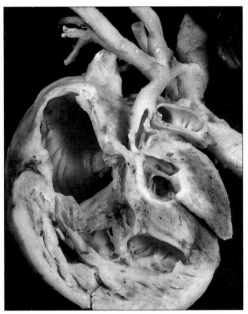

Fig. 7.37 This four chamber section shows hypoplasia of the left heart with aortic atresia.

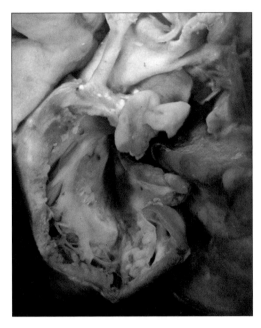

Fig. 7.38 In this heart, the atretic aorta arises from the morphologically right ventricle which is, in turn, connected to the left atrium. In other words, aortic atresia co-exists with congenitally corrected transposition.

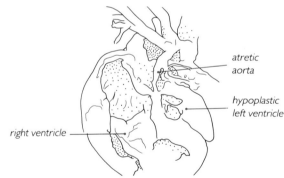

atretic aorta

hypoplastic left ventricle

right ventricle

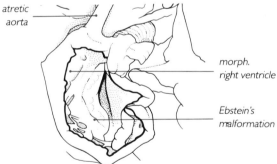

atretic aorta

morph. right ventricle

Ebstein's malformation

Fig. 7.39 This dissection shows the slit-like left ventricle found when aortic atresia is associated with absence of the left atrioventricular connexion.

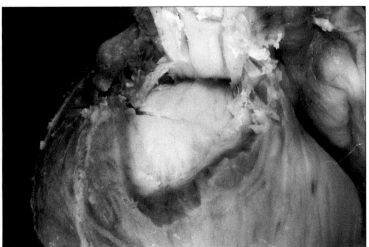

theless, there have been attempts to perform 'corrective' surgery, either by means of reconstructive procedures, or by transplantation. It is the much rarer cases in which aortic atresia co-exists with a ventricular septal defect which have a better chance of survival. Due to the ventricular septal defect, the left ventricle is much larger and can approach normal size (Fig. 7.40).

Irrespective of the atrioventricular and ventriculo–arterial connexions, an important consequence of aortic atresia will always be that the coronary arterial blood is supplied in retrograde fashion via the arterial duct and the aortic isthmus (Fig. 7.41). The arrangement of the great arteries often gives the impression that the descending aorta arises from the pulmonary trunk. In reality, the arterial duct is interposed between trunk and descending aorta, but the hypoplastic ascending aorta should not be misinterpreted as representing an anomalous coronary artery arising from the brachiocephalic artery in association with a common arterial trunk. The parlous state of the ductal-dependent circulation to the upper body and coronary arteries is usually further compromised by discrete coarctation at the site of the origin of the isthmus (Fig. 7.41).

Obstruction of the morphologically right ventricular outlet

The morphologically right ventricular outlet is almost always a complete muscular structure supporting the leaflets of its arterial valve. There is, therefore, considerable potential for the development of muscular subvalvar stenosis. Such infundibular obstruction is seen with great frequency in association with a ventricular septal defect, such as in tetralogy of Fallot (see Fig. 7.18) or in complete transposition or double-outlet right ventricle (see below). In these lesions, however, it is the deviation of the outlet septum which acts as the stimulus to formation of infundibular obstruction. Indeed, the obstruction can be so severe as to sequestrate the outlet part of the ventricle as a discrete chamber. When the ventricular septum is intact, muscular obstruction below the level of the valve is rare. We ourselves have not encountered isolated right ventricular infundibular stenosis, or seen it together with valvar stenosis and intact ventricular septum, except as a consequence of hypertrophic cardiomyopathy which obstructs the outlets of both left and right

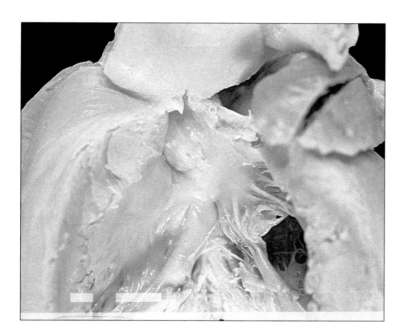

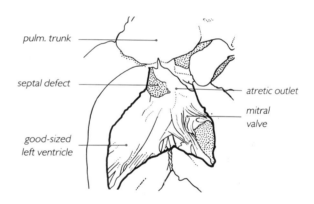

Fig. 7.40 In this heart with aortic atresia, there is a ventricular septal defect and a normal-sized left ventricle.

Fig. 7.41 This dissection of the aortic arch shows preductal coarctation co-existing with aortic atresia and the hypoplastic left heart syndrome.

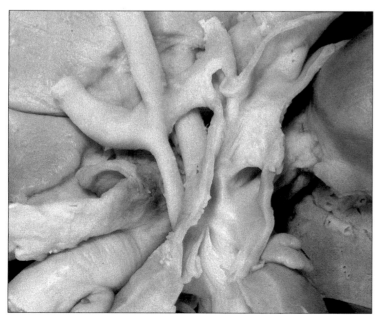

ventricles. Obstruction of the right ventricular outflow tract can rarely be produced at subvalvar level by herniation of huge aneurysms from fibrous structures, either an aneurysm of the membranous septum or from a valve guarding one of the venous connexions of the atrium (see Fig. 6.31).

Obstruction of the left ventricular outlet

Unlike the morphologically right ventricle, the outlet of the morphologically left ventricle is, in part, a muscular structure and, in part, composed of fibrous tissue (see Fig. 1.53). The anterior part is made up of the left ventricular aspect of the outlet septum, together with the left margin of the ventriculo–infundibular fold and the anterolateral muscle bundle of the left ventricle. The posterior part is composed of the extensive area of fibrous continuity between the leaflets of the arterial and mitral valves, with the left fibrous trigone and the central fibrous body at its two extremities (see Fig. 1.51). In very rare cases, there may be persistence of the ventriculo–infundibular fold in the left ventricle between arterial and atrioventricular valves.

This bar of muscle is small when there are concordant connexions, but can be more substantial with discordant ventriculo–arterial connexions. It is the overall anatomy of the outflow tract which dictates the nature of obstructive lesions as dynamic or fixed.

Dynamic obstruction is characterized by a muscular thickening of the septal surface. When minimal, the thickening merely produces a bulge and may not be of pathological significance. When extreme, its obstructive nature is no longer in doubt (Fig. 7.42). Indeed, it may also compromise the outflow tract of the right ventricle. Such muscular septal hypertrophy is almost always due to hypertrophic cardiomyopathy (see Section 5).

Fixed obstructive lesions can be divided into fibrous shelves, fibromuscular tunnels, aneurysmal tissue tags, anomalous insertion of tension apparatus of an atrioventricular valve, hypertrophy of the anterolateral muscle bundle, or deviation of the outlet septum in the presence of a ventricular septal defect.

A fibrous shelf is usually found on the septal surface, but can extend onto the facing leaflet of the mitral valve (Fig. 7.43). The lesion rarely forms a completely circular obstruction, but takes

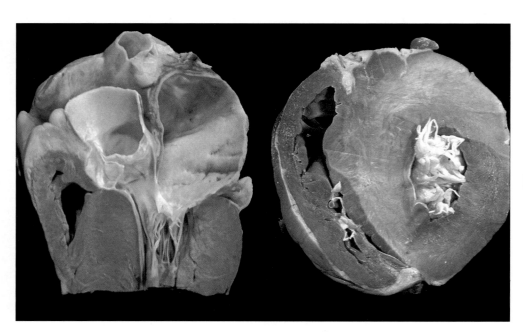

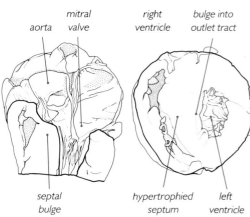

Fig. 7.42 These long axis and cross sections of the same heart show hypertrophic cardiomyopathy producing obstruction of the left ventricular outflow tract.

aorta *mitral valve* *right ventricle* *bulge into outlet tract* *septal bulge* *hypertrophied septum* *left ventricle*

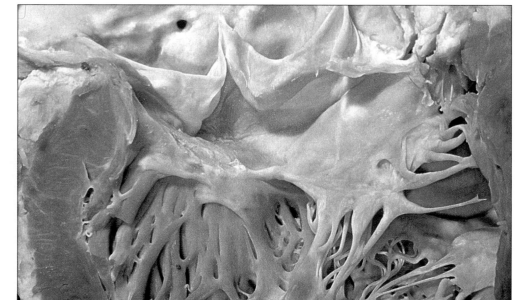

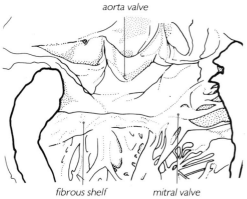

Fig. 7.43 In this heart, subaortic obstruction is produced by an extensive fibrous shelf.

aorta valve *fibrous shelf* *mitral valve*

more of the shape of a horseshoe. Fibromuscular tunnels are more severe examples of the discrete shelf, a much longer segment of stenotic outflow tract often being combined with a distinct septal bulge. Aneurysmal tissue tags may arise from the membranous septum, be it intact or partially formed; from the mitral valve (or the left valve in an atrioventricular septal defect); or from the tricuspid valve when there is a ventricular septal defect. They are most significant as obstructive lesions either when there is complete transposition, or when there is an atrioventricular septal defect (Fig. 7.44). Anomalous insertion of the tension apparatus of an atrioventricular valve is also most frequently a problem in association with atrioventricular septal defects, but can give problems in other circumstances, including

complete transposition. Hypertrophy of the anterolateral muscle bundle is seen most frequently when ventricular septal defects are associated with obstruction of the left ventricular outflow tract and interruption of the aortic arch, but we have seen one case where hypertrophy of the bundle was an isolated lesion (Fig. 7.45). More usually, it is deviation of the outlet septum, with insertion into the left ventricle, which produces the greatest obstruction (see Fig. 7.7).

As an aside before describing lesions of the arterial valves, it is pertinent to mention another rare malformation of the left ventricular outflow tract, namely, a tunnel from the left ventricle to the aorta. This structure extends from the cavity of the left ventricle and emerges to the right of the pulmonary trunk,

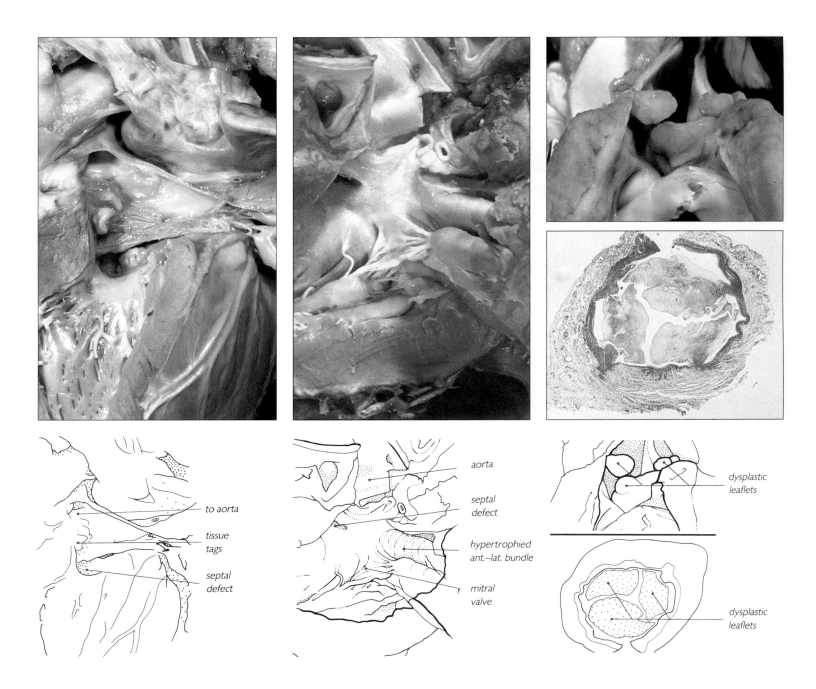

Fig. 7.44 In this heart with an atrioventricular septal defect, obstruction of the subaortic outflow tract is produced by fibrous tissue tags.

Fig. 7.45 In this heart, the obstruction of the subaortic outlet is due to hypertrophy of the antero-lateral muscle bundle.

Fig. 7.46 In this heart, obstruction at the level of the leaflets of the pulmonary valve is due to the dysplastic changes – shown grossly (above) and in section (below).

penetrating the aortic wall to communicate with its lumen. It is sinusoidal in its intramyocardial course, while its external part is arterial-like.

Lesions of the arterial valves

Abnormalities of the arterial valves are often associated with other congenital lesions within the heart, but valvar stenosis is by far the most common form of isolated stenosis of the outflow tract of either the right or left ventricles. Valvar aortic stenosis, while common in hearts with concordant ventriculo–arterial connexions, is exceedingly rare when the ventriculo–arterial connexions are discordant. Valvar stenosis, in contrast, is by far the most common cause of isolated pulmonary stenosis.

Stenosis can be produced either by dysplasia of the leaflets (Fig. 7.46) or by fusion along the commissures (Fig. 7.47). Dys-

plasia can affect the leaflets of either the aortic or pulmonary valves, and is the typical lesion in Ulrich–Noonan syndrome. Commissural fusion producing a dome-shaped stenosis usually affects the pulmonary valve, leaving a central pinhole meatus (Fig. 7.47). Commissural fusion in the aortic valve, in contrast, tends to affect two commissures while sparing the third; this produces the arrangement often described as unicuspid and unicommissural valve stenosis (Fig. 7.48). Evidence of the three leaflets initially present is provided by the two raphes that can usually be seen radiating from the keyhole orifice. Valves with two leaflets are the most common malformation. Although, in themselves, not intrinsically stenotic they frequently become the seat of pathological processes such as thickening and calcification. Having become stenotic (Fig. 7.49), they are then particularly susceptible to development of other pathological conditions such as infective endocarditis or prolapse. The two leaflets can be of

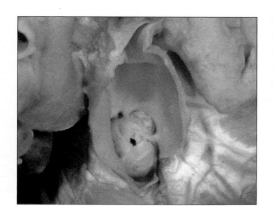

Fig. 7.47 This heart shows stenosis of the pulmonary valve with doming and a central pinhole meatus.

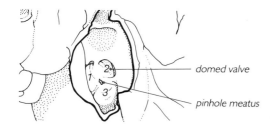

domed valve

pinhole meatus

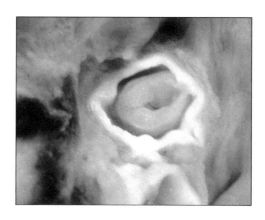

Fig. 7.48 In this heart with valvar aortic stenosis, two commissures are fused to the centre of the orifice leaving one patent commissure, hence the title "unicommissural and unicuspid stenosis".

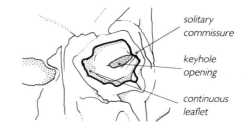

solitary commissure

keyhole opening

continuous leaflet

Fig. 7.49 This view of the aorta from above shows a stenotic valve with two leaflets.

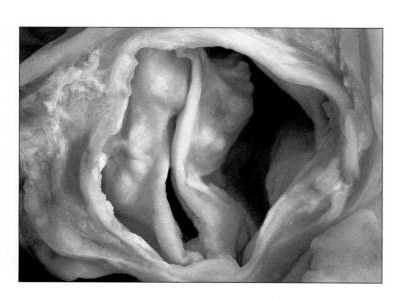

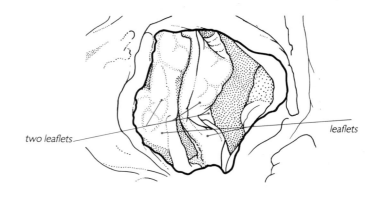

two leaflets

leaflets

equal size, but usually they are unequal. The larger leaflet then tends to have a shallow raphe in its middle part and is termed the conjoined leaflet (Fig. 7.50). The finding of a quadricuspid valve is, in general, of no functional signficance. Indeed, its finding in the pulmonary position (Fig. 7.51) is by no means uncommon. A quadricuspid aortic valve, in contrast, is extremely rare. It is of pathological significance only when a further change occurs, such as when the deformed leaflets obstruct the orifice of a coronary artery (Fig. 7.52).

Supravalvar arterial stenosis

Lesions of the ascending arterial trunks have a predilection for the aorta rather than the pulmonary trunk, and are described as occurring in hourglass, diaphragmatic, or tubular forms (Fig. 7.53). The tubular type is the rarest, but is also the most severe, since it tends to involve the aortic arch and its branches. In the other forms, there is a disorganized architecture of the arterial wall, termed a mosaic pattern. With any of these lesions, the

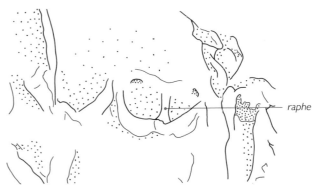

Fig. 7.50 In this opened aortic valve with two leaflets, the raphe is seen in the conjoined leaflet.

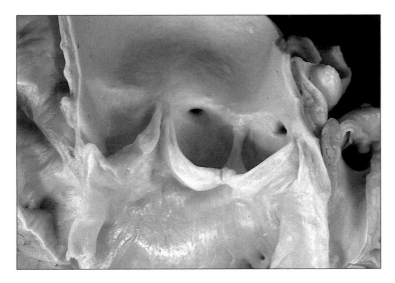

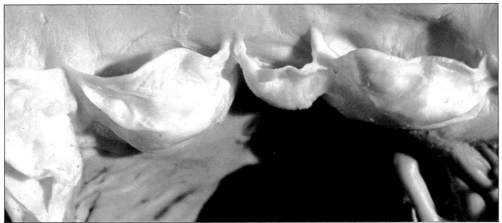

Fig. 7.51 This pulmonary valve has four leaflets.

Fig. 7.52 In this aortic valve with four leaflets, one of the leaflets encroaches upon the orifice of a coronary artery.

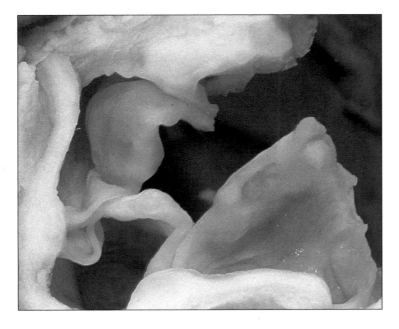

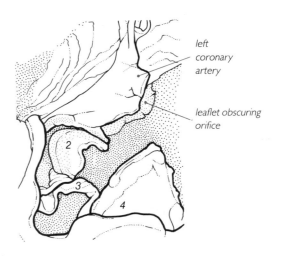

ascending aorta is divided into high-pressure proximal and low-pressure distal components. Since the coronary arteries arise proximal to the obstruction, they are part of the high-pressure system. Usually, therefore, they are dilated (Fig. 7.54) and run a tortuous course, showing premature atherosclerosis. This, in combination with ventricular hypertrophy, underlies the common occurrence of sudden death. Whatever the type of supravalvar aortic stenosis, the abnormality of the wall also involves the commissural attachments of the valvar leaflets while,

in the hourglass and the diaphragmatic lesions, a Venturi effect produces dilatation of the distal ascending aorta.

Before concluding the discussion on arterial trunks, it is convenient to describe here aneurysm of an aortic sinus, since this is also considered to be congenital in origin. Aneurysm of the left sinus is exceedingly rare. Expansion of the right sinus takes it into the right atrium or the outflow tract of the right ventricle, where it can produce severe obstruction (Fig. 7.55). Rupture is the most common complication, irrespective of the sinus involved, and occurs in approximatey 75% of cases.

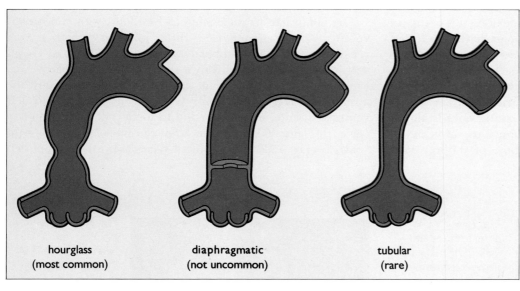

Fig. 7.53 This diagram shows how supravalvar aortic stenosis is divided into tubular, hourglass, and diaphragmatic forms.

hourglass
(most common)

diaphragmatic
(not uncommon)

tubular
(rare)

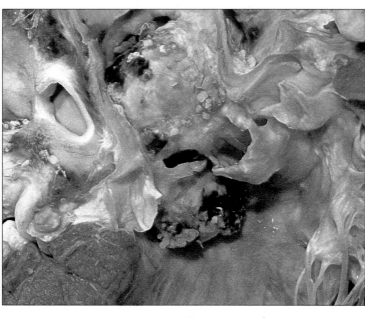

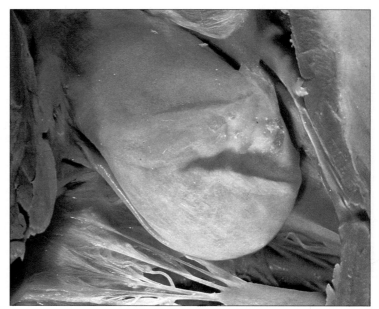

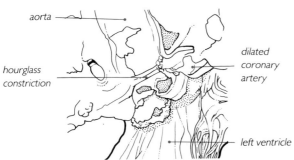

aorta

hourglass
constriction

dilated
coronary
artery

left ventricle

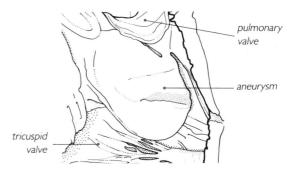

pulmonary
valve

aneurysm

tricuspid
valve

Fig. 7.54 In this heart with stenosis at the level of the sinutubular junction ("supravalvar" stenosis), the coronary arteries are dilated.

Fig. 7.55 This heart has gross dilatation of the right sinus of the aorta, obstructing the subpulmonary infundibulum.

ABNORMAL VENTRICULO–ARTERIAL CONNEXIONS

The abnormal ventriculo–arterial connexions to be given special consideration in this section are discordant ventriculo–arterial connexions in association with concordant atrioventricular connexions (complete transposition); double-outlet ventricles; and a common arterial trunk. The other variants of single outlet of the heart (namely solitary pulmonary trunk with aortic atresia and solitary aortic trunk with pulmonary atresia) have been discussed in a previous section, along with solitary arterial trunk in the absence of intrapericardial pulmonary arteries.

Before considering these abnormal connexions, it is pertinent to consider briefly the abnormal arrangements that can be found when the ventriculo–arterial connexions are concordant but the great arteries are abnormally related to each other and to the underlying ventricles. When concordant ventriculo–arterial connexions are found with concordant atrioventricular connexions and usual atrial arrangement, the aortic valve is almost always posterior and to the right of the pulmonary valve, and its leaflets are in fibrous continuity with those of the left-sided mitral valve; this is so-called 'normal relations'. In an individual with mirror-image atrial arrangement and concordant atrioventricular and ventriculo–arterial connexions, a mirror-image relationship of the arterial trunks is also found (see Fig. 7.6). In this latter situation, the aortic valve is posterior and left-sided and is in fibrous continuity with the right-sided mitral valve. In these arrangements, almost always, the pulmonary valve has a complete muscular infundibulum while the leaflets of the aortic valve are in fibrous continuity with those of the mitral valve. Only exceedingly rarely, as discussed above, are otherwise normal hearts found with muscular tissue interposed between the leaflets of the aortic and mitral valves.

The abnormal arrangements to be found with concordant ventriculo–arterial connexions differ in terms of both arterial relationships and infundibular morphology. The most frequently encountered abnormality is when, in those with usual atrial arrangement and concordant atrioventricular connexions, the aortic valve (Fig. 7.56) arises from the morphologically left ventricle in anterior position and to the left of the pulmonary valve, the latter taking origin from the morphologically right ventricle (Fig. 7.57). Both arterial valves are usually supported

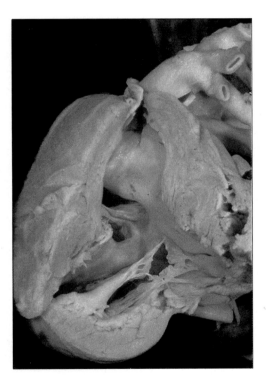

Fig. 7.56 The aorta arises from the left ventricle in this heart above a complete infundibulum, and anteriorly and to the left relative to the pulmonary trunk. This abnormal relationship with concordant connexions is sometimes called anatomically corrected malposition.

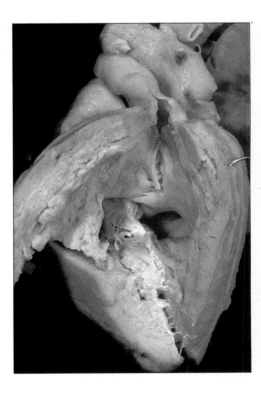

Fig. 7.57 This shows the other side of the heart seen in Fig. 7.56. The pulmonary trunk arises from the morphologically right ventricle.

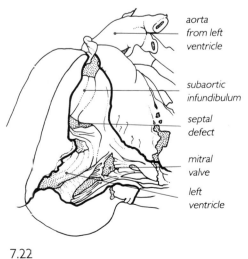

aorta
from left
ventricle

subaortic
infundibulum

septal
defect

mitral
valve

left
ventricle

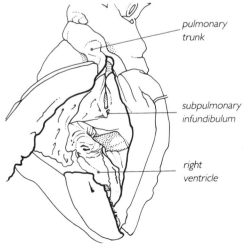

pulmonary
trunk

subpulmonary
infundibulum

right
ventricle

by complete muscular infundibular structures. This abnormal arrangement of the ventriculo–arterial junctions, often called 'anatomically corrected malposition', can exist with any atrial arrangement, and with any possible atrioventricular connexions, as long as there are separate morphologically right and left ventricles. Tricuspid atresia and juxtaposition of the atrial appendages are frequent accompaniments.

Other rare abnormal relationships can be found with concordant ventriculo–arterial connexions such as when, with discordant atrioventricular connexions, the aortic valve is posterior and right-sided and in fibrous continuity with the right-sided mitral valve. Although some might call this arrangement 'isolated ventricular inversion', our own preference when dealing with these very rare cardiac malformations is to describe fully the cardiac connexions and then separately detail both the abnormal relationships and the infundibular morphology.

Complete transposition

Complete transposition is the consequence of the specific combination of concordant atrioventricular with discordant ventriculo–arterial connexions. It can, therefore, be found either in hearts with usual or with mirror-image atrial arrangement (Fig. 7.58). There is marked heterogeneity in the morphology encountered in terms of relationships of the ventricles and the great arteries, as well as in the infundibular morphology. The arrangement can be further complicated by the existence of associated malformations such as ventricular septal defects, obstruction of the left ventricular outflow tract, and so on.

The variability encountered in the arterial relationships is considerable. When there is usual atrial arrangement, the aorta is typically found in anterior and right-sided position relative to the pulmonary trunk (Fig. 7.59). This, however, is by no means universal. The aorta may be directly anterior, or anterior and left-sided (Fig. 7.60) Indeed, the aorta may rarely be posterior

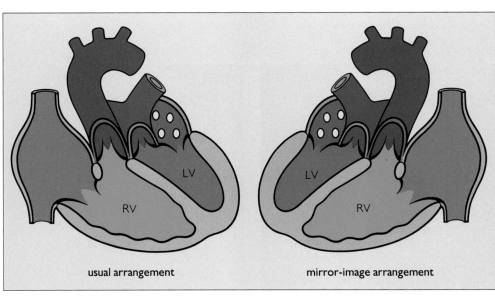

usual arrangement   mirror-image arrangement

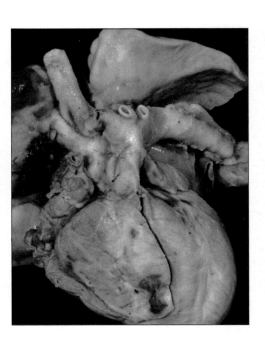

Fig. 7.58 This diagram shows the segmental arrangements which produce complete transposition.

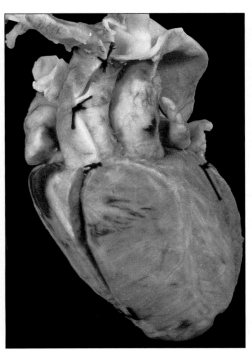

Fig. 7.59 This anterior view shows the typical anterior and right-sided location of the aorta in hearts with complete transposition.

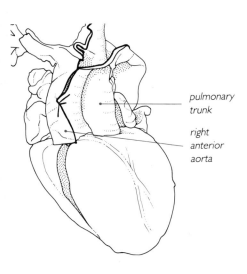

pulmonary trunk

right anterior aorta

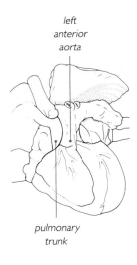

left anterior aorta

pulmonary trunk

Fig. 7.60 In this heart with usual atrial arrangement and complete transposition, the aorta is located anteriorly and to the left.

and right-sided relative to the pulmonary trunk – so-called 'normal relations' (Fig. 7.61). These findings, coupled with the fact that an anterior left-sided aorta is the usual finding when complete transposition exists in the mirror-image variant (see Fig. 6.3), point to the inadvisability of using the term 'd-transposition' as an overall name for this group of anomalies.

Considering infundibular morphology, the aortic valve is almost always supported by a complete muscular infundibulum (Fig. 7.62) while there is fibrous continuity between the leaflets of the pulmonary and mitral valves (Fig. 7.63). It is by no means unusual, however, to encounter hearts with a complete muscular infundibulum in both ventricles. Furthermore, in rare cases where an aorta arises in the posterior position from the morphologically right ventricle, it is usual to find fibrous continuity between the leaflets of the aortic and mitral valves through the roof of a co-existing ventricular septal defect (Fig. 7.64). The

leaflets of the pulmonary valve, in contrast, are supported by a complete muscular infundibulum.

The atrial chambers in complete transposition are usually normal, although any anomalous venous connexion can co-exist. Juxtaposition of the atrial appendages is a frequent accompanying lesion, while a defect of the atrial septum is the rule. Usually, this defect is within the oval fossa, and, in present times, the atrial septum is frequently found to be further ruptured at autopsy because of balloon atrial septostomy. Due to the virtually normal atrial morphology, the conduction tissues are positioned as in the normal heart.

The atrioventricular connexions are, by definition, concordant and the morphology of the tricuspid and mitral valves is virtually normal, although subtle differences are found in the arrangement of the tension apparatus and in the anatomy of the atrioventricular septum. The ventricular thicknesses are almost equal

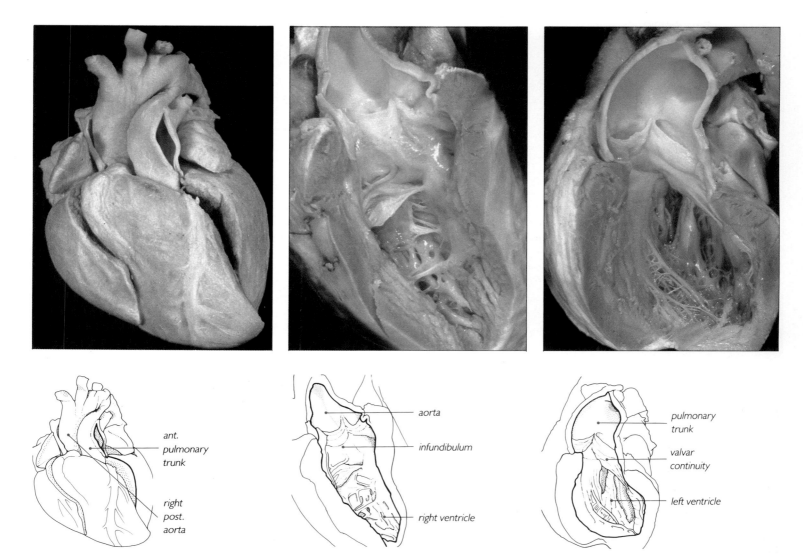

Fig. 7.61 In this heart with the segmental combinations producing complete transposition, the aorta is located posteriorly and to the right of the pulmonary trunk – so-called "normal relations".

Fig. 7.62 This view of the right ventricle shows the typical subaortic infundibulum of complete transposition.

Fig. 7.63 This view of the left ventricle of the heart shown in Fig. 7.62 shows the leaflets of the pulmonary and mitral valves in fibrous continuity.

at birth but, soon after, the morphologically right ventricle becomes dominant as it takes over the load of the systemic circulation. The most significant deviations in ventricular anatomy are found when there are associated malformations. A ventricular septal defect is frequently present. Such defects can show just as much variation as in the otherwise normally structured heart, but defects with malalignment between the outlet septum and the rest of the ventricular septum are frequent (Fig. 7.65). Such defects are in an immediately subpulmonary position, with the pulmonary valve overriding the crest of the muscular ventricular septum. Indeed, a series of anomalies is found between complete transposition and double-outlet right ventricle with subpulmonary defect (see below). These defects with malalignment of the outlet septum can either be perimembranous or have muscular posteroinferior rims. Their right ventricular aspect is frequently crossed by the tension apparatus of the tricuspid valve.

Although defects opening between the outlets are the rule, any type can be found in the setting of complete transposition, including perimembranous or muscular defects opening into the inlet of the right ventricle. Straddling and overriding tricuspid valve is particularly significant because then the septum does not extend to the crux. This produces a grossly abnormal arrangement of the axis of the conduction tissue (see Fig. 6.77). Straddling of the mitral valve can be found when there is a malalignment outlet defect. Apart from the arrangement with straddling tricuspid valve, the disposition of the conduction tissues is as anticipated for ventricular septal defects as seen in the otherwise normal heart.

As discussed above, any of the lesions that affect the outflow tract of the morphologically left ventricle can produce pulmonary stenosis in complete transposition. Valvar stenosis can exist in isolation but, most usually, it complicates subvalvar stenosis. Dynamic obstruction is often seen angiocardiographically but, when pressures across the outflow tract are measured during surgery, there is no significant gradient and none persists after operation. Fixed obstructions are, therefore, the major problem. Particularly significant are fibromuscular shelves or tunnels because of their relation to the atrioventricular conduction axis. Tissue tags are also found, with or without a ventricular septal

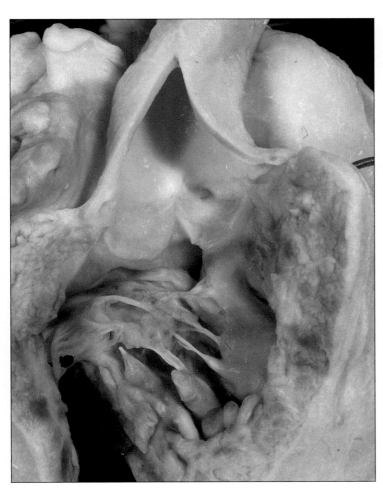

Fig. 7.64 In this heart with complete transposition and posterior aorta, there is fibrous continuity between the leaflets of the aortic and mitral valves in the roof of a perimembranous ventricular septal defect.

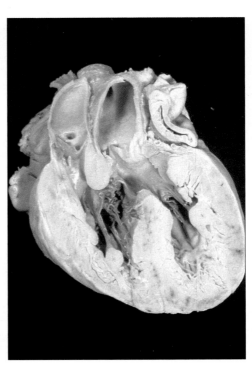

Fig. 7.65 This four chamber section shows the typical malalignment between the outlet septum and the rest of the septum when there is a subpulmonary ventricular septal defect.

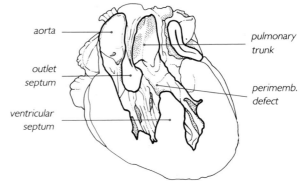

aorta

outlet septum

ventricular septum

pulmonary trunk

perimemb. defect

defect (Fig. 7.66). When the ventricular septum is deficient, the lesion most usually producing obstruction is deviation of the outlet septum into the left ventricle (Fig. 7.67). Subaortic obstruction is less common in complete transposition, and aortic valvar stenosis is exceedingly rare. When found, nonetheless, stenosis of the aortic outflow tract is almost always associated with coarctation, isthmal hypoplasia, and patency of the arterial duct. Persistent patency of the duct is a significant associated lesion in its own right and can be found in isolation or along with other anomalies.

Irrespective of the presence or absence of associated lesions, abnormalities in the epicardial course of the coronary arteries are frequent in complete transposition. These abnormalities in epicardial course, nonetheless, rarely affect the origin of the coronary arteries, which almost invariably arise from the two aortic sinuses adjacent to the pulmonary trunk (the 'facing' sinuses; Fig. 7.68). This is of great value to the surgeon, since it means that the coronary arteries can readily be transferred to the pulmonary trunk in the 'arterial switch' procedure. Although arising from the facing sinuses, however, there is marked variation in terms of which sinus gives rise to which artery. This is further compounded by variability in the relationships of the arterial trunks. In order to provide a simple system for naming the sinuses, therefore, it is best to consider them as being right-handed or left-handed from the stance of the observer positioned within the nonfacing sinus (Fig. 7.69).

Double-outlet ventricle

For us, double-outlet ventricle describes only a connexion between the ventricles and the great arteries. When there is overriding of an arterial valve, we assign it to the chamber connected to its greater part. Double-outlet ventricle can be defined, therefore, as the arrangement in which more than half of both arterial valves are connected to the same ventricle, which may be of right, left, or indeterminate morphology. These ventriculo–arterial connexions can be found with any type of atrioventricular connexions, but double outlet in the setting of discordant atrioventricular connexions and with double inlet ventricle, as well as with isomerism of the atrial appendages, has already been discussed. This section, therefore, is primarily concerned with the most common types of double-outlet ventricle, namely double-outlet right or left ventricle in association with usual atrial arrangement and concordant atrioventricular connexions.

Double-outlet right ventricle

There are some who define double-outlet right ventricle only in the presence of bilaterally complete infundibular structures. There seems little logic in this, since a bilateral infundibulum is not used as a criterion of double outlet when the ventriculo–arterial connexions are discordant. Others distinguish tetralogy

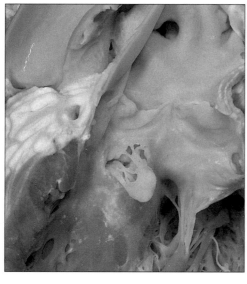
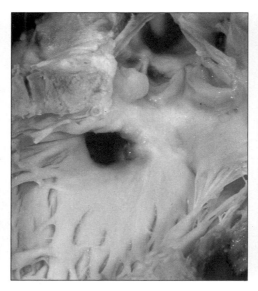
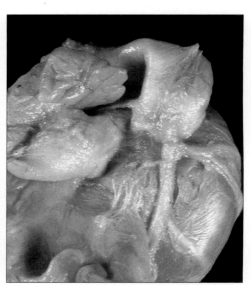

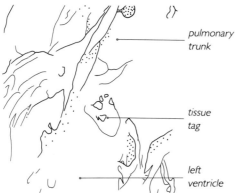

Fig. 7.66 In this view of the left ventricle in complete transposition, subpulmonary obstruction is produced by a tissue tag herniated through a ventricular septal defect from the tricuspid valve.

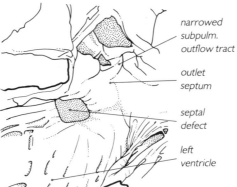

Fig. 7.67 In this view of the left ventricle in complete transposition, subpulmonary obstruction is due to posterior deviation of the outlet septum.

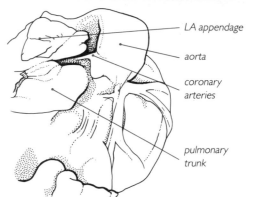

Fig. 7.68 The aorta is retracted forward in this example of complete transposition, showing the origin of the coronary arteries from the sinuses which face the pulmonary trunk.

of Fallot from double outlet even when, in the presence of the morphology typical for tetralogy, most of the circumference of the aortic valve, together with that of the pulmonary valve, is attached within the right ventricle. Again, we see little merit in this convention. Double outlet describes a type of ventriculo–arterial connexion, while tetralogy is defined according to intra-cardiac anatomy. We have no problems in describing the co-existence of the morphology of tetralogy of Fallot with double-outlet ventriculo–arterial connexion.

Thus, definition of double-outlet right ventricle as a ventriculo–arterial connexion unifies an otherwise grossly heterogeneous group of malformations. This heterogeneity must then be distinguished in terms of the position and morphology of the ventricular septal defect (which is almost universally present), the interrelationships of the arterial trunks, the infundibular morphology, and the presence of associated malformations. In any given heart, it is possible that any variation in one of these features can co-exist with any possible variation in others, thus giving a myriad of patterns. Despite this, it is clear that there is a certain predictability that permits categorization of double-outlet right ventricle.

In general terms, the relationships of the great arteries can be fitted into one of three patterns. These are, first, with the aorta more or less normally related to the pulmonary trunk; second, with the aorta anterior and to the right; or, third, with the aorta anterior and to the left.

When the great arteries are more or less normally related, the ventricular septal defect is most usually beneath the posteriorly located aortic outflow tract (Fig. 7.70). The attachment of the malaligned outlet septum separates the subpulmonary outflow tract from the defect. The proximity of the aortic valve depends on the extent of the ventriculo–infundibular fold. With an extensive subaortic infundibulum, the valve is further from the defect than when there is fibrous continuity between the aortic and the atrioventricular valves. The relationship of the conduction tissue to the edge of the defect depends upon whether the defect is perimembranous (Fig. 7.71) or whether the posterior limb of the septomarginal trabeculation fuses with the ventriculo–infundibular fold. As with isolated defects, the bar of muscle produced by the latter arrangement protects the axis of conduction tissue. Perimembranous defects with basically normally related great arteries can extend into the inlet septum. This

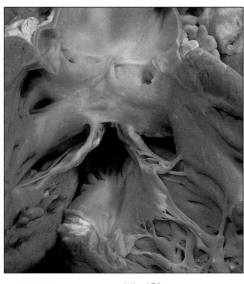

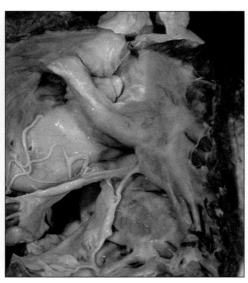

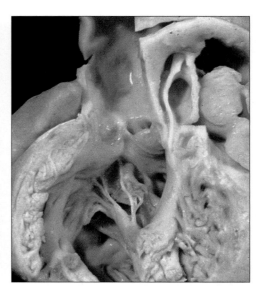

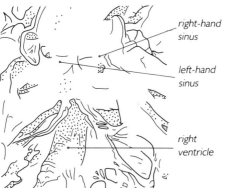

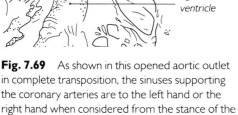

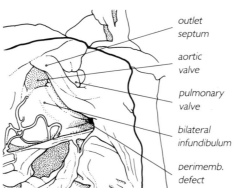

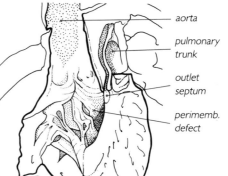

Fig. 7.69 As shown in this opened aortic outlet in complete transposition, the sinuses supporting the coronary arteries are to the left hand or the right hand when considered from the stance of the observer within the non-facing sinus.

Fig. 7.70 This heart with double outlet right ventricle and an extensive bilateral infundibulum has a subaortic and perimembranous ventricular septal defect.

Fig. 7.71 In this heart with double outlet right ventricle and a subaortic perimembranous defect, the defect is much closer to the aortic valve because the leaflets of this valve are in fibrous continuity with those of the mitral valve.

feature also takes the defect further away from the aorta (towards becoming noncommitted).

A less-common type of defect with basically normally related great arteries is the doubly committed and juxtaarterial defect. This can also be perimembranous or can have a muscular postero-inferior rim (Fig. 7.72). Noncommitted muscular inlet defects are rare, and we have not seen a subpulmonary defect with a 'normal' arrangement of the arterial trunks. Subpulmonary obstruction, in contrast, is frequent, and mitral atresia due to an imperforate valve is by no means rare.

The second pattern of great arteries is for the aorta to be side-by-side or anterior and right-sided, the arrangement more usually found in complete transposition. The defect in this setting is most frequently in subpulmonary position (Fig. 7.73). Indeed, a series of anomalies is found between double-outlet and complete transposition, depending on the precise connexion of the pulmonary valve. The entire spectrum is often described as the Taussig–Bing anomaly. The defect, clasped between the limbs of the septomarginal trabeculation, is in subpulmonary position because the outlet septum fuses with the posterior limb of the trabeculation, and, usually, also with the ventriculo–infundibular fold. The defect, therefore, usually has a muscular posteroinferior rim that protects the conduction tissues, but it can extend to become perimembranous. In these circumstances, the defect can extend into the inlet septum and become noncommitted (Fig. 7.74). The proximity of the pulmonary valve to the defect

again depends on the extent of the ventriculo–infundibular fold. We have not observed either a subaortic or a doubly committed defect when the aorta is right-sided and anterior. With the defect in the typical subpulmonary position, it is frequent to find obstructive lesions of the aortic arch, straddling of the mitral valve, or a combination of these two lesions.

The final group of hearts with double-outlet right ventricle are those with an anterior and left-sided aorta. This is, by far, the rarest group. The defect is frequently subaortic, but it may be doubly committed, subpulmonary, or noncommitted. The same variability exists in terms of the morphology of the defect itself, and the integrity of the ventriculo–infundibular fold, as with other forms. Juxtaposition of the atrial appendages is a frequent accompanying lesion, as is subpulmonary stenosis. When the latter is present, a major coronary artery is frequently found crossing the obstructive outflow tract, a feature also found with an anterior right-sided aorta and a subpulmonary defect.

Double-outlet left ventricle

As with double-outlet right ventricle, double-outlet left ventricle is a heterogeneous malformation and must be analysed in terms of the position and morphology of the ventricular septal defect, the relationships of the great arteries, the infundibular morphology, and the presence of associated malformations. All of these are as variable as found with double-outlet right ventricle.

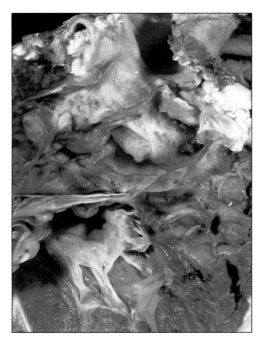

Fig. 7.72 This heart with double outlet right ventricle has a doubly committed ventricular septal defect with a muscular postero-inferior rim.

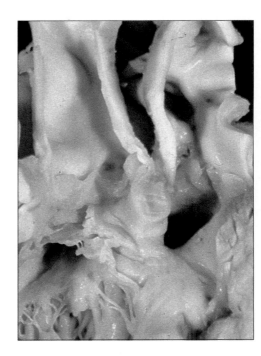

Fig. 7.73 In this heart with double outlet right ventricle, the defect, with a muscular postero-inferior rim, is subpulmonary.

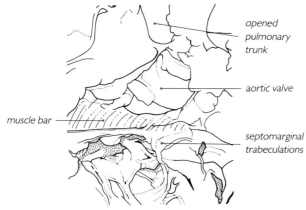

opened pulmonary trunk

aortic valve

muscle bar

septomarginal trabeculations

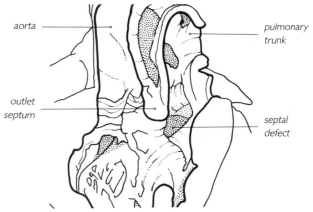

aorta

outlet septum

pulmonary trunk

septal defect

Common arterial trunk

The ventriculo–arterial connexion of single outlet of the heart has four variants, of which only one, a common trunk, is to be discussed here. We define a common trunk as one exiting from the heart through a solitary arterial valve and supplying directly the coronary, at least one pulmonary, and the systemic arteries. As with the other ventriculo–arterial connexions, a common arterial trunk can be found with any atrioventricular connexions. Here, description is confined to cases with usual atrial arrangement and concordant atrioventricular connexions.

The first variable to consider is the ventricular connexion of the trunk. Usually, the truncal valve overrides the septum, being attached within both ventricles (Fig. 7.75). It can, however, be exclusively connected to either the morphologically right (Fig. 7.76) or the left ventricle. When the trunk is exclusively connected to one or other ventricle then, as with double-outlet ventricle, the ventricular septal defect is the only exit for one ventricle. If the trunk arises exclusively, or even predominantly, from the right ventricle, there can be problems in surgical correction if the defect is restrictive. The second important variable, therefore, is the morphology of the ventricular septal defect.

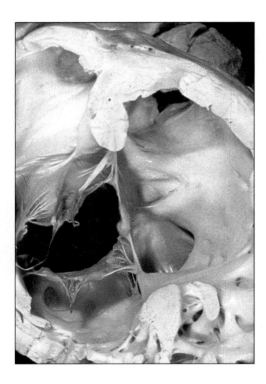

Fig. 7.74 The defect in this heart with double outlet right ventricle is perimembranous and noncommitted.

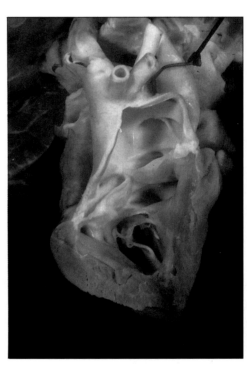

Fig. 7.75 This heart has a common arterial trunk which overrides the ventricular septum.

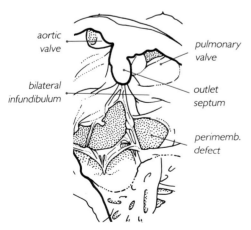

aortic valve

pulmonary valve

bilateral infundibulum

outlet septum

perimemb. defect

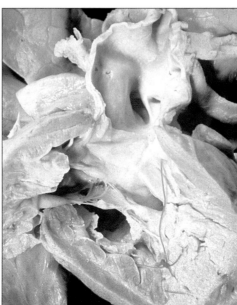

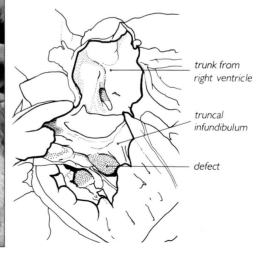

Fig. 7.76 In this heart, a common arterial trunk arises exclusively from the right ventricle with a complete subtruncal infundibulum.

trunk from right ventricle

truncal infundibulum

defect

Virtually always, there is a communication above the ventricular septum during ventricular systole but, occasionally, the septum can be so well formed that, during diastole, the leaflets of the truncal valve fall back onto the septal crest, thus obstructing the interventricular communication. Usually, however, there is a defect during diastole as well as systole. The defect is clasped between the limbs of the septomarginal trabeculations but varies according to whether the posterior limb fuses with the ventriculo–infundibular fold (Figs 7.77 and 7.78). The axis of atrioventricular conduction tissue is more closely related to the edge of the defect in a perimembranous defect but, in both perimembranous and muscular defects, the part related to the anterior limb of the septomarginal trabeculation is the safe area for resection during surgery. Muscular inlet or trabecular defects can, very rarely, be found in association with a common arterial trunk.

There is usually a trileaflet truncal valve, but quadrifoliate valves are found with some frequency, and valves with two leaflets are not uncommon. Valves with five or six leaflets have been reported but are rare. The leaflets frequently exhibit dysplasia, particularly in patients dying in infancy. The dysplastic features render them either stenotic or incompetent. The leaflets of the truncal valve are usually in fibrous continuity with the leaflets of the mitral valve, but there may be a complete subtruncal infundibulum, most often when the trunk is exclusively connected to the morphologically right ventricle (see Fig. 7.76).

Another variability of common arterial trunk is that by which it has most frequently been categorized, namely, the morphology of the aortic and pulmonary arterial branches. In terms of pulmonary arterial pattern, it is usual for the right and left arteries to arise from the left posterior aspect of the trunk very close to each other. Less frequently, there may be a well-formed common pulmonary channel which then divides into right and left branches. The variant with origin of the right and left pulmonary arteries from the sides of the trunk is exceedingly rare. The lesion with complete absence of intrapericardial pulmonary arteries is also rare. When seen, it is better categorized as solitary rather than common arterial trunk (see Fig. 7.27). One pulmonary artery, however, can have a separate origin from an arterial duct and still satisfy the criterion for presence of a common trunk, but the variant in which one pulmonary artery arises from the ascending aorta and the other from the right ventricle (sometimes called 'hemitruncus') is unequivocally not an example of a common trunk.

The major variability in an aortic pattern depends upon whether or not the aortic arch is interrupted. Most frequently, there is no interruption and, in these circumstances, it is unusual to find either an arterial duct or ligament unless there is severe coarctation. In a minority of cases, the transverse aortic arch is interrupted at some point and the descending aorta, together occasionally with the arteries to the head or arms, is supplied via a patent arterial duct (Fig. 7.79). A right aortic arch is frequent.

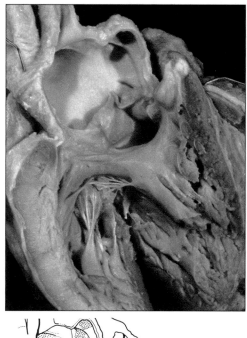
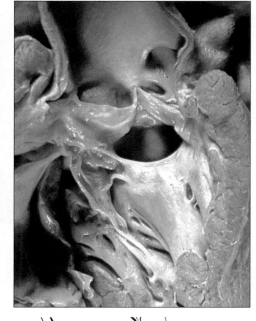
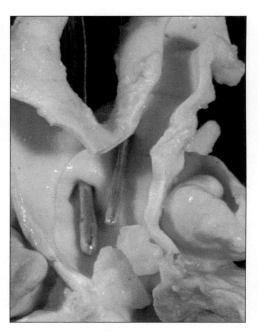

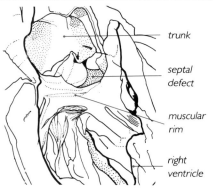

trunk

septal
defect

muscular
rim

right
ventricle

trunk

septal
defect

truncal–
TV continuity

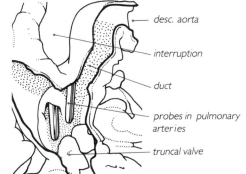

desc. aorta

interruption

duct

probes in pulmonary
arteries

truncal valve

Fig. 7.77 The ventricular septal defect in this heart with a common arterial trunk has a muscular postero-inferior rim.

Fig. 7.78 In this heart with common arterial trunk, the ventricular septal defect is perimembranous.

Fig. 7.79 There is interruption of the aortic arch in this example of common arterial trunk, the descending aorta being fed through the arterial duct.

ANOMALIES OF THE GREAT ARTERIES

This section is concerned with anomalous communications between, and abnormal branching patterns of, the great arterial trunks. Thus, in terms of communications, the various forms of aortopulmonary windows are described, and the arterial duct and its pathology are considered. With regard to abnormal patterns of branching, stenotic lesions (coarctation) and complete interruption in the aortic arch, along with the more complex arrangements generally termed vascular rings, are described. On the pulmonary side, the vascular sling (anomalous origin of one pulmonary artery from the other with bronchial compression) is considered, and crossed pulmonary arteries and anomalous origin of one pulmonary artery are briefly mentioned.

Aortopulmonary window

An aortopulmonary window (or fenestration) is a defect between the ascending portions of the aortic and pulmonary trunks. The major feature that distinguishes such a window from a common arterial trunk is the presence of separate orifices for the aortic and pulmonary valves. The size of the defect can vary considerably, from small circumscribed lesions (Fig. 8.1) to extensive communications running almost from the valvar leaflets to the pulmonary bifurcation (Fig. 8.2). The hole is usually simply a window between the trunks, but sometimes a more extensive tubular communication is found. Windows are often found along with other lesions such as a right aortic arch or anomalous origin of one coronary artery from the pulmonary trunk. Found most

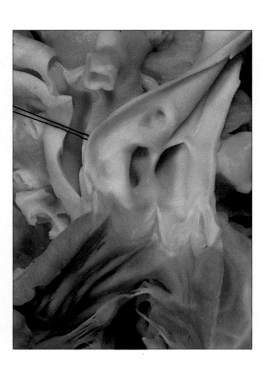

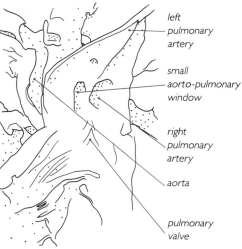

left pulmonary artery

small aorto-pulmonary window

right pulmonary artery

aorta

pulmonary valve

Fig. 8.1 This shows a small window between the ascending components of the aorta and pulmonary trunk, and demonstrates the separate aortic and pulmonary valvar orifices.

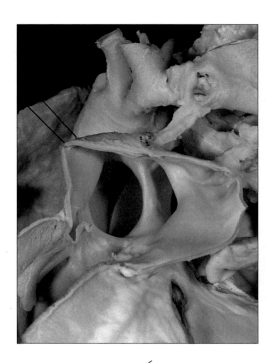

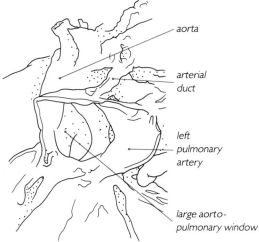

aorta

arterial duct

left pulmonary artery

large aorto-pulmonary window

Fig. 8.2 In this specimen, the aorto-pulmonary window is consideraby larger (compare with Fig. 8.1).

frequently with two patent arterial valves, the windows can also exist with aortic or pulmonary atresia. Association with an interrupted arch poses particular problems in clinical diagnosis, but should be easily recognized at autopsy.

The arterial duct

The arterial duct is a vital part of the normal fetal circulation, permitting the deoxygenated blood returning from the head to be conveyed via the right ventricle to the descending aorta and thence to the placenta for reoxygenation (see Fig. 7.51). Pathology of this pathway can take several forms. One is for the duct to persist as an integral part of the circulation when there is atresia or stenosis of one or other arterial trunk. There is even the possibility that two ducts may be present since, during embryonic development, the duct is a bilateral structure. It is not, however, the pathology of the duct in those situations with which we are concerned. Here, we are specifically concerned with pathology of the duct in an otherwise normal circulatory system. The anomalies to be considered are premature closure, persistent patency, and aneurysmal dilatation.

Premature closure of the duct during fetal life is a rare but significant finding in autopsies of stillborns and neonates. The duct has a diminished external diameter (Fig. 8.3) and, although the histology of the wall is normal (see below), the ductal lumen is narrowed, a feature best seen from the aortic side.

Persistent patency must be distinguished from delayed closure of the duct. Although the duct is a significant pathway in the fetal circulation, it has no role in normal postnatal life. Its structure is such that it permits rapid closure after birth, since it has muscular walls in comparison to the elastic walls of the aorta and pulmonary trunk (Fig. 8.4). Over the five weeks before birth, major changes occur within these walls which prepare the duct for closure. There is fragmentation of the internal elastic

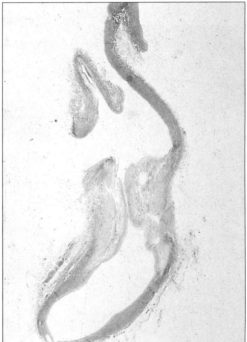

Fig. 8.4 This histological section, stained with the trichrome technique, shows the differing structure of the arterial duct relative to the aorta and the pulmonary trunk.

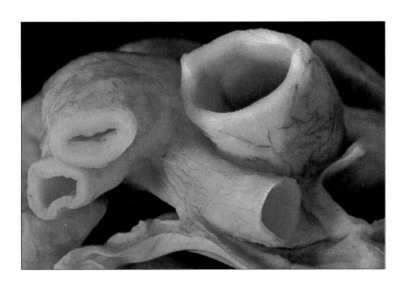

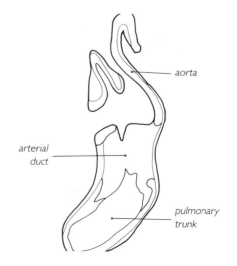

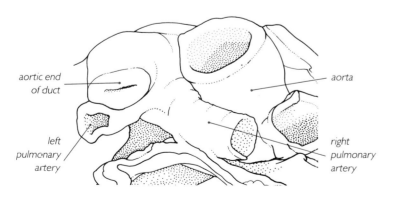

aortic end of duct

aorta

left pulmonary artery

right pulmonary artery

arterial duct

aorta

pulmonary trunk

Fig. 8.3 There is premature closure of the arterial duct in this heart from a stillborn neonate.

lamina, formation of 'cushions' in the intimal layer, and aggregation of mucoid lakes within the inner part of the medial layer. At birth, the normal constriction of the muscular walls in response to increased oxygen tension, prostaglandins, and other factors, produces functional closure. Thereafter, definitive closure is the consequence of secondary intimal fibrosis and proliferation. Delayed closure of the duct is, thus, a usual finding in premature infants or infants born by caesarean section, since the anatomical and physiological preparations for closure will not all have taken place. True persistent patency, in contrast, is itself a congenital malformation. Histological examination of such ducts has shown preservation of an intact internal elastic lamina (Fig. 8.5). This is, nonetheless, a histological diagnosis. The distinction of

delayed and persistent patency during life is made by waiting for the duct to close, or else encouraging its closure with inhibitors or prostaglandins, such as indomethacin. It is exceedingly rare nowadays to find isolated persistent patency in the autopsy room. It is even rarer to find complications such as pulmonary vascular disease, bacterial endocarditis, or dissecting aneurysms.

Although dissecting aneurysms are now rare, it may be possible to encounter a congenital aneurysm of the duct. Such aneurysms, when found in infants, usually have a closed pulmonary and an opened aortic end. Most aneurysms found in childhood or later, in contrast, are open at both ends (Fig. 8.6). Death with a congenital ductal aneurysm is usually the consequence of a complication, such as rupture, dissection, thrombosis, or infection.

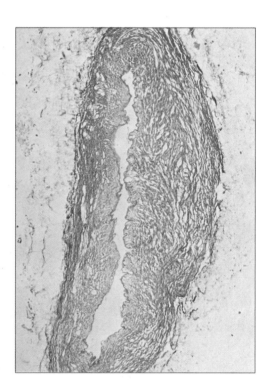

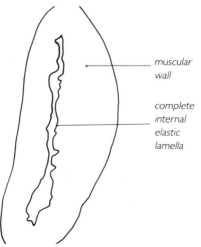

muscular wall

complete internal elastic lamella

Fig. 8.5 This section, also stained with the trichrome technique, shows an intact internal elastic lamina in a persistently patent duct.

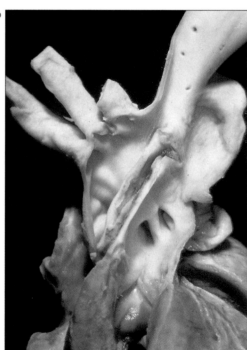

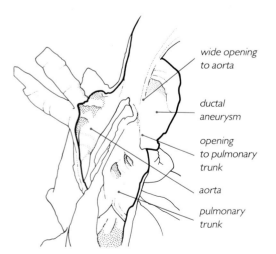

wide opening to aorta

ductal aneurysm

opening to pulmonary trunk

aorta

pulmonary trunk

Fig. 8.6 The arterial duct is aneurysmal in this heart.

Coarctation of the aorta

Coarctation, literally, means a 'drawing together'. Two types of obstructive lesions of the aortic arch can be described under this heading. Although the two varieties can co-exist, it is preferable to distinguish between them. Most commonly, there is a discrete shelf-like lesion at some point within the arch, with a gradual tapering of the proximal arch to the obstructive lesion (Fig. 8.7). Alternatively, but much more rarely, an entire segment of the arch can be uniformly narrow, usually the isthmus but sometimes the segment between left common carotid and subclavian arteries. This second arrangement is termed tubular hypoplasia (Fig. 8.8).

Although discrete coarctation has been the subject of many and varied classifications, a classification that takes account of the site of the lesion, the patency of the duct, and the presence or absence of associated malformations, particularly of the subclavian arteries, caters for most needs.

Most usually, a discrete coarctation lesion is found between the isthmus and the descending aorta (see Fig. 8.7). In this typical variety, the isthmus inserts into the major pathway of flow from the duct (which is usually patent) to the descending aorta. In specimens from infants, when the duct is patent in this fashion, it can be seen that a cushion of ductal tissue encircles the orifice of the isthmus (Fig. 8.9). In older children, or when the duct is closed, this encircling arrangement of ductal tissue is less obvious. A preductal location of the obstructive lesion, nonetheless, is by far the most common. The shelf can, however, be opposite the mouth of an open duct, or even postductal. Coarctation can also be found within the thoracic or abdominal aorta.

As stated, the duct is most usually patent. When this is so, there are usually other lesions within the heart which serve to divert the blood away from the aorta during fetal life, such as obstruction of the ventricular septal defect in hearts with univentricular atrioventricular connexion to a dominant left ventricle together with discordant ventriculo–arterial connexions. Coarctation with a closed duct is far more likely to be an isolated lesion. In these cases, there is a high frequency of aortic valves with two leaflets. When isolated, the stenotic lesion itself is more

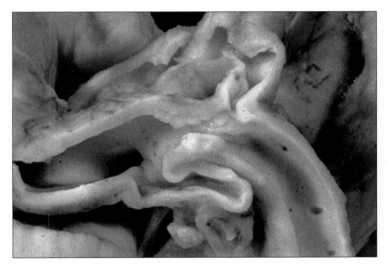

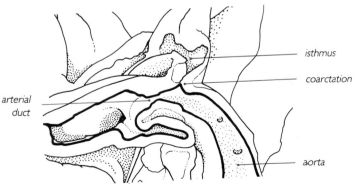

Fig. 8.7 This section of the aortic arch shows a discrete shelf lesion of coarctation due to ductal tissue encircling the orifice of the isthmus.

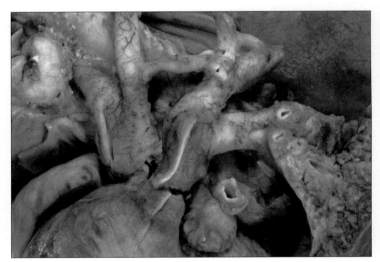

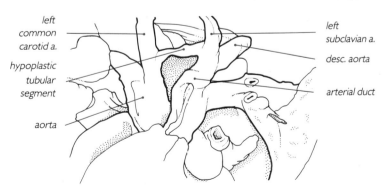

Fig. 8.8 This arch shows tubular hypoplasia of the segment between the left common carotid and subclavian arteries.

an indrawing of the walls of the aorta, the so-called waist lesion, as opposed to a shelf. Poststenotic dilatation of the aorta is seen when coarctation is found with a closed duct (Fig. 8.10). The development of collateral circulation is also of significance when the arterial duct is closed. It is the enlargement of the intercostal

arteries in this circumstance which produces the characteristic rib notching seen on the chest radiograph. Retroesophageal origin of the right subclavian artery can occur in any type of coarctation (Fig. 8.11).

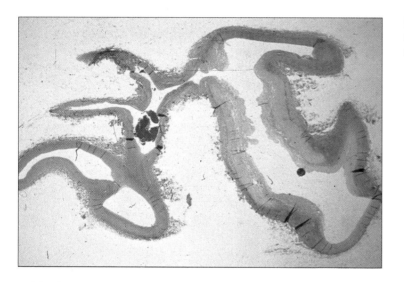

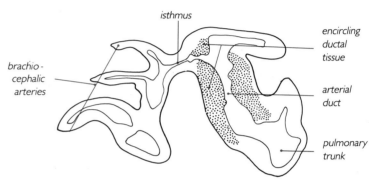

Fig. 8.9 This histological section, stained with the trichrome technique, shows the ductal tissue encircling the orifice of the isthmus in a shelf-like coarctation.

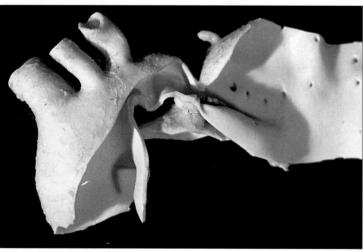

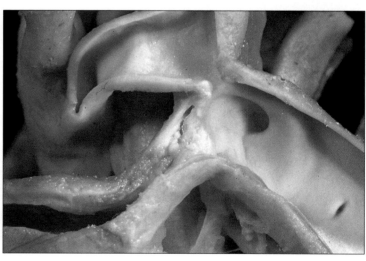

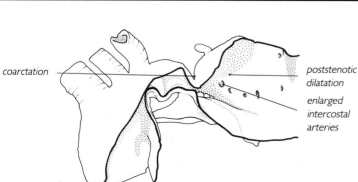

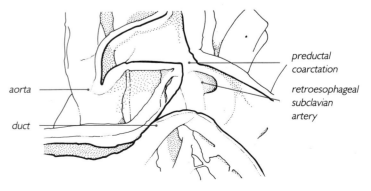

Fig. 8.10 This example shows a waist-like coarctation with dilatation of the descending aorta when the arterial duct is closed and ligamentous.

Fig. 8.11 In this arch, the retrooesophageal right subclavian artery takes origin distal to the preductal coarctation lesion.

Interruption and atresia of the aortic arch

Interruption and atresia of the aortic arch are two malformations best considered as a continuation of the pathological process seen in tubular hypoplasia. In tubular hypoplasia, an entire segment of the arch is thinned and narrowed. In atresia of the arch, the lumen of the narrowed segment is obliterated and the arch is represented as a fibrous cord. As with tubular hypoplasia, this is found either at the isthmus (Fig. 8.12) or between the left common carotid and subclavian arteries. Almost without exception, atresia is accompanied by other malformations, including a duct supplying the descending aorta.

Interruption of the arch is the continuation of the process described above in that the atretic cord has disappeared and there is no connexion whatsoever, either patent or atretic, between the ascending and descending portions of the aorta. Interruption of the arch is seen most frequently at the isthmus or between the left subclavian and left common carotid arteries, but can rarely be found between the carotid arteries (Fig. 8.13).

All of these varieties can be found with normal origin of the right subclavian artery from the brachiocephalic artery (Fig. 8.14) or with retroesophageal origin from the descending part of the aorta (Fig. 8.15). Almost always, interruption is associated with an arterial duct feeding the descending aorta, but there have been several well-documented examples of isolated interruption with the descending aorta fed via collateral circulation. When a ventricular septal defect is present, it is often associated with deviation of the outlet septum producing obstruction of the subaortic outflow tract (see Fig. 7.7). The defect can also be doubly committed and juxtaarterial (Fig. 8.16), or even centrally placed without producing obstruction to subaortic flow. The other commonly associated lesion is an aortopulmonary window.

Vascular rings and their aortic malformations

During embryonic development, the system of aortic arches is symmetrical. The various malformations persisting in postnatal

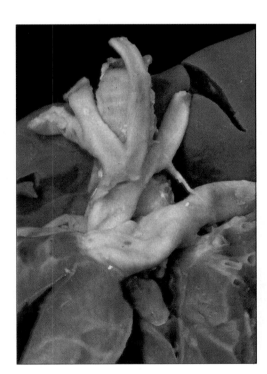

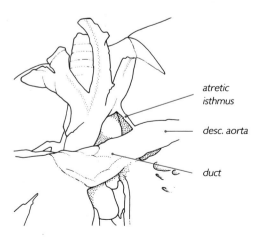

atretic isthmus

desc. aorta

duct

Fig. 8.12 This arch has atresia of the isthmus.

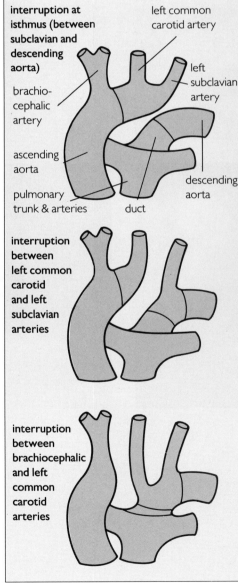

interruption at isthmus (between subclavian and descending aorta)

left common carotid artery

brachio-cephalic artery

left subclavian artery

ascending aorta

descending aorta

pulmonary trunk & arteries

duct

interruption between left common carotid and left subclavian arteries

interruption between brachiocephalic and left common carotid arteries

Fig. 8.13 These diagrams show the different sites at which interruption can occur within the aortic arch.

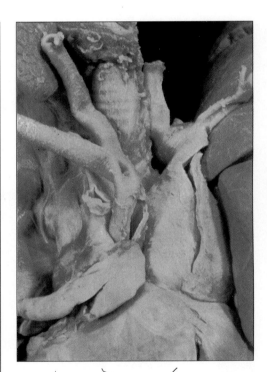

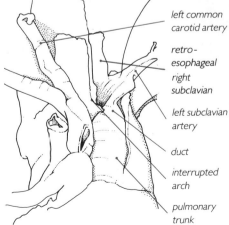

left common carotid artery

retro-esophageal right subclavian

left subclavian artery

duct

interrupted arch

pulmonary trunk

Fig. 8.14 This heart has interruption of the aortic arch between the left common carotid and subclavian arteries, but with retrooesophageal origin of the right subclavian artery.

life can readily be explained on the basis of retention in its entirety or in part of this double arrangement. In the model of the perfect double arch (Fig. 8.17), both right and left arches encircle the tracheoesophageal pedicle and fuse posteriorly to form the descending aorta. The transverse component of each arch gives rise to a subclavian and a common carotid artery, while a duct on each side connects the arches to the right and left pulmonary arteries, respectively, Although rarely seen in such perfect form, the various malformations thus far described are easily explained as persistence in part of this prototype.

Probably the simplest malformation, which does not in itself produce problems, is a right aortic arch. A right arch is found when its transverse component crosses over the right instead of the left bronchus, irrespective of the side of the descending aorta, which may itself be right- or left-sided. A right arch is usually associated with a mirror-image pattern of branching of the arteries to the head and arms. The brachiocephalic artery is then left-sided and supplies the left subclavian and left common carotid arteries. Perhaps surprisingly, a duct, when present in a right arch, is usually a left-sided structure, taking origin from the left brachiocephalic artery. A right-sided arch occurs most frequently in association with tetralogy of Fallot, where it is found in perhaps 25% of cases, or with common arterial trunk, where it is found in as many as 50%. In these circumstances, the left-sided transverse component of the double arch will have involuted.

The pattern of a right arch can also exist with persistence of the greater part of the left-sided transverse arch. These arrangements are more complicated. When found without any associated intracardiac defects, almost always it is retroesophageal origin and course of the left subclavian artery which represents the left-sided components of the double arch. The comparable arrangement with a left arch is represented by retroesophageal origin and course of the right subclavian artery. Such an artery originates as the last branch of the descending aorta (Fig. 8.15). With this arrangement of persistence of parts of both transverse components of a double arch, the tracheoesophageal pedicle becomes encircled by vascular structures.

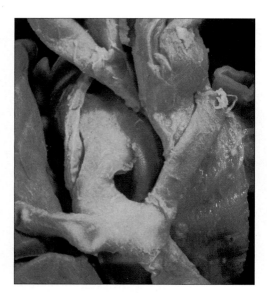

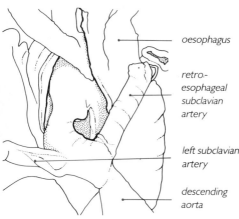

Fig. 8.15 This posterior view shows the retrooesophageal origin of the right subclavian artery shown in Fig. 8.14.

oesophagus

retro-esophageal subclavian artery

left subclavian artery

descending aorta

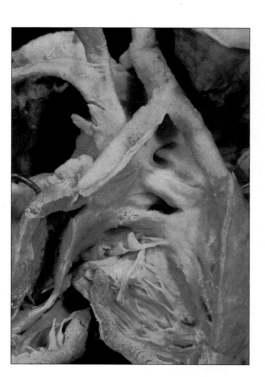

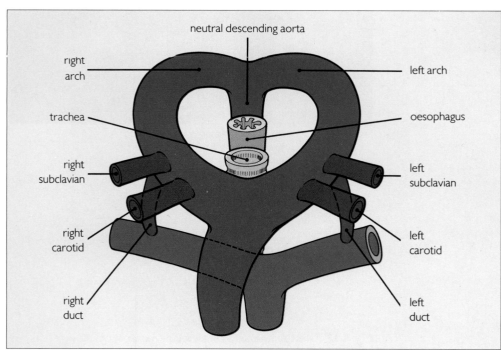

neutral descending aorta

right arch

left arch

trachea

oesophagus

right subclavian

left subclavian

right carotid

left carotid

right duct

left duct

Fig. 8.17 This diagram shows the arrangement of the perfect double aortic arch.

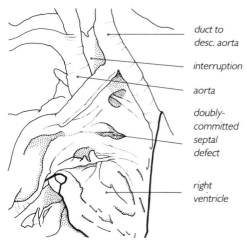

duct to desc. aorta

interruption

aorta

doubly-committed septal defect

right ventricle

Fig. 8.16 In this heart, interruption of the aortic arch is accompanied by a doubly committed and juxtaarterial ventricular septal defect.

In the case illustrated with a retroesophageal subclavian artery, the vascular ring produced is incomplete. In its complete form, the vascular ring persists as two transverse arches, both patent, which encircle the tracheoesophageal pedicle and fuse posteriorly to form the descending aorta (Fig. 8.18). It is double arches of this type which are more likely to produce dysphagia but, even with a perfect double arch, this symptom is not uniformly present. It is rare with such a double arch for the two transverse components to be of comparable size. More usually, it is the right arch that is the wider arterial pathway. As with other malformations of the aortic pathways, double arches usually accompany intracardiac lesions.

Anomalies of the pulmonary arteries

Although the branching of the pulmonary trunk is much less complex than that of the aorta, abnormal patterns of branching do occur. Thus, one pulmonary artery can take an anomalous origin from the other pulmonary artery, from the ascending portion of the aorta, or from some part of the aortic system via an arterial duct.

Anomalous origin of the left from the right pulmonary artery usually occurs in such a way that it courses to the left hilum by passing between the oesophagus and the trachea (Fig. 8.19). Closely related in terms of anatomy, but not encircling or passing behind the trachea, is the arrangement where the pulmonary trunk branches in such a way that the right pulmonary artery originates in advance of the left, and the two arteries then cross each other as they run to their respective lungs. Such crossed pulmonary arteries are exceedingly rare.

When one pulmonary artery arises from a systemic source, the lung it supplies receives systemic arterial rather than systemic venous blood. This can occur in partial or complete forms. An example of partially anomalous arterial supply is seen in the scimitar syndrome, where the arterial supply and the pulmonary venous return are abnormal, the latter being connected to the inferior caval vein.

Totally anomalous pulmonary arterial supply to one lung is a more severe malformation. This arrangement is often called 'absent pulmonary artery', but it is rare for the artery that is supplying the afflicted lung to be completely absent. Rather, the 'absent' artery is isolated from the pulmonary trunk, usually

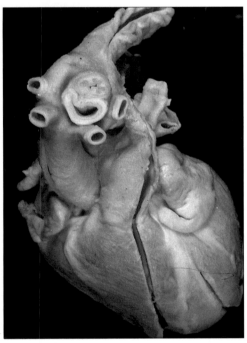

Fig. 8.18 This double aortic arch encircles the tracheooesophageal pedicle.

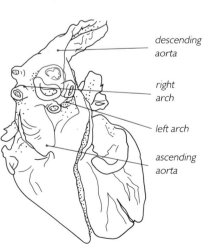

descending aorta

right arch

left arch

ascending aorta

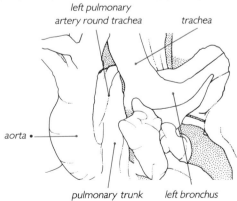

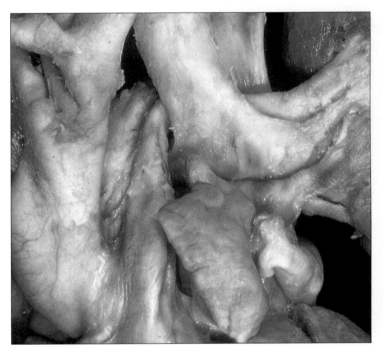

left pulmonary artery round trachea trachea

aorta

pulmonary trunk left bronchus

Fig. 8.19 This heart has origin of the left pulmonary from the right pulmonary artery with encirclement of the trachea – the so-called pulmonary arterial sling.

being supplied from the aortic arch via an arterial duct, which may be left- or right-sided and which, when seen, may be ligamentous. Alternatively, as often occurs in tetralogy with pulmonary atresia, the isolated lung may be supplied via major aortopulmonary collateral arteries. In extreme cases, one lung may be supplied by a duct and the other by collateral arteries (Fig. 8.20), the intrapericardial arteries being absent, and the trunk arising from the heart being best described as a solitary arterial trunk (see Fig. 7.27). There is then one further possibility, namely the pulmonary artery arising directly from the ascending aorta. This arrangement has been termed 'hemitruncus' but such a term is not recommended since it is most often found when the other pulmonary artery arises from the right ventricle, an arrangement that does not produce a common arterial trunk (Fig. 8.21).

ANOMALIES OF THE SUBSYSTEMS

In this final section on congenital lesions, those that afflict the walls of the heart, together with the coronary arteries and conduction tissues that supply and activate them, are considered briefly. Discussion of malformations of the arteries and conduction tissues is confined to primary malformations of these structures, thus avoiding discussion of anomalies that co-exist with other congenital malformations. These will have been dealt with largely in the section devoted to the specific lesion.

The myocardium

Some congenital lesions that affect the myocardium have already been mentioned in previous sections. Probably the most severe anomaly is hypertrophic cardiomyopathy which, although often not presenting until relatively late in life, almost certainly has a congenital background. This entity is discussed at length in Section 5 , where the more recently discovered cardiomyopathy that affects infants and presents with arrhythmias in the first two years of life, namely foamy transformation of the myocardium of infancy, is also described. Congenital absence of the myocardium of the morphologically right ventricle has also been discussed previously (Uhl's malformation – see Fig. 7.13).

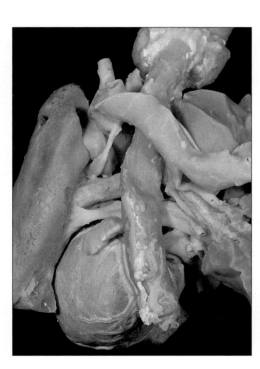

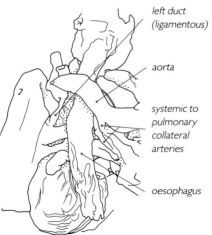

Fig. 8.20 In this heart with a solitary arterial trunk (see Fig. 7.27), the supply to the left lung was initially supplied by the arterial duct, which has become ligamentous, while the supply to the right lung is through systemic-to-pulmonary collateral arteries.

left duct (ligamentous)

aorta

systemic to pulmonary collateral arteries

oesophagus

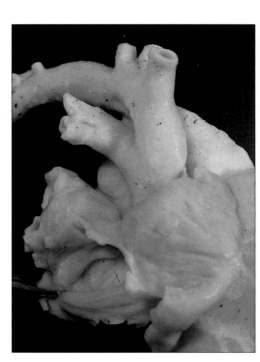

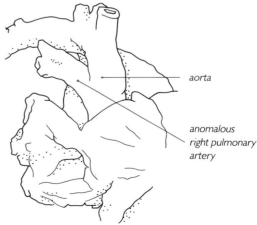

Fig. 8.21 This view of the ascending aorta shows an anomalous origin of the right pulmonary artery, the left pulmonary artery coming from the right ventricle.

aorta

anomalous right pulmonary artery

The endocardium

Isolated congenital abnormalities affecting the endocardium are rare. By far the most significant is primary, or idiopathic, endocardial fibroelastosis. This is a porcelain-like thickening of the endocardium which, as an isolated lesion, almost always affects the left ventricle (Fig. 8.22). Such thickening is seen most frequently as a secondary finding, particularly in the hypoplastic left heart syndrome occurring with mitral stenosis rather than atresia (see Fig. 6.87).

Primary endocardial fibroelastosis is found in contracted and dilated forms, the latter being much more common. In the dilated form, the entire trabecular zone of the left ventricle is dilated, and the thickened endocardium covers the entire surface like a blanket. The myocardium is thinned because of the dilatation, but is histologically normal. Due to the dilatation, the mitral valve seems to be hypoplastic, but this is also a secondary effect (Fig. 8.23). In the contracted form, the cavity of the left ventricle is grossly hypoplastic, but the outflow tract to the aorta, and the aortic valve, are relatively spared (Fig. 8.24).

The pericardium

Congenital lesions of the pericardium are rare. Congenital absence is most frequent as part of a pleuropericardial defect, which may be partial or complete. When partial, it is usually the left side that is affected and, when small, the left atrial appendage may herniate through the deficiency and become strangulated. More frequently, the defect is larger and does not produce symptoms (Fig. 8.25). Congenital anomalies of either the heart or lungs are found in approximately one-third of cases. Defects in the diaphragmatic part of the pericardium are exceedingly rare. The other congenital malformations warranting mention are cysts and diverticulums.

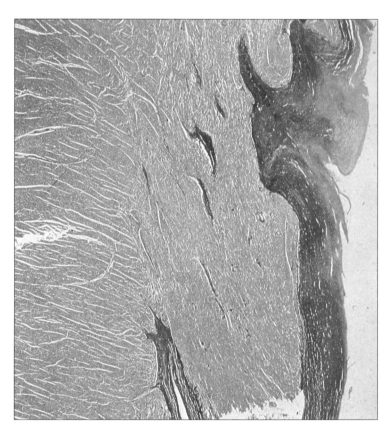

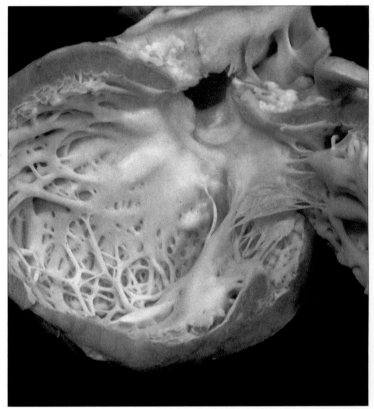

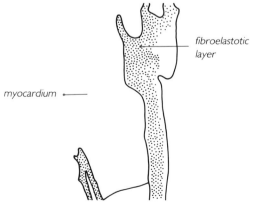

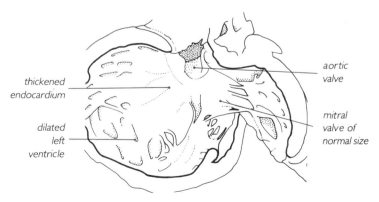

Fig. 8.22 This histological section, stained to show elastic, shows a dense fibroelastotic layer on the surface of the left ventricle.

Fig. 8.23 In this heart, the dilated left ventricle is lined by a layer of fibroelastosis.

Malformations of the coronary arteries

Congenital anomalies of the coronary arteries make up a hetero-geneous group of anomalies that usually are of little or no clinical significance but which can be life-threatening. The over-all incidence in otherwise normal hearts is approximately 1%, but they are seen more frequently when searched for actively. According to the morphology, they can be divided into four main groups: first, there are variations in the number of orifices of the arteries; second, is the variation to be found in the level of origin of the arteries relative to the sinuses; third, there may be variations in the site of origin; and fourth, abnormal communications can occur between the coronary arteries and other structures.

In terms of the number of arterial orifices, the most significant anomaly is a single artery. This itself can take two forms. A single coronary artery can follow the normal course of the right coronary artery but then cross the crux, encircle the mitral orifice, and terminate as the anterior interventricular coronary artery. Even more rarely, the circumflex artery may feed the right coronary artery. More frequently, a single artery divides immediately into right and left branches, the left branch then sometimes encircling the pulmonary trunk before dividing into circumflex and anterior interventricular arteries (Fig. 8.26). Multiple orifices of either the right or left coronary arteries are of no functional significance other than occasionally leading to erroneous interpretation of coronary angiograms. Dual orifices of the right coronary artery, or even triple orifices, occur frequ-

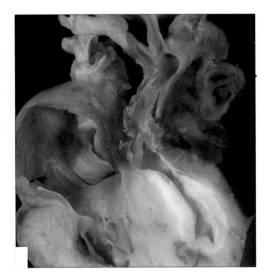

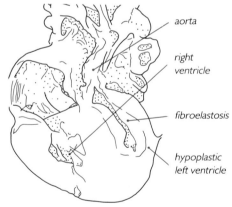

Fig. 8.24 In this heart, the fibroelastosis is found within a hypoplastic left ventricle with a patent aortic root.

aorta

right ventricle

fibroelastosis

hypoplastic left ventricle

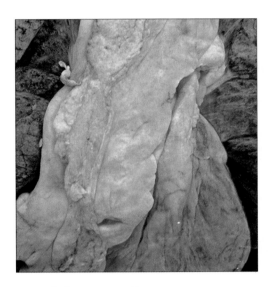

Fig. 8.25 This heart has congenital absence of the left side of the pericardial cavity.

no left-sided pericardium

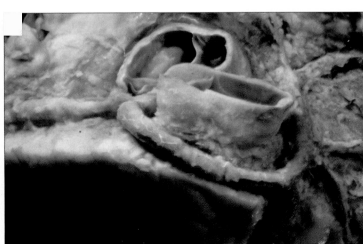

Fig. 8.26 All coronary arteries in this heart arise from one orifice in the right hand facing aortic sinus. Note the course of the left coronary artery in front of the pulmonary trunk.

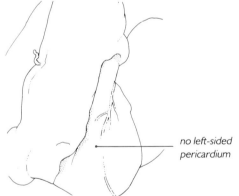

single coronary artery

right coronary artery

pulmonary trunk

left coronary artery

ently. Separate orifices for the branches of the left coronary artery (Fig. 8.27), in contrast, are very rare.

The usual site of the orifice of a coronary artery is at, or just below, the line of junction between the sinusal and tubular parts of the aorta. When an artery arises more than 1 cm above the bar, it is considered abnormal. Although of no functional significance in itself, the oblique take-off of the artery in this circumstance could induce orificial narrowing. An abnormal origin of the coronary arteries, therefore, can occur from either the aorta or from the pulmonary trunk, the latter being more

significant. It is usually the left coronary artery which arises anomalously (Fig. 8.28, upper). Collateral supply from the normally attached coronary artery can produce a 'steal' situation (Fig. 8.28, lower), and this can exacerbate the myocardial ischaemia and infarction produced by the anomalous origin of the artery from the pulmonary trunk. Dilatation and fibrosis of the left ventricle (Fig. 8.29) are not a feature in hearts of patients who die in the neonatal period. In those who survive the critical neonatal period, however, it is these subsequent changes which can produce the trigger for sudden death during adolescence.

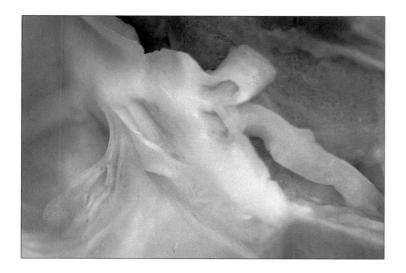

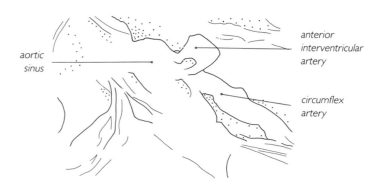

Fig. 8.27 This heart has origin of the circumflex and anterior interventricular arteries by separate orifices within the left hand facing aortic sinus.

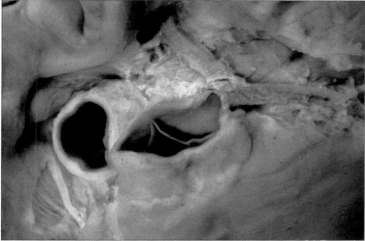

Fig. 8.28 This heart has anomalous origin of the left coronary artery from the pulmonary trunk (upper) with the potential to "steal" by collateral vessels from the normally connected right coronary artery (lower).

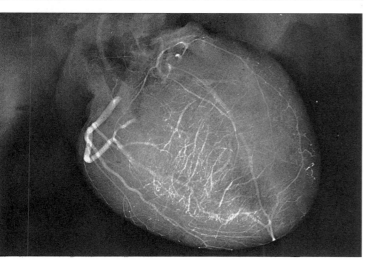

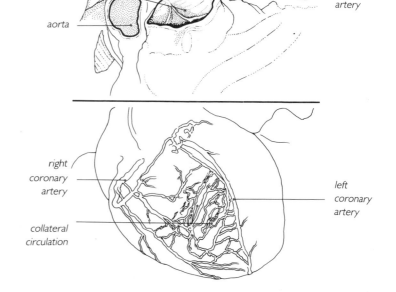

In some cases, it is only the anterior interventricular branch of the left coronary artery that has an aberrant pulmonary origin. Aberrant pulmonary origin of the right coronary artery can also lead to ischaemia, but is much rarer and, usually, has no clinical significance. Anomalous origin of both coronary arteries from the pulmonary trunk is an even rarer finding which, unless treated surgically, will result in death in the neonatal period.

An anomalous course of the coronary arteries relative to the aortic root is of much less clinical significance. Many patterns exist, the most common being the origin of the left circumflex artery from either the right aortic sinus or the right coronary artery (Fig. 8.30). More noteworthy are anomalous courses which result in the main stem of the left coronary artery being sandwiched between the aorta and the pulmonary trunk (Fig. 8.31). This arrangement can result in myocardial ischaemia, but probably as a consequence of the oblique anomalous origin of the artery rather than compression between the two great arterial trunks.

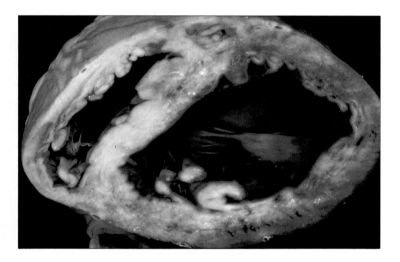

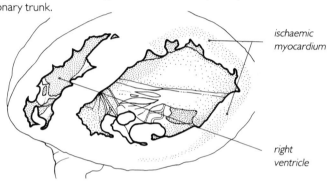

Fig. 8.29 This cross section shows the dilated and fibrotic left ventricle resulting from anomalous origin of the left coronary artery from the pulmonary trunk.

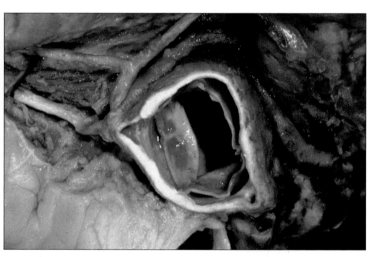

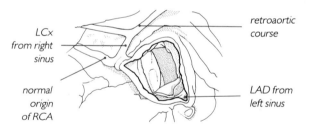

Fig. 8.30 In this heart, the circumflex artery arises from the right coronary artery and runs behind the aorta.

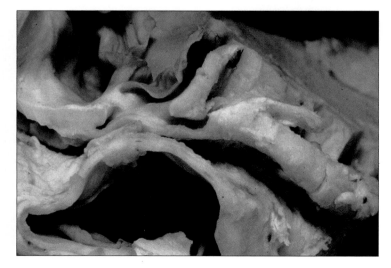

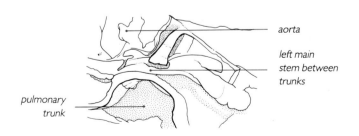

Fig. 8.31 This dissection shows an oblique origin of the left coronary artery between the aorta and the pulmonary trunk.

Fistulous connexions with the coronary arteries are most frequently found in cases with either aortic or pulmonary atresia when the ventricular septum is intact (see Fig. 6.32). Fistulous connexions can, much more rarely, exist in isolation. The sites of drainage, in decreasing order of frequency, are the right ventricle, right atrium, pulmonary trunk, and left atrium. Rarer sites also occur, such as the peripheral branches of the pulmonary arteries.

The conduction system

Congenital lesions that affect the conduction system in an otherwise normally structured heart can be considered under the headings of congenitally complete heart block and ventricular pre-excitation.

In the normal heart, the only muscular connexion that crosses the plane of atrioventricular insulation is the penetrating atrioventricular bundle (the bundle of His). If this axis of atrioventricular conduction is interrupted, complete heart block will result. This can occur as a consequence of disruption of the axis (nodoventricular discontinuity), encasement of the axis in fibrous tissue with absence of the atrioventricular node (atrial-axis dis-

continuity), or isolation of the ventricular bundle branches (Fig. 8.32). Although this section is only concerned with the findings in otherwise normal hearts, congenitally complete heart block is found with some frequency in patients with congenitally corrected transposition and in those with isomerism of the left atrial appendages. When found in an otherwise normal heart, the most frequent pattern is discontinuity between the axis and the atrial myocardium (Fig. 8.33). This is the pattern found in infants born to mothers with systemic lupus erythematosus, and is almost certainly due to destruction of the atrioventricular node by antigens crossing the placenta from the mothers. It is much rarer to find cases where the atrioventricular node and bundle branches are well formed in the atrial and ventricular myocardial segments, respectively, but with no connexion between them across the septal atrioventricular junction (Fig. 8.34). The final type, with isolation of the bundle branches, is even rarer, although it does have a familial inheritance.

Ventricular pre-excitation results from congenital lesions that produce alternate pathways of conduction from atrial to ventricular myocardium other than by the usual route through the axis of atrioventricular conduction tissue. The reason for the axis of atrioventricular conduction tissue being insulated from

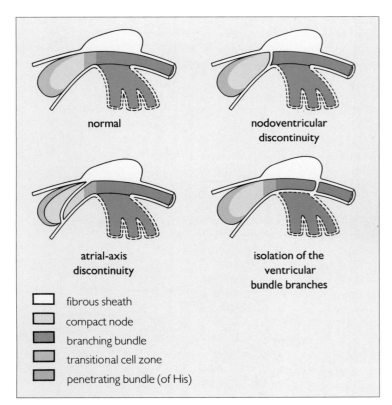

Fig. 8.32 This diagram shows, compared to normal, the different patterns of complete atrioventricular block.

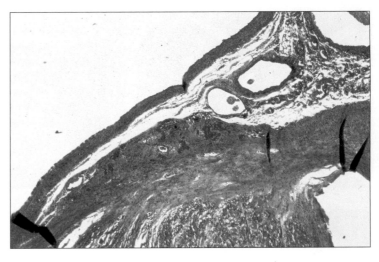
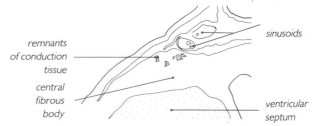

Fig. 8.33 This section through the anticipated site of the atrioventricular node, stained with the trichrome technique, shows the pattern of atrial-axis discontinuity typically found in infants of mothers with systemic lupus erythematosus.

the myocardium is so that the atrioventricular node can induce a delay in conduction, giving time for the ventricular conduction system to distribute the wave of activation from the ventricular apices (Fig. 8.35, upper). Ventricular pre-excitation can be produced by several anomalous pathways that short-circuit this normal pathway of activation (Fig. 8.35, lower).

The most common type of pre-excitation is the so-called Wolff–Parkinson–White syndrome. Characterized electrocardiographically by a short PR interval and a broad QRS complex with a delta wave, it is produced by an anomalous muscular connexion between atrial and ventricular musculatures which circumvents entirely the nodal delay. Such accessory muscular connexions can be found at any point round the atrioventricular junctions. Left-sided pathways usually skirt a well-formed fibrous junction and pass through the epicardial fat pad in close approximation to the origin of the leaflet of the mitral valve. They are composed of ordinary working atrial myocardium (Fig. 8.36).

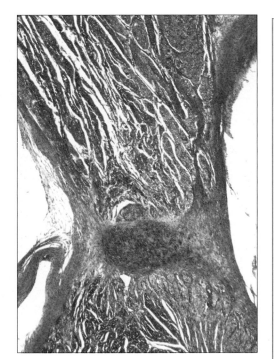

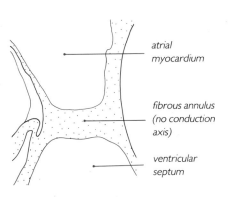

atrial
myocardium

fibrous annulus
(no conduction
axis)

ventricular
septum

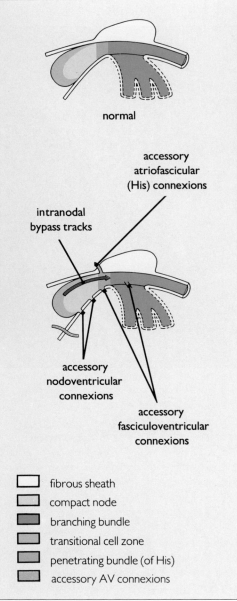

normal

accessory
atriofascicular
(His) connexions

intranodal
bypass tracks

accessory
nodoventricular
connexions

accessory
fasciculoventricular
connexions

☐ fibrous sheath

☐ compact node

☐ branching bundle

☐ transitional cell zone

☐ penetrating bundle (of His)

☐ accessory AV connexions

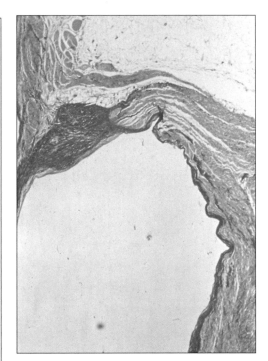

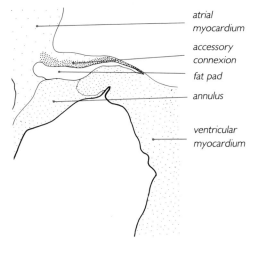

atrial
myocardium

accessory
connexion

fat pad

annulus

ventricular
myocardium

Fig. 8.34 This section, again stained with the trichrome technique, shows absence of continuity in a case of nodal-axis discontinuity.

Fig. 8.35 This diagram shows the potential pathways which may produce ventricular pre-excitation, compared with the normal arrangement.

Fig. 8.36 This section, stained with an elastic technique, shows a left-sided accessory atrioventricular connexion from a patient with Wolff– Parkinson–White syndrome.

Right-sided connexions can also pass through the epicardial fat pad, but can penetrate closer to the endocardial surface, the tricuspid valve never having such well-formed fibrous support as does the mitral valve. These pathways are usually composed of working myocardium, but they can originate in node-like tissue (Fig. 8.37). Septal pathways can be found at any point in the septum outside the tissues of the atrioventricular junctional area. The only such connexion we discovered ran from the tip of the right atrial myocardium and passed across the atrioventricular groove to join the ventricular myocardium; it was made of ordinary working myocardium (Fig. 8.38). Accessory muscular atrioventricular connexions are usually single, but multiple pathways may be present.

The other pathways that can potentially produce pre-excitation lack solid anatomico-clinical correlations. An accessory atriofascicular pathway has been identified in one case with a short PR interval and a normal QRS pattern (Lown–Ganong–Levine syndrome). It is also possible that anomalous pathways within the atrioventricular node, or even a congenitally small node, could produce this electrocardiographic pattern. The remaining postulated anomalous pathways pass from either the atrial part of the specialized junction (nodoventricular fibres) or from the ventricular conduction tissues themselves (fasciculoventricular fibres) to join the septal ventricular myocardium. These fibres, if functional, would short-circuit the part of delay that is produced as the impulse passes through the insulated segments of the ventricular conduction pathways. The pathways would produce an atypical pattern of pre-excitation with a short PR interval together with a broadened QRS complex and a delta wave. The entire groups of these fibres are described as Mahaim fibres. They are to be found in all hearts during fetal development but, at this time, they do not function as bypass tracts. They can also be found in hearts from children and adults who, as far as can be known, had no electrocardiographic evidence of instability of cardiac rhythm. More correlative studies are needed to establish the natural history of these connexions between the conduction axis and the ventricular septum (Fig. 8.39), and to establish their role, if any, in the production of ventricular pre-excitation.

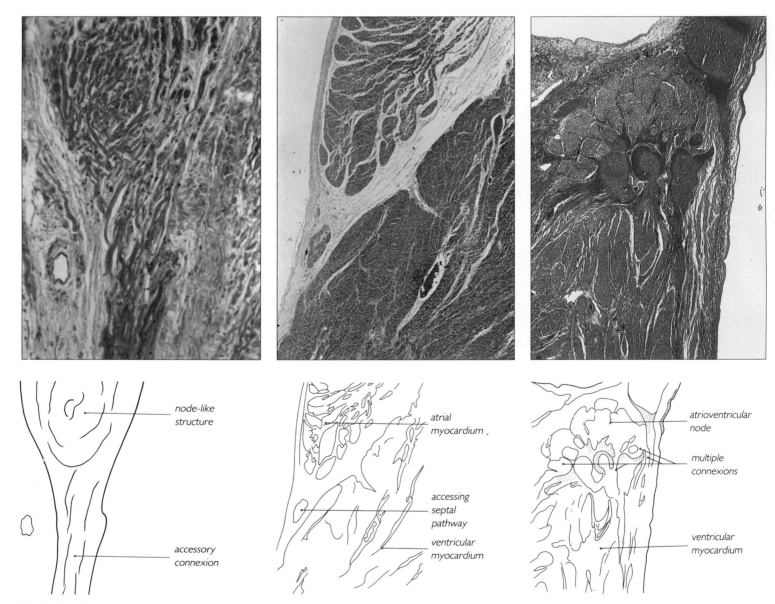

Fig. 8.37 This section, stained with the trichrome technique, shows a specialized right-sided atrioventricular connexion from a patient with Wolff–Parkinson–White syndrome.

Fig. 8.38 This section, stained with the trichrome technique, shows a septal accessory connexion from a patient with Wolff–Parkinson–White syndrome.

Fig. 8.39 This section, stained with an elastic technique, shows multiple connexions extending through the central fibrous body – so-called Mahaim fibres.

Acquired conditions primarily affecting contractility

INTRODUCTION

A variety of diseases primarily affect the function of the heart as a pump, and in the Western world, ischaemic heart disease is by far the most common, the underlying pathology being obstructive coronary arterial disease. Myocardial ischaemia and necrosis may also be found, nonetheless, as complications of conditions that primarily affect the pressure or volume load on the heart (see Chapter 13), as well as in most forms of congenital heart disease. Furthermore, all other diseases that primarily

affect myocardial contractility, which although in themselves are basically not ischaemic in nature, may become complicated by ischaemia despite the minimal degree and extent of obstructive coronary arterial disease. In general, all circumstances that produce an imbalance between myocardial demand for oxygen and its consumption may initiate myocardial ischaemia and, hence, infarction.

---

9   ISCHAEMIA

ISCHAEMIC HEART DISEASE

Coronary atherosclerosis

Coronary arteries, because of their small size, are particularly susceptible to luminal narrowing by atherosclerotic plaques. Pathological studies reveal that once atherosclerotic disease is present, the plaques are usually widely distributed throughout

the coronary arterial tree (Fig. 9.1). Plaques are rarely limited to a single spot, despite the fact that patients clinically may present with localized stenosis in a single artery.

These aspects are relevant to the interpretation of clinical coronary angiograms, since a severe proximal stenosis may influence the imaging of the distal segments and, hence, the overall interpretation of the severity of the disease.

Atherosclerotic lesions in coronary arteries are either eccentric

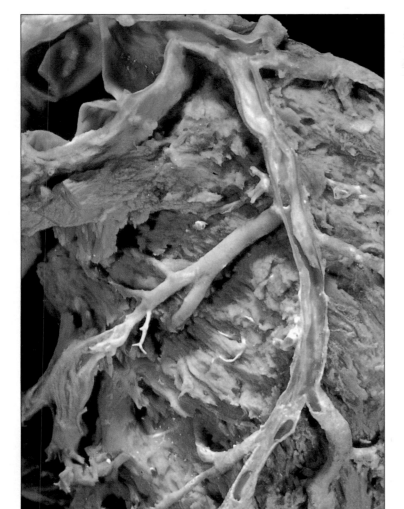

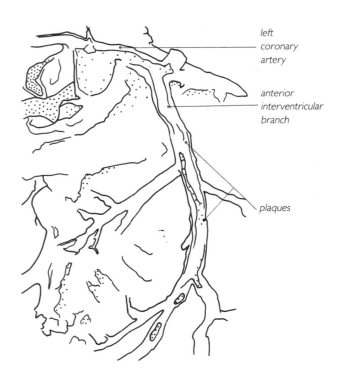

Fig. 9.1   Dissection of a left anterior descending artery showing various atherosclerotic plaques.

left coronary artery

anterior interventricular branch

plaques

(Fig. 9.2) or concentric (Fig. 9.3), eccentric lesions being by far the most common. From a histological point of view, the architecture and composition of atherosclerotic plaques may vary markedly. A correlation exists between clinical presentation and the type of plaque. In patients with classical effort angina, distinct obstructive coronary arterial lesions are usually present (Fig. 9.4); the atherosclerotic plaque in this clinical setting is described as 'stable', being characteristically composed almost

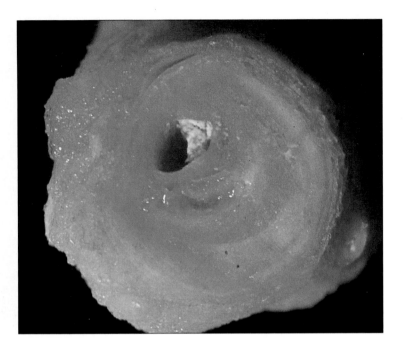

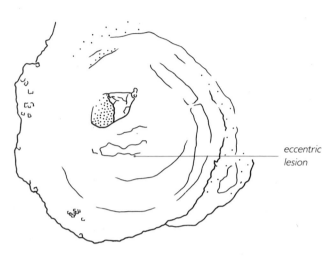

Fig. 9.2 Cross-section through a coronary artery showing an eccentric sclerotic lesion.

eccentric lesion

Fig. 9.4 Post-mortem coronary angiogram showing dominant left coronary artery.

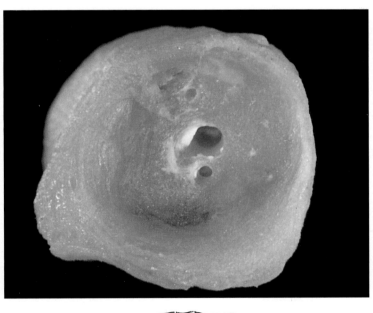

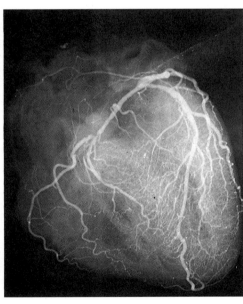

wall irregularities

stenosis

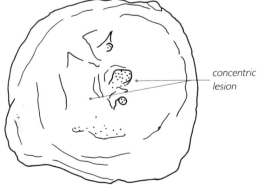

concentric lesion

Fig. 9.3 Cross-section through a coronary artery showing a concentric sclerotic lesion.

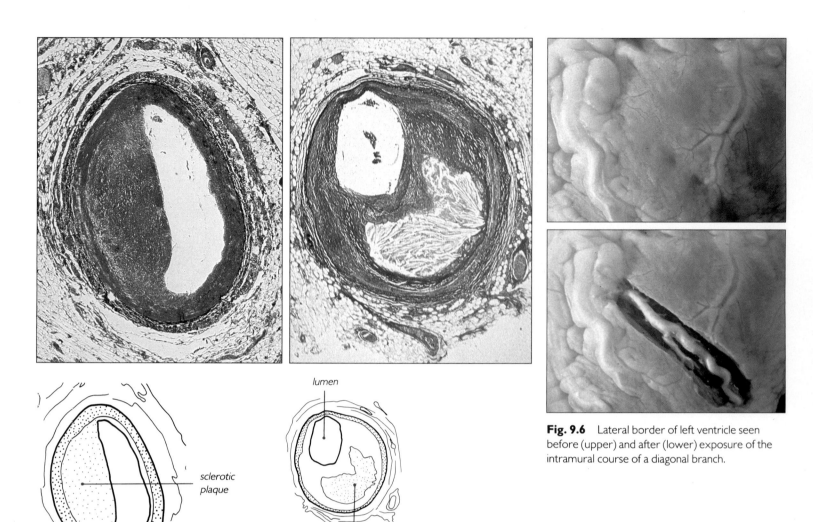

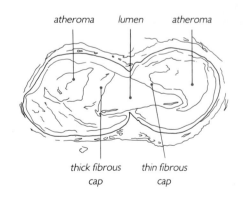

Fig. 9.6 Lateral border of left ventricle seen before (upper) and after (lower) exposure of the intramural course of a diagonal branch.

Fig. 9.5 Histological section of coronary artery showing obstructive atherosclerotic lesion mainly composed of dense collagen (left). Section through major stenosis in LAD (right) exhibits classical atherosclerotic plaque. E-VG stain.

Fig. 9.7 Cross-section through a coronary artery at a branching point. The relatively thick fibrous cap on the left hand side contrasts with the rather thin fibrous cap on the right.

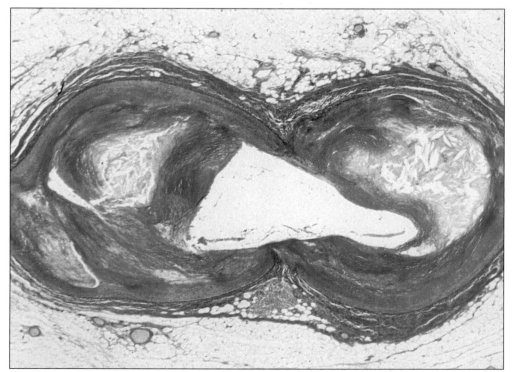

Acquired Conditions Primarily Affecting Contractility

exclusively of dense collagen (Fig. 9.5, left), or as having a firm fibrous cap separating the atheromatous debris from the lumen (Fig. 9.5, right). In some patients, classical effort angina, and occasionally myocardial infarction, can be due to the 'milking effect' of myocardial bridges; the anterior descending coronary artery and its main branches are most commonly affected (Fig. 9.6). Narrowing of the intramural segment during cardiac systole by the myocardial bridges has been incriminated as the underlying cause of unexpected and sudden death in apparently healthy subjects.

In contrast, the underlying obstructive coronary atherosclerosis usually shows a different pattern in those presenting with unstable angina. The lesion in this setting contains a large atheromatous pool, and the overlying fibrous cap is attenuated (Fig. 9.7). Platelets may aggregate at the luminal side and minute thrombi made up of platelets and fibrin may be present (Fig. 9.8). Such atherosclerotic plaques are considered 'at risk' and have been named collectively as 'unstable'. A spectrum evidently exists between 'stable' and 'unstable' plaques.

Another aspect that may play a role in unstable angina is an increased vasomotor tone of the affected coronary arterial segment. In almost all instances, the presence of an atherosclerotic plaque leaves the medial wall intact, so that the anatomical substrate for vasoconstriction is still present (Fig. 9.9). Changes in the autonomic nervous regulation, and decreased production of the endothelial-derived relaxation factor, all due to the atherosclerotic lesion, may play a role in vasoconstriction under these circumstances. It is also important to realize that a minor degree of contraction may have a profound effect on the surface area of the arterial lumen (Fig. 9.10).

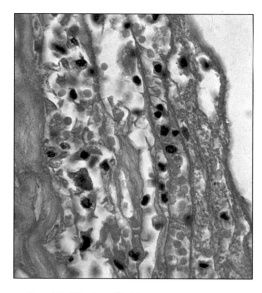

Fig. 9.8 Detail of platelet–fibrin aggregate at surface of fibrous cap. H&E stain.

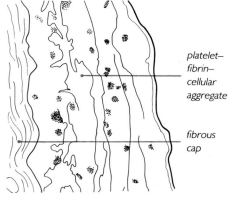

platelet–fibrin–cellular aggregate

fibrous cap

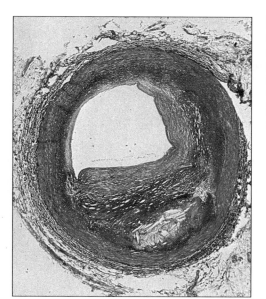

Fig. 9.9 Histological section of coronary artery showing atherosclerosis with intact medial layer. Vasospasm may easily be conceived. E-VG stain.

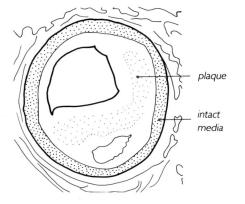

plaque

intact media

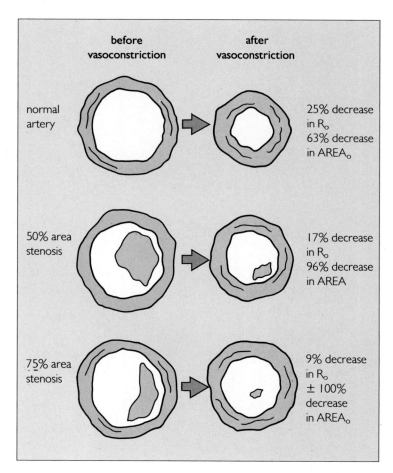

before vasoconstriction

after vasoconstriction

normal artery — 25% decrease in R_o 63% decrease in $AREA_o$

50% area stenosis — 17% decrease in R_o 96% decrease in AREA

75% area stenosis — 9% decrease in R_o ± 100% decrease in $AREA_o$

Fig. 9.10 The effects of vasoconstriction on sections with differing degrees of stenosis.

At present, it is well established that the vast majority, if not all, patients with myocardial infarction, will have, at least temporarily, total occlusion of the principal coronary artery. The underlying pathology is thrombosis superimposed on complex malformations of the atherosclerotic plaque (Fig. 9.11). This observation provides the rationale for thrombolytic or myo-cardial infarction. The plaque is usually fissured (Fig. 9.12), a so-called cracked plaque. Alternatively, the fibrous cap may show marked attenuation without a distinct and localized fissure, but rather with exposure of a large area of the atheromatous debris to the lumen (Fig. 9.13). It is now well accepted that fissuring of the plaque may most likely occur as part of unstable

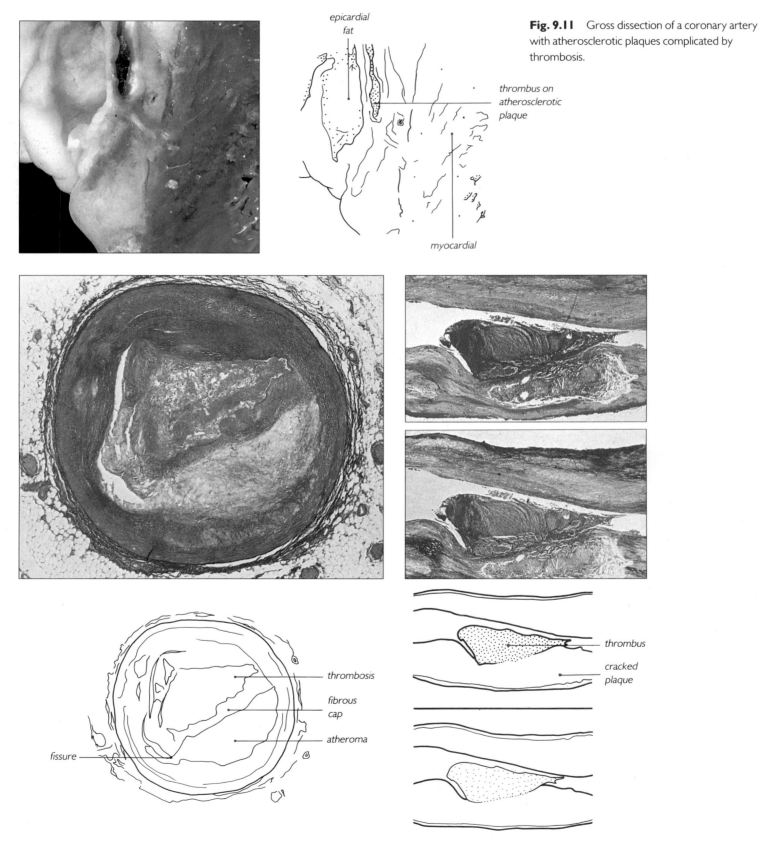

Fig. 9.11   Gross dissection of a coronary artery with atherosclerotic plaques complicated by thrombosis.

Fig. 9.12   Cross-section through a coronary artery showing a plaque fissure with thrombus occluding the lumen.

Fig. 9.13   Longitudinal histological section through coronary artery with occluding thrombus adherent to atherosclerotic 'cracked' plaque. (Upper) H&E, (lower) E-VG stains.

angina, but does not necessarily lead to total occlusion of the affected arterial segment. Under such circumstances, the fissure may heal, and such healing may then be the mechanism underlying progression of the atherosclerotic lesion (Fig. 9.14).

Coronary arterial thrombosis should be distinguished from the relatively rare occurrence of thromboembolism (Fig. 9.15).

Thromboembolic lesions are usually found peripherally in epicardial arteries, often at the site of branching, and lack a distinct relation to atherosclerotic plaques. Calcific and cholesterol emboli (Fig. 9.16) are usually of such a small size that they lodge in intramural branches.

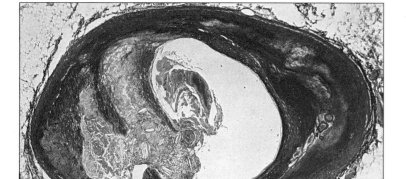

Fig. 9.14 Histological section of coronary artery with stratified atheroma.. The superficial atheroma exhibits a cracked plaque. E-VG stain.

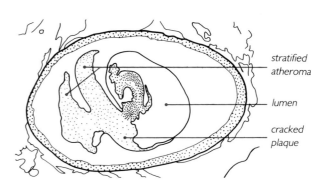

stratified atheroma

lumen

cracked plaque

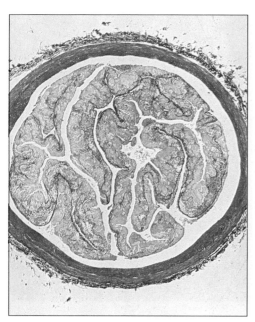

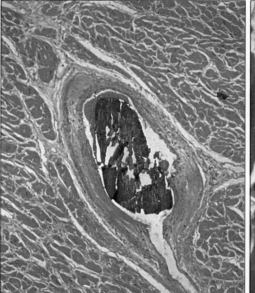

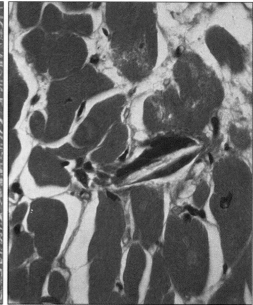

Fig. 9.15 Histological section showing thromboembolus in coronary artery. E-VG stain.

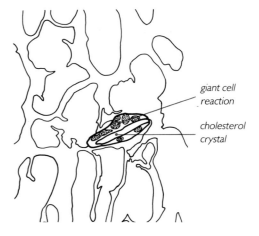

giant cell reaction

cholesterol crystal

Fig. 9.16 Histological sections of mural coronary artery showing (left) calcific embolus derived from calcified aortic valve (AoV); (right) cholesterol embolus with giant cell reaction obstructing small intramural coronary arteriolar branch. H&E stains.

Longstanding coronary arterial thrombosis will eventually lead to plugging of the lumen by fibrous tissue (Fig. 9.17). Occasionally, extensive revascularization may occur (Fig. 9.18), in some cases to the extent of effective restoration of flow.

Aneurysms of coronary arteries are yet another complication of atherosclerosis, almost always indicating far-advanced disease. They usually present as localized saccular aneurysms (Fig. 9.19), filled for their greater part with thrombus. Multiple fusiform aneurysms occasionally occur, often in association with atherosclerotic aneurysms of the abdominal aorta. Other diseases, such as Kawasaki's disease, may underlie coronary arterial aneurysms in adults, but are relatively rare in the Western world. Dissecting aneurysm of the coronary arteries, as a disease entity, is extremely rare; Marfan's syndrome, nonetheless, may be complicated by laceration of the coronary arterial wall and subsequent dissection. Dissections of coronary arteries are otherwise complications of other conditions such as surgical trauma, percutaneous transluminal coronary angioplasty, or are an extension of an aortic dissecting haematoma.

Obstructive coronary atherosclerosis can be associated with growth of the affected vessel wall, thus compensating in part for the luminal narrowing induced by the plaque, and with the development of collateral circulation (Fig. 9.20). The extent and quality of collateral circulation is highly variable among patients with obstructive coronary arterial disease. In general, the intensity of collateral arteries increases with time and with the severity of the obstructive disease, although little is known about the rapidity of this development. There is good evidence to suggest that such collateral supply may prevent myocardial necrosis, at least when effective perfusion develops rapidly following the onset of ischaemia. Collateral supply may also limit the extent of infarction once irreversible ischaemia has occurred. On the other hand, the presence of collateral arteries in themselves is insufficient to prevent infarction. Collateral supply occurs less frequently in patients with an acute infarct leading to death or rupture than in patients with similar-sized infarcts who die of 'simple' pump failure.

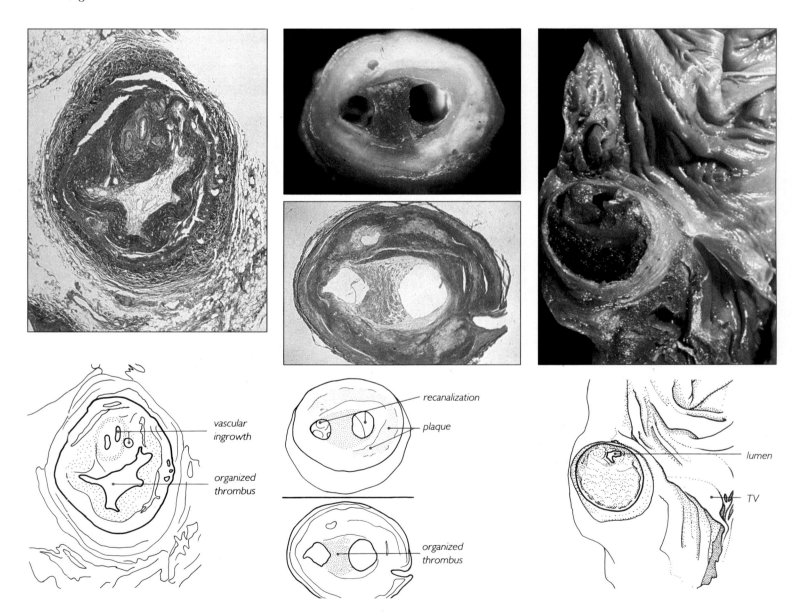

Fig. 9.17 Histological section of coronary artery with fibrous occlusion as end result of thrombosis. E-VG stain.

Fig. 9.18 Recanalized organized thrombosis of coronary artery: (upper) gross appearance; (lower) histology. E-VG stain.

Fig. 9.19 Cross-section through right atrioventricular junction showing atherosclerotic aneurysm of right coronary artery largely filled with thrombus.

Obstruction to coronary arterial perfusion can also be caused by atherosclerosis of the ascending aorta which obstructs the orifice of the coronary arteries (Fig. 9.21). Occasionally, the tip of the catheter may lacerate the site of origin of a coronary artery, generally at the site of an atherosclerotic plaque. Due to the pre-existent weakening of the walls, the coronary arteries are particularly at risk in Marfan's syndrome. Other external factors, such as compression of coronary arteries by a dissecting aneurysm of the aorta, should be included among the rare causes of myocardial ischaemia and necrosis. It would also be inappropriate to conclude this section without a brief discussion of small-vessel disease, or intramyocardial coronary arteriosclerosis. Introduced initially as an 'escape' to explain the occurrence of myocardial infarction without obstructive coronary atherosclerosis, it is now evident that small-vessel disease is a true rarity. Nevertheless, cases do occur in which the majority of intramyocardial arteries exhibit various degrees of intimal thickening, usually caused by fibrocellular proliferation (Fig. 9.22). The underlying injury that triggers this response is unknown. Similar vascular changes may occur in the left ventricular papillary muscles, in the base of the ventricular septum of elderly patients, and in hypertrophic cardiomyopathy, suggesting a mechanical effect. Such changes, nonetheless, are confined to these sites.

Obstructive coronary arterial disease is rare in infancy and childhood, but may occur either as early, but otherwise classical atherosclerosis (as seen in patients with the homozygous form of type II hyperbetalipoproteinaemia) or as a diffuse fibromuscular proliferation that usually affects both medial and intimal layers of the coronary arteries. Such diffuse proliferation may occur following viral infections in pregnancy, but may also accompany systemic metabolic disorders such as mucopolysaccharidoses. Calcification may ensue and, hence, lead to a condition known as 'idiopathic infantile arterial calcification'.

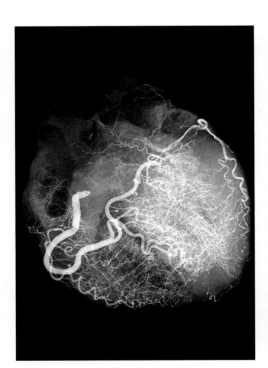

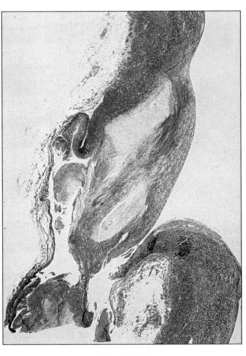

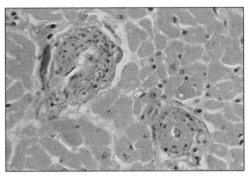

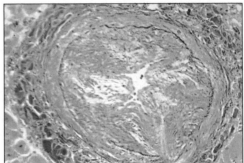

Fig. 9.20 Post-mortem coronary angiogram showing extensive collateral filling of left coronary artery system following injection of right coronary artery only.

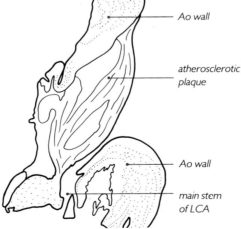

Fig. 9.21 Histological section showing coronary ostial narrowing due to severe obstruction by atherosclerotic plaque. E-VG stain.

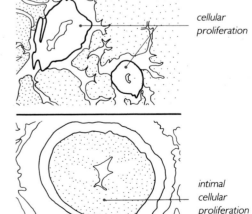

Fig. 9.22 Histological sections showing small-vessel disease of intramural coronary arteries: (upper) cellular proliferation in small arterioles; (lower) large-calibre artery with excessive cellular intimal proliferation. E-VG stain.

ISCHAEMIA VERSUS INFARCTION

Myocardial ischaemia is the condition in which myocardial cells have developed a deficit between the demand for consumption of oxygen, the process being potentially reversible. Infarction is death of cells, considered classically to be due to prolonged ischaemia. The morphology of these conditions is diverse. At least two major types of myocardial necrosis are recognized; both share ischaemia as an aetiological factor, but the pathogenetic mechanisms leading to death of the cells are different.

Ischaemia

In the majority of instances, ischaemia has no detectable morphological substrate, despite the fact that, once it is induced, it may rapidly be followed by electrical disturbances. Indeed, sudden death due to ventricular fibrillation can occur as a consequence of ischaemia. On the other hand, it is well established that ischaemia rapidly disregulates metabolism of the cell. Anaerobic glycolysis ensues, which leads to depletion of supplies of adeno-

sine triphosphate and to acidosis of the cell, both of which interfere with the efficacy of the sodium pump. As a consequence, cellular osmolarity changes and there is an excessive influx of water. The morphology of this change is known as hydropic cell swelling (Fig. 9.23). The cells are characterized by peripheral displacement of myofibrils, giving the cell an empty appearance.

Hydropic cell swelling accompanies classical infarction and has a preference for the subendocardial layers (Fig. 9.24). Zones of swollen cells can also surround intramyocardial arteries inside the zone of infarction (Fig. 9.25), as well as occurring in the transitional zone between the infarct and viable myocardium. These observations suggest that cells in these locations are less affected by prolonged ischaemia than are neighbouring cells. Indeed, in old infarcts, a small rim of viable cells usually occurs on the subendocardial side of the scar, while almost isolated cuffs of viable cells surrounding blood vessels may occur amidst dense areas of collagen. Hydropic cell swelling thus appears to be a potentially reversible process. It, nevertheless, renders the cell vulnerable not only to prolonged ischaemia but also to restored perfusion (see below).

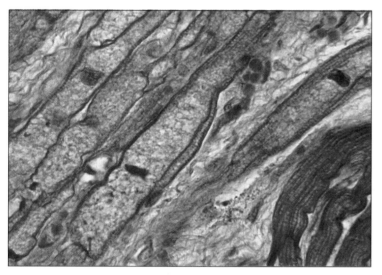

Fig. 9.23 Histological section of myocardium showing hydropic cell swelling. Mallory's phosphotungstic acid-haematoxylin (PTAH) stain.

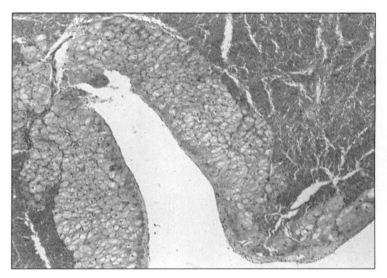

Fig. 9.24 Histological section showing hydropic cell swelling in subendocardial zone bordering classical infarct. H&E stain.

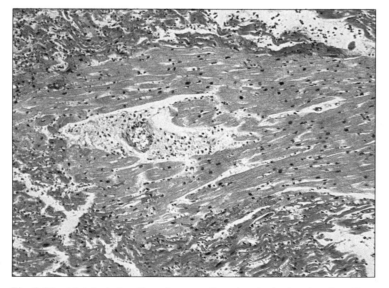

Fig. 9.25 Histological section of myocardium showing hydropic cell swelling around intramural coronary artery inside classical infarct. H&E stain.

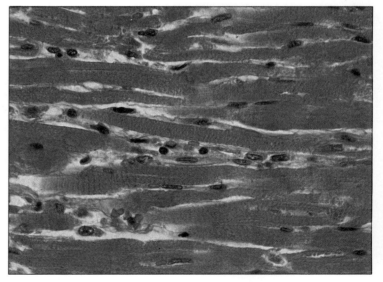

Fig. 9.26 Histological section of myocardium showing early coagulation necrosis. Z-bands are still identifiable but are farther apart. Some fibres show waviness. H&E stain.

Infarction

The leading morphological feature in classical myocardial infarction is coagulation necrosis. It has been shown, nonetheless, that a second type of myocardial necrosis may occur, namely contraction band necrosis. Proper distinction of these two entities adds to the understanding of the various pathophysiological mechanisms underscoring impaired myocardial perfusion.

Coagulation necrosis

Cells exhibiting coagulation necrosis are characterized by cytoplasmic eosinophilia and nuclear pyknosis (Fig. 9.26). Cross-striation is preserved initially, but close observation will reveal that the Z-bands are further apart than usual. Swelling of mitochondria, and changes in the structural characteristics of the sarcolemma, are the early alterations seen with the electron microscope. These morphological changes are the expression of intracellular acidosis and deficiency of the calcium pump, leading to loss of contractility.

The changes explain why, in the beating heart, myocardial fibres affected by prolonged ischaemia may become attenuated, giving a wavy appearance in histological sections. The waviness is a nonspecific alteration which is not restricted to ischaemia.

Contraction band necrosis

The second type of myocardial cell death, contraction band necrosis, is characterized by clumping of contractile elements which, under the light microscope, are seen as accumulations of eosinophilic material (Fig. 9.27). Ultrastructural studies show the contraction bands to consist of electron-dense material. The sarcomeres are shortened with an excessively scalloped sarcolemma (Fig. 9.28). The myofilaments continue into the contraction bands and, in these areas, exhibit marked disarray (Fig. 9.29).

The appearances suggest that the cell is in a hypercontracted state, the contraction bands representing accumulations of Z-band material. These changes may vary considerably in degree and extent and, unless carefully searched for, can be easily missed. Contraction bands are always found in cells exhibiting

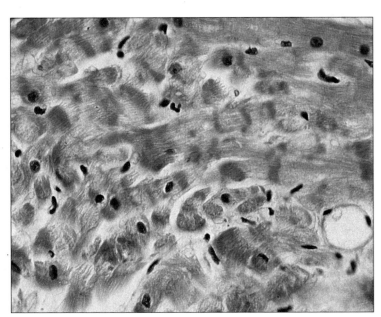

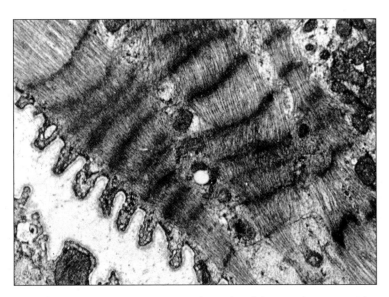

Fig. 9.28 Myocardial contraction bands consist of electron-dense material resembling Z-bands. EN, × 12,400. By courtesy of Dr K.P. Dingemans.

Fig. 9.27 Histological section of myocardium showing contraction band necrosis characterized by clumping of eosinophilic material. H&E stain.

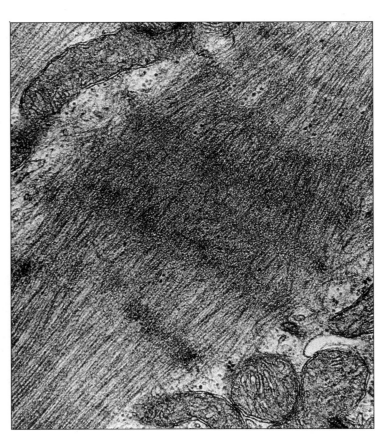

Fig. 9.29 Myofilaments are in continuity with the abnormal band and display marked disarray. EM, × 40,760. By courtesy of Dr K.P. Dingemans.

hydropic cell swelling (Fig. 9.30), although again they are not always readily apparent and occur under diverse circumstances. Although widely dispersed, they can be seen in the zone of potentially viable cells directly adjacent to other cells affected by coagulation necrosis, as in classical infarcts (Fig. 9.31). This phenomenon most likely relates to collateral perfusion in the zone at risk (see below).

Contraction bands are the morphological substrate of the 'stone heart' (see also complications of coronary bypass surgery, page 9.32) as well as the myocardial lesions that occur with phaeochromocytomas and increased intracranial pressures. These associations suggest that catecholamines may be one of the causative factors. The link with ischaemia, nonetheless, is well established. Experimental studies have shown that restoration of flow following a critical period of cellular ischaemia induces the appearance of contraction bands. This phenomenon is accompanied by accumulation of calcium by the mitochondria.

It was once believed that contraction band necrosis occurred only in cells destined to die; this opinion has now been challenged. Sudden perfusion can act as a critical event in a cell with potentially reversible ischaemic damage. Prior to a certain time, a cell may benefit from reperfusion. Beyond this critical period, however, reperfusion adds insult to injury. This concept has implications concerning myocardial preservation, be it in cardiac surgery or in the setting of acute myocardial infarction. If restoration of flow is to be beneficial, it should be established shortly following the onset of infarction. Alternatively, the metabolic demand of the myocardium should be depressed to such an extent that late reperfusion, be it natural or artificial, occurs at an early stage in terms of metabolism of the cell. These considerations suggest that thrombolysis as a treatment for myocardial infarction should be employed early following its onset.

MYOCARDIAL INFARCTION: GENERAL ASPECTS

Myocardial infarction can be classified in at least three ways: firstly, as regional or diffuse according to the relationship to the coronary artery involved; secondly, as anterior, lateral, inferior/ posterior, or septal according to its position (or a mixture of these); and thirdly, as transmural or subendocardial according to the mural extent of the infarction. These classifications highlight different aspects of infarction and, hence, are often used in combination.

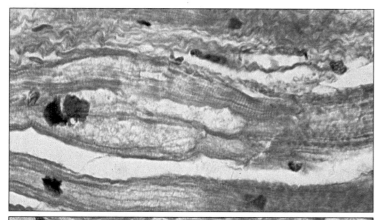

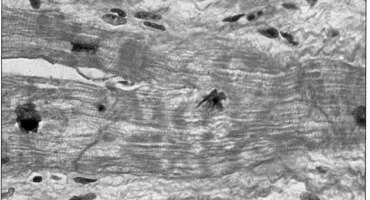

Fig. 9.30 Histological sections of myocardium showing (upper) hydropic cell swelling only; (lower) this change in association with contraction bands. H&E stains.

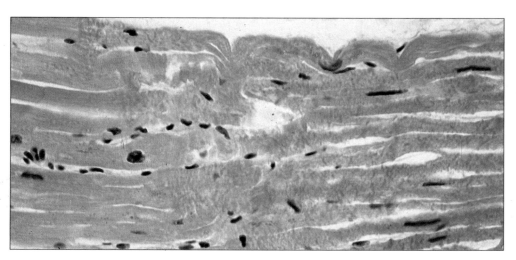

Fig. 9.31 Histology of myocardium showing detail of border zone of infarct: on the left-hand side of the picture there is hydropic cell swelling and on the right-hand side there is attenuation and coagulation necrosis with a tendency to waviness. In the transitional area between there is an abundance of contraction bands. H&E stain.

Regional infarction is confined to an area of the ventricular wall supplied by one of the main coronary arteries (Fig. 9.32, left). Diffuse infarction presents a patchy distribution extending beyond the limits of individual arterial supply (Fig. 9.33).

Mixtures of these two basic types are common, and factors beyond the coronary arteries often play a role in their genesis; for instance, in the acute stage of regional transmural infarction, a rise in left ventricular end-diastolic volume and pressure may lead to subendocardial ischaemia, inducing necrosis with preference for the subendocardial zone, a situation also known as 'spreading of the infarct' (Fig. 9.34). In the chronic stage, when patients have survived an initial regional infarct but are left with a seriously inadequate left ventricle, often in the presence of multifocal obstructive coronary arterial disease, re-infarction can occur due to the same basic mechanisms (Fig. 9.35).

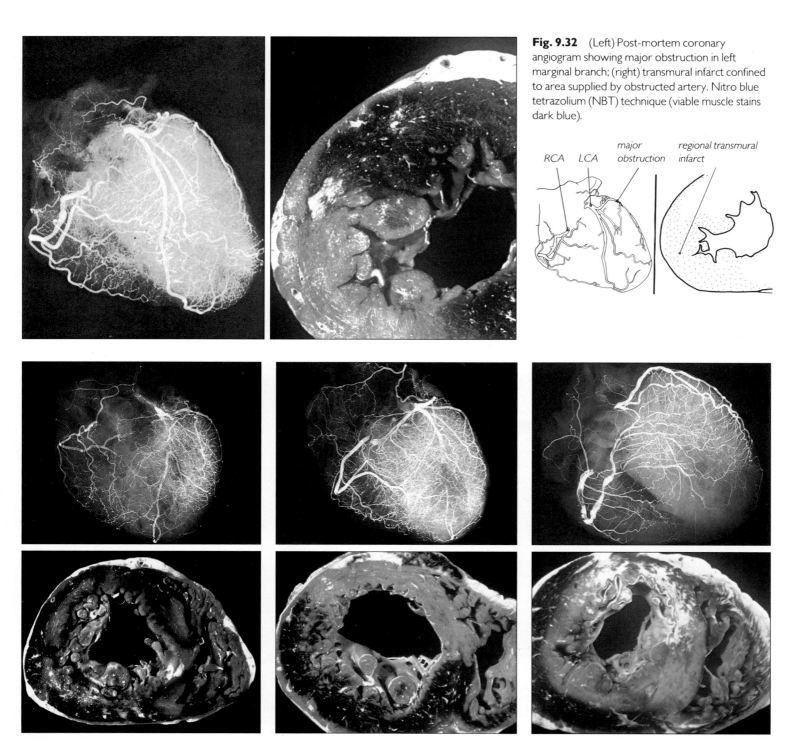

Fig. 9.32 (Left) Post-mortem coronary angiogram showing major obstruction in left marginal branch; (right) transmural infarct confined to area supplied by obstructed artery. Nitro blue tetrazolium (NBT) technique (viable muscle stains dark blue).

Fig. 9.33 (Upper) Post-mortem coronary angiogram showing multifocal obstructive disease in all three main arteries; (lower) extensive patchy discolouration, indicative of infarction, is not restricted to a single artery. Bright white patches are due to injected barium. NBT technique.

Fig. 9.34 (Upper) Post-mortem coronary angiogram showing occlusion of LAD; (lower) regional anteroseptal infarct with subendocardial circumferential spread. Such pronounced right ventricular extension is unusual. NBT technique.

Fig. 9.35 Reinfarction: (upper) post-mortem coronary angiogram showing total occlusion of LAD and multiple stenoses in dominant right coronary artery; (lower) anteroseptal scar and recent circumferential infarct transmurally in septum and subendocardially in left ventricle free wall. NBT technique.

Extension of a left ventricular infarct into the right ventricular wall is a common finding (Fig. 9.36). The clinical significance of this event remains, as yet, unknown. Anteroseptal infarcts usually present little or no right ventricular extension, whereas infarction of the inferior wall of the left ventricle shows a much higher incidence of right ventricular involvement. Indeed, in the setting of a dominant right coronary artery with stenosis proximal to the right marginal branch, extensive infarction of the right ventricular wall may complicate a left ventricular infarct of relatively small size. Additional complications, such as involvement of the group of the posteromedial papillary muscles, either totally or partially, with dysfunction of the papillary muscle as

a result, may aggravate the haemodynamic consequences produced by loss of right ventricular muscle. Right ventricular failure may then ensue as the predominant haemodynamic problem, particularly in the setting of an elevated pulmonary vascular resistance.

Pure right ventricular infarction (that is, infarction not due to extension of a left ventricular infarct) is extremely rare. It generally only occurs in patients with severe and longstanding pulmonary hypertension, usually due to pulmonary parenchymal disease and marked right ventricular hypertrophy and dilatation (Fig. 9.37). The proper recognition of right ventricular infarction, whether 'pure' or as an extension of a left ventricular

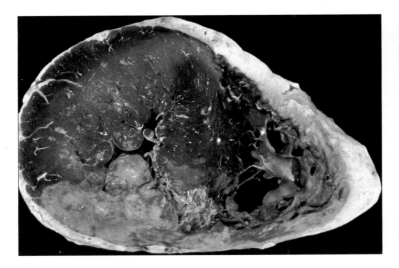

Fig. 9.36 Marked extension of recent left ventricle inferior wall infarct into right ventricle inferior wall, which shhows hypertrophy. Septal rupture has occurred. NBT technique.

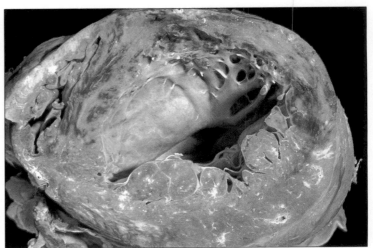

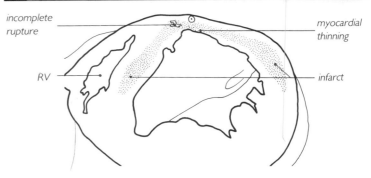

Fig. 9.38 Extension of anteroseptal infarct characterized by pronounced wall-thinning. Incomplete rupture is present.

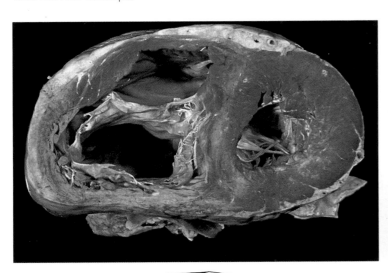

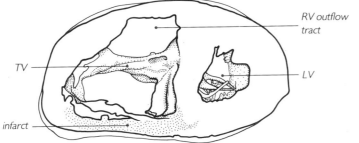

Fig. 9.37 Marked right ventricular hypertrophy and dilatation. A recent infarct does not extend into the left ventricle.

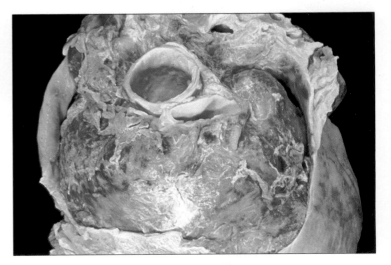

Fig. 9.39 Pericarditis, characterized by fibrinous exudation, in the setting of acute transmural infarction.

infarct, is of considerable therapeutic importance.

Expansion of acute myocardial infarction is another clinically important morphological feature. Expansion is characterized by mural thinning at the site of infarction (Fig. 9.38), and may develop within a few hours of the onset of infarction. Echocardiographic identification of expansion at the acute stage of infarction presages a poor prognosis.

Pericarditis is yet another phenomenon that often accompanies the acute state of infarction. When present, it is an almost definitive sign of transmural infarction. The pericardial friction rub that it produces is due to a fibrinous exudate (Fig. 9.39). When congestive heart failure complicates acute myocardial infarction, excessive fluid may accumulate within the pericardial sac. As a rule, the pericardial rub that occurs in association with acute myocardial infarction disappears within a few days, leaving no morphological residue. Occasionally, for instance in the case of imminent rupture, the two pericardial layers may be 'glued' together and fibrous encasement may eventually result. The mere possibility of the existence of false aneurysms following myocardial infarction (see page 9.26) depends on this phenomenon.

Identification and histological dating

Following irreversible cellular damage, an inflammatory response will ensue which results eventually in a myocardial scar. Dating of infarctions by pathologists is based on the anticipated changes that occur with time. In general, the first week is dominated by an acute inflammatory reaction. During the second week, there is a shift towards the chronic type of cellular inflammatory response; and in the third week, there is active proliferation of connective tissue. Marked variations occur, however, within this basic framework.

Oedema is one of the earliest changes that occurs. The first reliable sign of this change is reactive hyperaemia in the peripheral zone of the infarct, accompanied by an increased density and margination of polymorphonuclear leucocytes. This phenomenon is usually present within 12 hours, but its identification may require careful study. Grossly, the area of infarction may show as a pale, glossy, and soft region, but otherwise there is no indication. It is in these instances that the nitro-blue tetrazolium technique may prove helpful. With this method, fresh, unfixed slices of the heart are tested for the presence or absence of coenzymes necessary to produce a formazan. Areas of infarction, with leakage of enzymes, remain pale, whereas areas with vital myocardium at the time of death are dark blue (see Fig 9.32, right). Extravasation of polymorphonuclear leucocytes occurs within 12 hours (Fig. 9.40, upper) and reaches its peak on the third day (Fig. 9.40, lower). The intense cellularity thus produced will remain until approximately the sixth or seventh day following the onset of infarction. Degeneration of polymorphonuclear leucocytes and disintegration of myocytes run an almost parallel time course.

An infarct of 3–5 days' duration is usually identified grossly because of its yellowish colour and its peripheral zone of hyperaemic reaction (Fig. 9.41). The reparative response is clearly defined along the epicardial surface and lateral borders of the infarct, but is usually less well defined at the endocardial side, where the response may be totally absent. The number of polymorphonuclear leucocytes decreases while the number of lymphocytes, plasma cells, and tissue macrophages increases, the latter reaching their peak concentration in the second week. At the same time, there is a proliferation of cells producing connective tissue. Necrotic myocardial cells are actively removed and the whole picture changes from that of an active inflammatory response to one of replacement by scar tissue (Fig. 9.42).

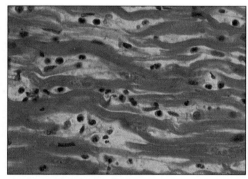
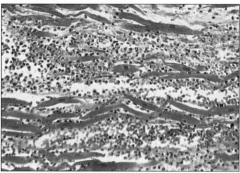
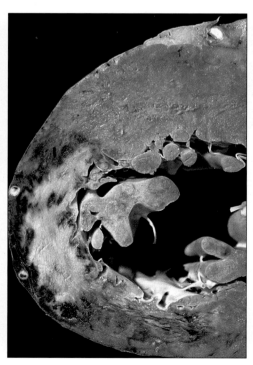
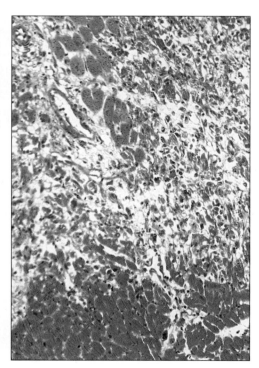

Fig. 9.40 Histological sections of myocardium: (upper) oedema and early extravasation of polymorphs; (lower) massive infiltration with leucocytes. H&E stains.

Fig. 9.41 Left ventricular transmural infarct of approximately 5–7 days; note adjacent scar from previous infarct.

Fig. 9.42 Histological section of myocardial infarct of 2–3 weeks. Necrotic muscle cells are actively removed. There is a mixed cellular infiltrate but macrophages dominate. H&E stain.

Reperfusion dilates pre-existent capillaries, accentuating the similarity to granulation tissue (Fig. 9.43). At this stage, there is a dramatic change in the gross appearance of the infarct. Usually, the wall is markedly thinned and is composed of a watery pale-staining tissue that collapses on the cut surface of a fresh section (Fig. 9.44). From the second and third week onwards, the number of inflammatory cells decreases further. Macrophages laden with haemosiderin often remain as the last conspicuous components of this episode (Fig. 9.45). Eventually, the cellular connective tissue (Fig. 9.46, left) changes into a sclerotic and almost acellular scar (Fig. 9.46, right). At this stage, the gross appearance is unmistakeably that of a scar. It is identified as greyish-white tissue, often surrounded by other tissue that has a darker colour because of the increased vascularity, representing the remaining token of past events (Fig. 9.47).

The time span over which these events take place may differ from one individual to another. Necrotic muscle often remains present for a long time and, in some instances, it may never disappear completely. The size of the infarct and the ability to perfuse the surrounding viable myocardium and pericardium probably play a key role in achieving an adequate tissue response and, hence, repair.

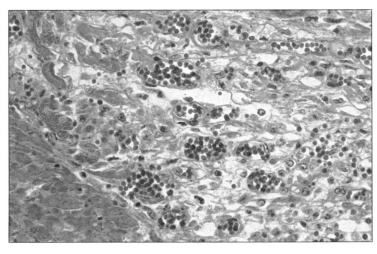

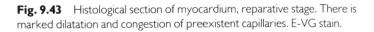

Fig. 9.43 Histological section of myocardium, reparative stage. There is marked dilatation and congestion of preexistent capillaries. E-VG stain.

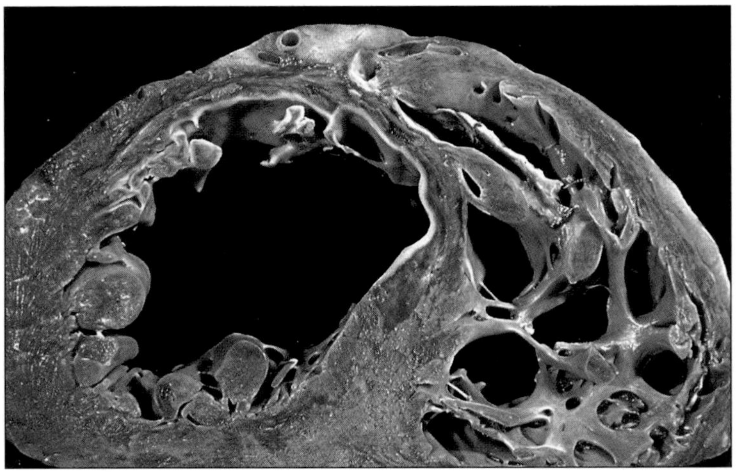

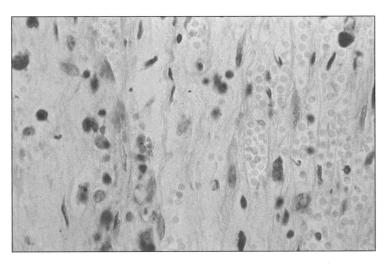

Fig. 9.44 Transmural anteroseptal infarct of approximately 2–3 weeks with marked wall-thinning and replacement of myocardium by soft watery tissue. Note endocardial thickening.

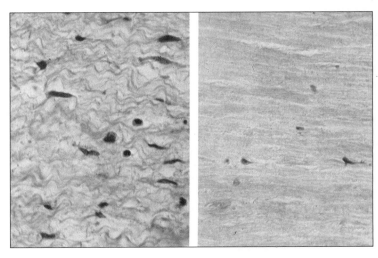

Fig. 9.45 Histological section of myocardium, reparative stage. Iron-laden macrophages are conspicuous by their blue colour. Perls' stain.

Fig. 9.46 Histological section of myocardium: (left) cellular connective tissue which gradually transforms into a sclerotic acellular scar (right). H&E stains.

MYOCARDIAL INFARCTION: COMPLICATIONS

The majority of complications of myocardial infarction belong either to the category of pump failure or to that of electrical disturbances. These features can, of course, appear in combination, the development of electrical failure in the setting of pump failure being particularly well recognized.

Pump failure

At present, pump failure is the most important cause of hospital mortality in patients with acute myocardial infarction.

Myocardial loss

Extensive myocardial loss is the most frequent pathology underlying this complication (Fig. 9.48). Infarcts that involve 40% or more of the left ventricular myocardium fall into this category. Two distinct clinical syndromes are recognized, namely cardiogenic shock and refractory congestive heart failure. Both have in common the presence of severe obstructive disease of the anterior descending coronary artery. Obstruction proximal to the first septal branch is particularly significant. Patients with cardiogenic shock also usually have disease over long segments of the remaining main coronary arteries. In contrast, patients

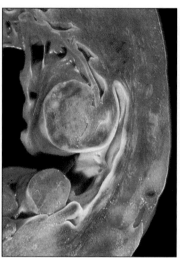
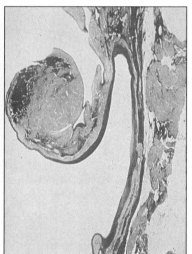

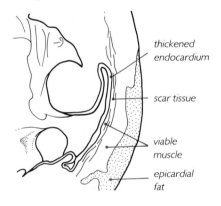

Fig. 9.47 End result of an infarct: (left) band-like scar separated from a thickened endocardium by a small rim of viable muscle. The epicardial side shows remaining myocardium and fat. E-VG stain.

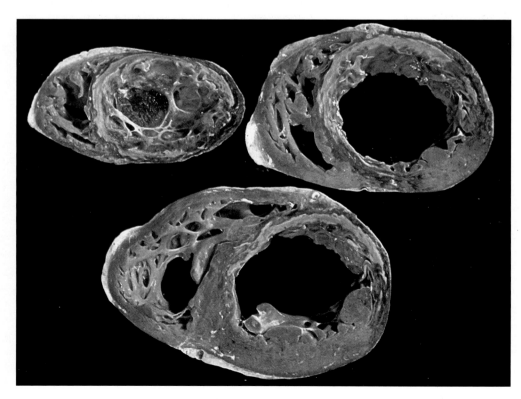

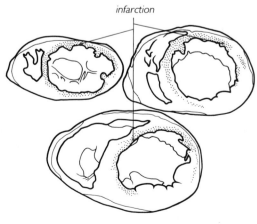

Fig. 9.48 Transverse slices of heart with extensive recent myocardial infarct involving more than 40% of preexistent left ventricle myocardium; the patient died of progressive pump failure.

with refractory congestive heart failure tend to have a lower incidence of severe obstruction in the right and circumflex coronary arteries. Refractory pump failure, nonetheless, can occur when small infarcts are complicated by dysfunction of the papillary muscles (Fig. 9.49). In these cases, a discrepancy can exist between the size of the infarct, as determined clinically, and the haemodynamic situation.

Myocardial rupture

Rupture of myocardium is the second most frequent cause of pump failure, being responsible for approximately 20% of all deaths due to pump failure in the setting of acute myocardial infarction. The majority of such patients have a rupture of the free wall with cardiac tamponade. The ventricular septum and

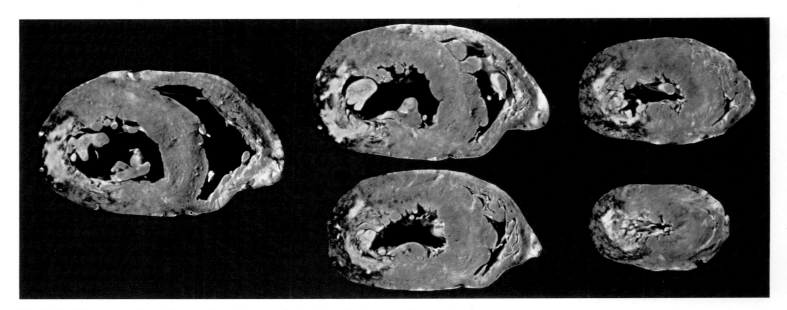

Fig. 9.49 Transverse slices of heart with relatively small-sized lateral infarct but with extension into both papillary muscle groups; refractory pump failure with mitral valve insufficiency ensued.

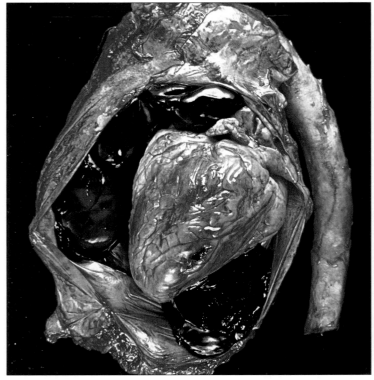

Fig. 9.50 Cardiac tamponade tue to rupture of left ventricle free wall following acute infarction. By courtesy of Dr J.E. Edwards.

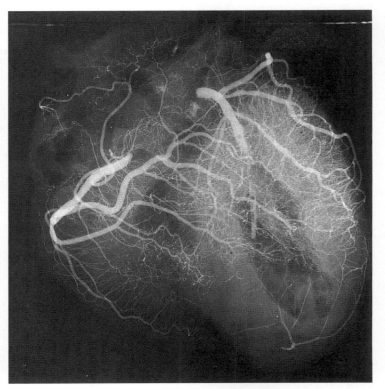

Fig. 9.51 Post-mortem coronary angiogram showing single vessel disease with total occlusion of LAD in a case of cardiac rupture.

papillary muscles can also be involved, each rupturing in approximately 1–2% of fatal cases.

Rupture of the free wall

Rupture of the free wall rapidly results in extravasation of blood into the pericardial sac and, hence, cardiac tamponade (Fig. 9.50). Usually, 300–400ml of blood are recovered. As a general rule, tamponade occurs under particular circumstances; the patients are elderly (60 years or more) and have no previous history of myocardial infarction. Postmortem coronary angiograms show single-vessel disease with a localized obstruction (Fig. 9.51), and thrombotic occlusion at the site of obstruction is frequent. Collaterals are poorly developed; this lack of collateral supply is statistically significant when compared with patients who die of otherwise uncomplicated pump failure.

Approximately 50% of all ruptures of the free wall occur within 24 hours of the onset of infarction. Of the remaining cases, approximately 30% occur within the first week and 20% occur over a time span that may extend as long as 12 weeks. The site of rupture is usually central within the infarct (Fig. 9.52). Sites of preference relative to the ventricular landmarks are the anterior and posterior insertions of the septum (Fig. 9.53). The myocardium at the site of rupture often shows expansion (Fig. 9.54). Such marked thinning of the infarcted wall can occur within 12 hours (see also p.9.14). The degree and extent of expansion,

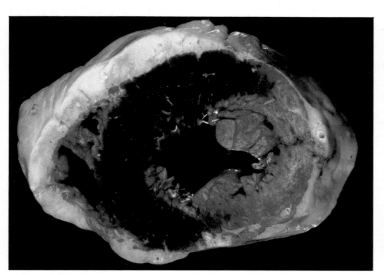

Fig. 9.52 Rupture of free lateral wall; the tear runs through the centre of the infarct. NBT technique.

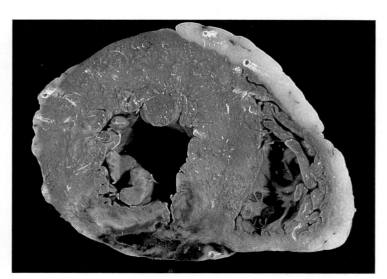

Fig. 9.53 Inferior wall infarct: rupture has occurred adjacent to septal insertion.

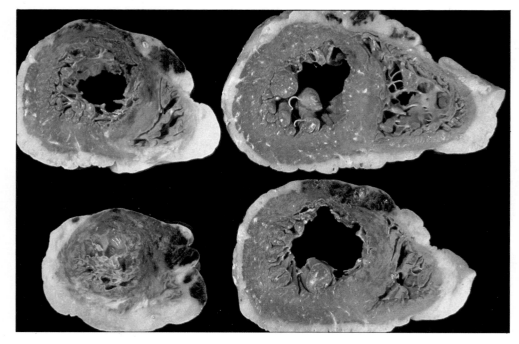

Fig. 9.54 Transverse slices of heart with ruptured anteroseptal infarct through area of marked expansion.

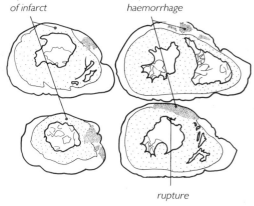

expansion of infarct

epicardial haemorrhage

rupture

however, is the same in patients who die of uncomplicated pump failure, raising a question over its role in pathogenesis.

From a morphological point of view, two basic types of rupture occur. In most cases, the tear is slit-like and well delineated (Fig. 9.55). This is the usual morphology in ruptures that occur either within 24 hours of onset of infarction, or several weeks later in cases with extreme wall thinning and cardiac dilatation (Fig. 9.56). The second, less-common, type is characterized by extensive erosion of infarcted myocardium (Fig. 9.57). This type of rupture tends to occur in the second and third week of infarction, although it can occur within 24 hours. The erosive type exhibits a distinct preference for the sites of septal insertion. The erosion

may be so extensive that the epicardial breakthrough is over the right ventricular surface (Fig. 9.58), thus erroneously suggesting right ventricular rupture.

The epicardium may occasionally withstand the pressure of cardiac rupture for a considerable time. This may then lead to extensive epicardial bleeding (Fig. 9.59) and may underlie the rare instances of incomplete rupture. Eventually, a 'false aneurysm' may develop. Indeed, there is good evidence that, in some instances, considerable time may elapse between the onset of rupture and the final breakthrough that leads to cardiac tamponade. The onset of rupture may even occasionally be the first sign of underlying myocardial infarction.

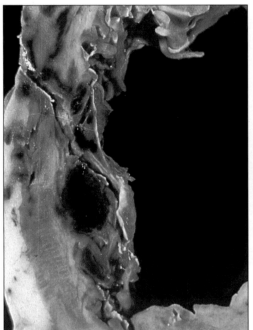
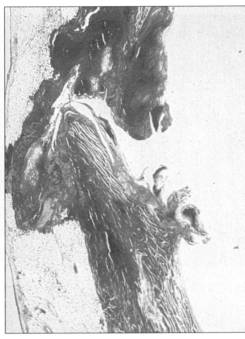

Fig. 9.55 Tear through expanded infarct zone: (left) gross aspect; (right) histology. H&E stain.

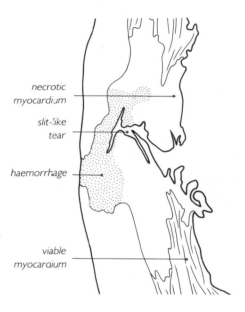

Fig. 9.56 Rupture with slit-like tear 28 days after onset of infarction: left ventricle dilatation and extreme wall-thinning with intramural haemorrhage.

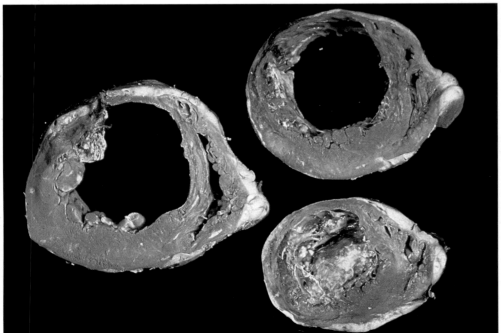

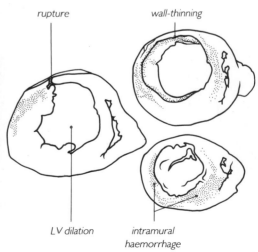

Septal rupture

Septal ruptures tend to occur more frequently with infarctions of the anterior wall than with those located inferiorly. The obstructive lesions are usually more extensive and particularly affect the anterior descending and the right coronary arteries. The septum is usually much attenuated (Fig. 9.60), similar to the degree of expansion in ruptures of the free wall. Ruptures at the site of ventricular septal insertions are often associated with concomitant rupture of the free wall. Multiple septal defects can also be produced. Septal ruptures occur most commonly in the setting of a large infarct with massive involvement of the septum. The rupture leads, theoretically, to an overload of both right and left ventricles, but heart failure is most likely due to the extent of infarction rather than to the rupture itself. Right ventricular failure, however, may be enhanced when there is

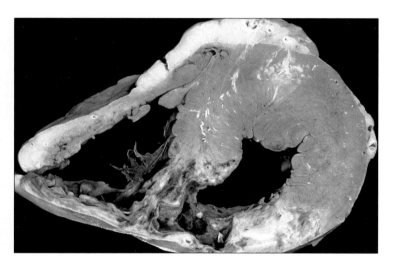

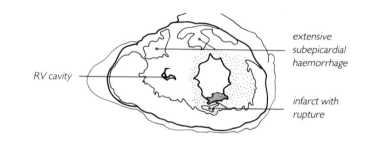

Fig. 9.57 Inferoseptal infarct with extensive erosion and rupture leading to tamponade.

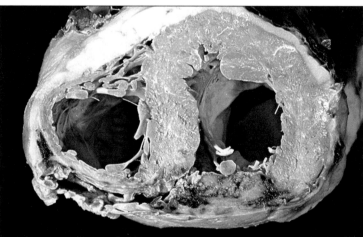

Fig. 9.58 Infarct of inferior wall with erosion of necrotic myocardium and rupture leading to dissection of right ventricle inferior wall.

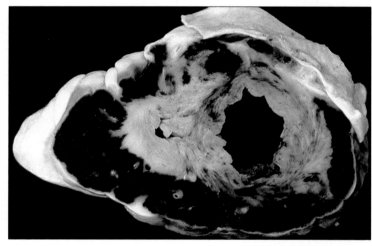

Fig. 9.59 Left ventricle free wall rupture with initial extensive bleeding limited by epicardium.

Fig. 9.60 Rupture of ventricular septum with marked extension.

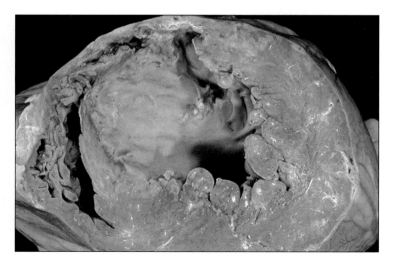

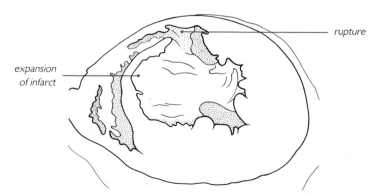

concomitant rupture of the papillary muscles of the tricuspid valve (Figs 9.61, 9.62). Approximately 50% of the patients with ventricular septal rupture die within one week; only less than 10% are alive after one year.

Rupture of papillary muscles

The more frequent finding of rupture of the posteromedial than the anterolateral group may relate to the peripheral distribution of the dominant right and left circumflex coronary arteries. In approximately half of all hearts, the group of posteromedial papillary muscles is within the 'watershed' zone between the peripheral ramifications of these systems. As with septal ruptures, the extent of obstructive coronary arterial disease is not usually limited to a single vessel.

Two major types of ruptures of papillary muscles occur (Fig. 9.63). Complete rupture at the base of the trunk of a papillary muscle is a major catastrophy (Fig. 9.64, left). Since each papillary muscle supports half of both overlying leaflets of the mitral valve, massive prolapse (Fig. 9.64, right) and regurgitation result. Occasionally, particularly in the group of posteromedial muscles, which tends to have multiple muscle heads blended with the ventricular wall, partial rupture can occur (Fig. 9.65). Under these circumstances, the patient may survive the sudden onset of mitral insufficiency, whereas the chances of survival are very poor in patients with complete rupture. Of the patients with

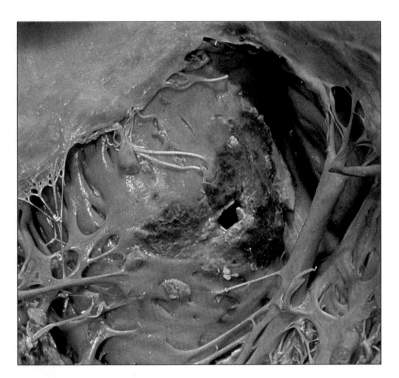

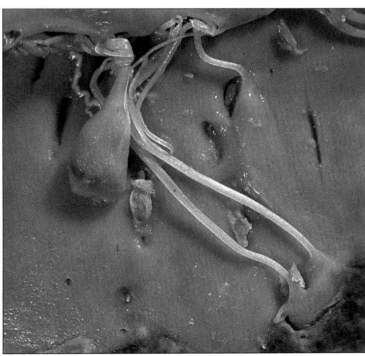

Fig. 9.61 Right ventricular aspect of ventricular septal infarction with rupture of both septum and papillary muscle.

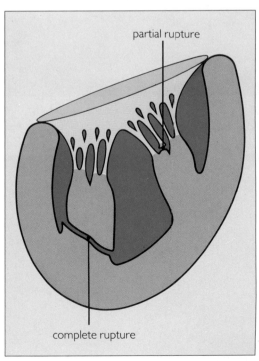

Fig. 9.62 Detail of Fig. 9.61 showing ruptured papillary muscle of tricuspid valve.

Fig. 9.63 Diagram of the two major forms of papillary muscle rupture: complete and partial.

rupture of papillary muscles, 70% die within 24 hours and only approximately 10% are alive after two months. The prognosis depends not only on the degree of insufficiency, but also on the remaining capacity of the left ventricle and, hence, on the size of the initial infarct. These considerations are very much similar to those for septal rupture.

Mural thrombosis

Mural thrombosis is a common complication in patients suffering from pump failure in the setting of an acute myocardial infarct (Fig. 9.66). Mural thrombosis may also develop in the acute stage in the absence of pump failure. Thromboembolic complications are a known hazard mitigated by anticoagulant treatment in the acute phase of the infarction.

Electrical disturbances

Disturbances of rhythm, such as extrasystole, tachycardia, and fibrillation, whether originating in the atria or ventricles, are common in the setting of acute infarction. Indeed, there is good evidence that a large proportion of patients with sudden and unexpected death die of ventricular fibrillation as an immediate consequence of infarction; sudden ventricular fibrillation, however, is not necessarily associated with infarction. There is, to date, no conclusive morphological evidence on these early disturbances of rhythm. Much more can be said about the morphological substrates of specific disturbances of conduction in the setting of acute infarction. A major distinction must be made between posteroinferior and anteroseptal infarcts. In the former, it is common for temporary complete or incomplete atrioventricular block to occur. This may persist for a few hours or days, but complete restoration of normal rhythm will usually be obtained within a week. This phenomenon most likely relates to the underlying vascular pathology since the right coronary artery is most commonly involved. Hence, infarcts may spread on the inferior wall of the right ventricle and adjacent atrial tissues, including the atrioventricular node. Recovery is most likely due to the relatively high resistance of conduction tissue to hypoxia.

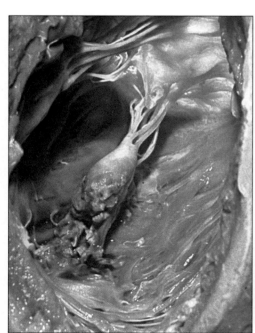
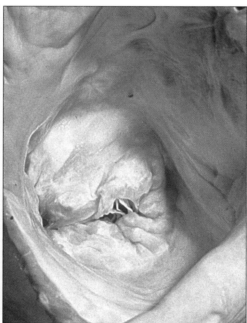

Fig. 9.64 Rupture of trunk of posteromedial papillary muscle of left ventricle: (left) left ventricular view; (right) left artery view showing prolapse of valve leaflets around posteromedial commissure.

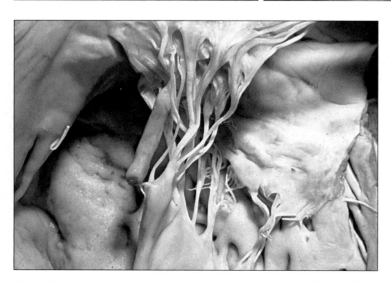

Fig. 9.65 Partial rupture of one head of a tethered posteromedial papillary muscle group.

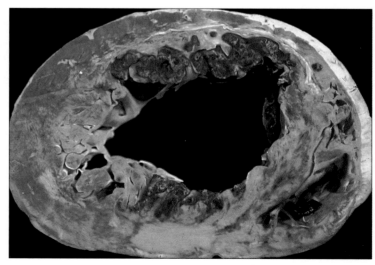

Fig. 9.66 Transverse slice of heart with extensive old and recent infarction with mural thrombosis in dilated chamber. The patient died of pump failure.

The development of conduction disturbances in patients with anteroseptal infarcts has a markedly different outlook. The proximal bundle branches are usually affected by ischaemia (Fig. 9.67), but necrosis of conduction tissues is relatively rare (Fig. 9.68). The atrioventricular node and bundle do not appear to be involved in these patients. The changes observed suggest a potentially reversible process. This finding supports the concept that the prognosis of acute anteroseptal infarction relates primarily to the extent of infarction rather than to necrosis of conduction tissues (Fig. 9.69).

Miscellaneous complications

There are complications of myocardial infarction which cannot readily be classified as either pump failure or electrical disturbances, although they often give rise to one or both.

Cardiac aneurysms

Defined as a distinct outward bulging of the ventricular wall, although not always readily identified either clinically or patho-

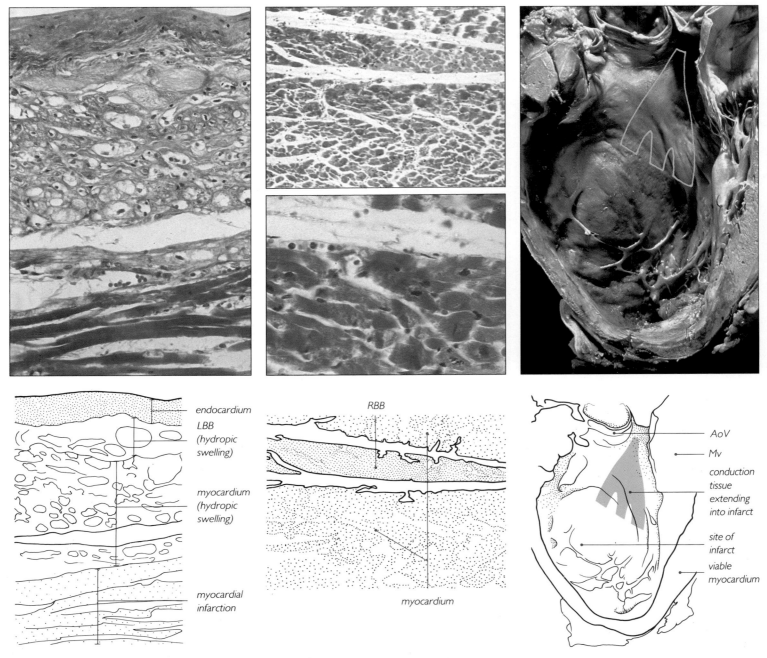

Fig. 9.67 Histological section showing hydropic swelling of proximal left bundle branches. H&E stain.

Fig. 9.68 Histological sections of right bundle branches within ventricular septum in a case with extensive anteroseptal infarction: (upper) low-power view; (lower) detail showing necrosis of parts of cellular constituents. H&E stain.

Fig. 9.69 Left ventricular aspect of extensive anteroseptal myocardial infarct sufficiently large to produce atrioventricular block.

logically, aneurysms can occur as either an early or late complication of acute myocardial infarction. In some instances, the aneurysm develops progressively from the very onset of infarction (Fig. 9.70), often leading to pump failure. In other instances, this situation is further complicated by bouts of tachycardia and

ventricular fibrillation which originate from the area of the aneurysm. The study of resected specimens reveals that dead and viable muscle often intermingle in these areas, rendering as obsolete the concept that the aneurysmal wall is devoid of viable myocardium, (Fig. 9.71).

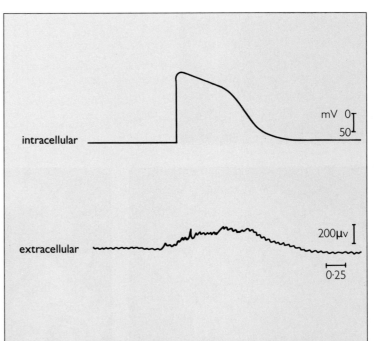

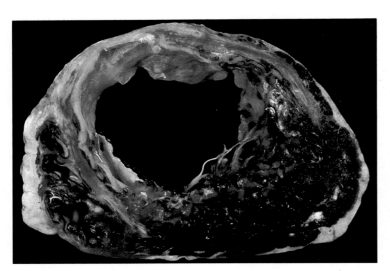

Fig. 9.70 Left ventricular aneurysm of anterior wall as early complication of acute infarct. NBT technique.

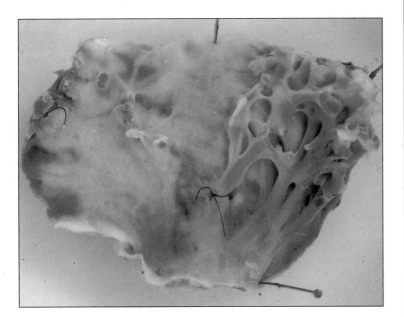

Fig. 9.71 (Left) A surgically resected specimen of a left ventricular aneurysm following myocardial infarction due to ventricular rhythm disorders. (Right) Recorded intra- and extra-cellular action potentials (upper), indicating that viable myocardial cells are still present amidst scar tissue (lower). (Slide provided by M.J. Janse.)

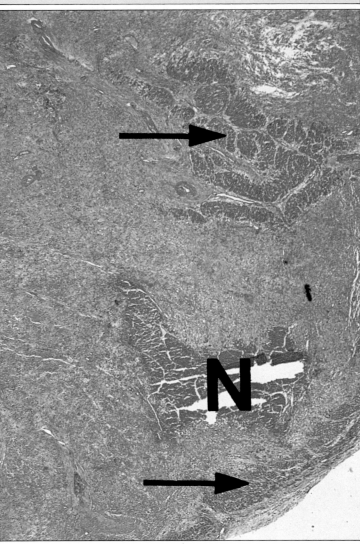

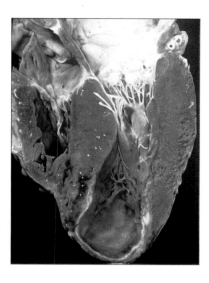

Fig. 9.72 Left ventricle apical aneurysm: the aneurysm wall is composed of scar tissue and endocardial layer is porcelain-like.

Aneurysms developing later have a slightly different morphology in that more scar tissue has been produced. In some instances, the aneurysmal wall is composed in its entirety of dense collagen, and the inner layer has a porcelain-like appearance (Fig. 9.72) composed of layered collagen and elastin fibres, so-called aorticization. In such instances, there is usually no mural thrombosis. In other cases, however, the aneurysms may be partially filled with thrombus and then usually lack the aortic-like lining (Fig. 9.73). The presence or absence of thrombus becomes clinically relevant when the size of the aneurysm is determined from angiograms. In terms of function of the myo-

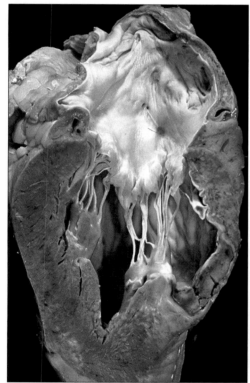

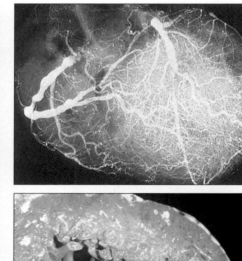

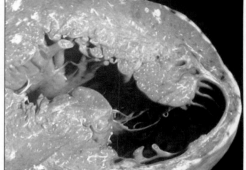

Fig. 9.74 Huge anteroseptal and apical left ventricle aneurysm. Pump failure was the leading symptom.

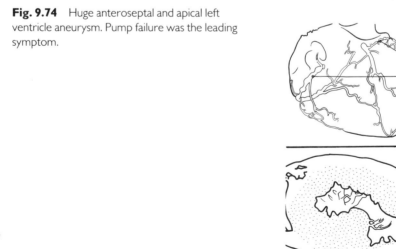

aneurysm
thrombus
posteromedial papillary muscle

Fig. 9.73 Inferior wall aneurysm partially filled with thrombus.

multifocal obstruction

aneurysm

Fig. 9.75 (Upper) Post-mortem coronary angiogram with multifocal obstructive lesions in main coronary arteries; (lower) old lateral wall infarction with aneurysm.

cardial pump, the significance of ventricular aneurysms is largely determined by their location and size (Fig. 9.74). In particular, their presence in the posterior wall may lead to dysfunction of papillary muscles (Fig. 9.73), despite the fact that such aneurysms are usually small in size. On the other hand, infarcts of the anterior wall tend to be large and, hence, may easily lead to pump failure because of direct loss of actively pumping myocardium.

In the usual instance of a ventricular aneurysm, the underlying coronary arterial pathology is not confined to a single vessel but tends to be of a more generalized nature (Fig. 9.75). Ventricular aneurysms may eventually become calcified (Fig.

9.76), sometimes to the extent that the aneurysm can be seen directly on a chest radiograph.

False ventricular aneurysms also occur, not only as a consequence of penetrating injuries but also as a secondary event of myocardial infarctions. The usual configuration of a false aneurysm is that of a saccular outbulging that communicates with the ventricular lumen via a narrow neck. In the majority of cases, the false aneurysm is almost completely filled with thrombus. Rupture of the wall, with confinement of the bleeding due to epicardial compression, is often considered the underlying pathogenetic mechanism (Fig. 9.77). False aneurysms may

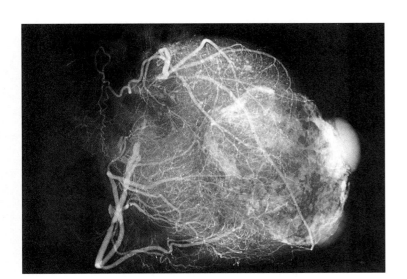

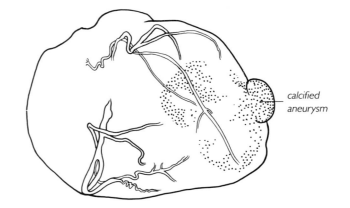

Fig. 9.76 Post-mortem radiograph following injection of coronary arteries shows heavily calcified left ventricle apical aneurysm.

calcified aneurysm

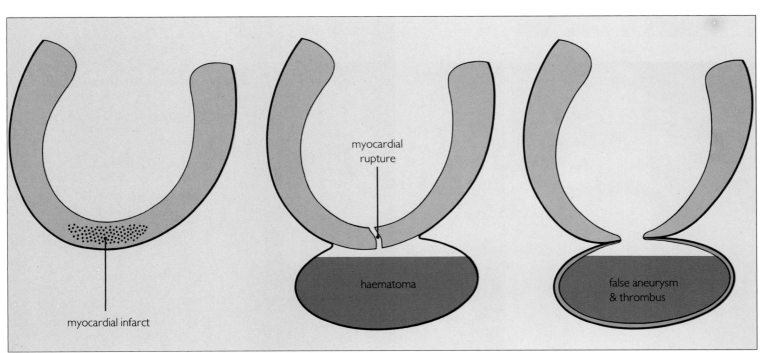

myocardial rupture

myocardial infarct

haematoma

false aneurysm & thrombus

Fig. 9.77 Diagram of the usual pathogenesis of false ventricular aneurysms following infarction: (left) infarction; (middle) rupture with epicardial limitation; (right) progression to false aneurysm with narrowed neck.

occasionally be present in the septum (Fig. 9.78), most likely as a consequence of incomplete rupture following acute infarction.

On rare occasions, ventricular aneurysms may be complicated by infection. The pathogenesis of this complication is not fully understood, but it is likely that infective thrombus adherent to the site of the aneurysm is the causative factor. This process may lead to the formation of abscesses in the ventricular wall (Fig. 9.79) and to purulent pericarditis.

Postmyocardial infarction syndrome

Postmyocardial infarction syndrome, also known as Dressler's syndrome, is rare (see Chapter 14). Constrictive pericarditis has been described as its leading sign.

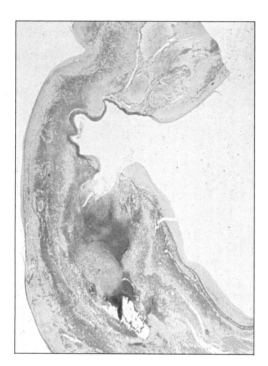

Fig. 9.78 Frontal section through ventricular septum: histology ('E-VG alcian blue stain).

PATHOLOGICAL ASPECTS OF CORONARY ANGIOPLASTY

Percutaneous transluminal coronary angioplasty is presently an important therapeutic tool in the symptomatic treatment of obstructive coronary arterial disease. The procedure does, however, have limitations. In approximately 25% of patients, restenosis occurs following an initially successful procedure and, usually, within six months following the initial procedure. Moreover, the attempt to dilate the obstructed segment may occasionally cause an acute complication, usually accompanied by thrombosis and sudden total occlusion of the diseases artery. In these latter circumstances, the pathology is that of a lacerated atherosclerotic plaque that usually has the morphological characteristics of a plaque 'at risk' (see Fig. 9.7). In case of 'late' restenosis, the pathology is that of fibrocellular tissue response (Fig. 9.80). Histological evaluation of the arterial segments involved reveals several forms of laceration induced by the procedure of dilatation. In eccentric lesions, the sites of preference for laceration are the free wall of the plaque (Fig. 9.81) and the border zones between the free wall and the atherosclerotic plaque. Dissections may occur at the latter sites, usually along the plane of the internal elastic lamina, thereby exposing either smooth-muscle cells of the pre-existent media or cells within the musculoelastic layer bordering on the plaque. In concentric atherosclerotic plaques, the injury caused by the dilatation is usually located at the thinnest site of the plaque.

The proliferative lesion is caused by smooth-muscle cells that originate either from the pre-existent medial wall or from the musculoelastic layer of the plaque itself. The precise pathogenetic mechanisms involved in initiating this proliferative response remains, as yet, unsettled. Deposition of fibrin and platelets is almost invariably present at the site of the early lesions, but the obstructive lesion causing late restenosis is not simply due to organized thrombosis. These aspects may explain why attempts to prevent thrombosis following angioplasty have little effect on the incidence of restenosis.

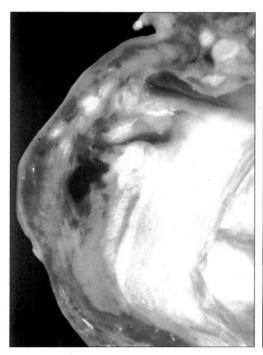
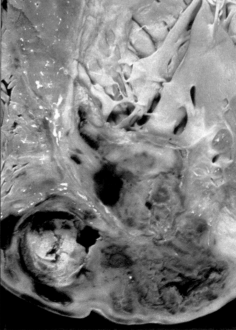

Fig. 9.79 Apical left ventricular aneurysm with secondary salmonellae infection and abscess formation.

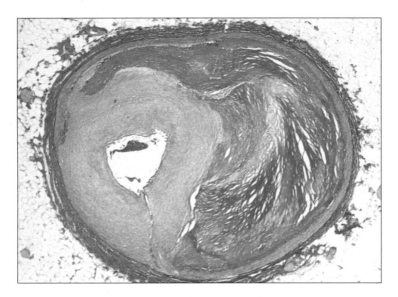

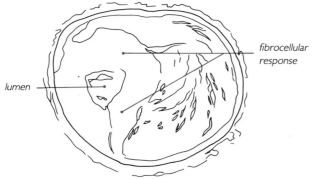

Fig. 9.80 Fibrous cellular response following PTCA.

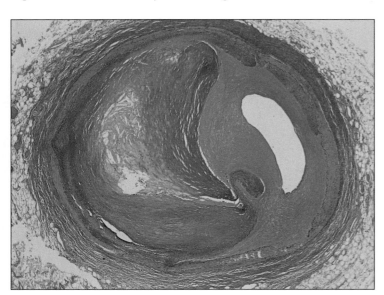

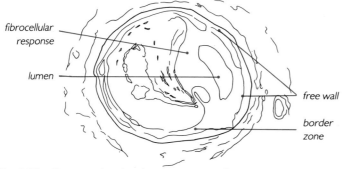

Fig. 9.81 Cross-section showing damage to wall.

PATHOLOGICAL ASPECTS OF CORONARY ARTERIAL BYPASS SURGERY

The main objective of surgery is to bypass the sites of obstruction by implanting a graft between the aorta and the distal non-diseased segment of a coronary artery. For the graft, the surgeon will usually see either the internal mammary (internal thoracic) artery or veins. Venous grafts are most commonly used, the veins being obtained from the patient's own legs. Single grafts can be constructed, but more usually, multiple grafts are placed (Fig. 9.82). The number of grafts may be almost unlimited. The same graft can be implanted into different coronary arteries using several side-to-side anastomoses and is then known as a jump graft (Fig. 9.83). The veins are always inserted in reverse to avoid the obstructive effect of venous valves. It is significant

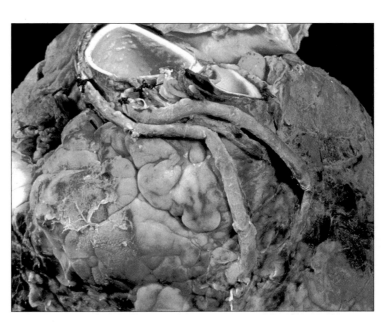

Fig. 9.82 Two venous grafts inserted between ascending aorta and LAD with oblique branch.

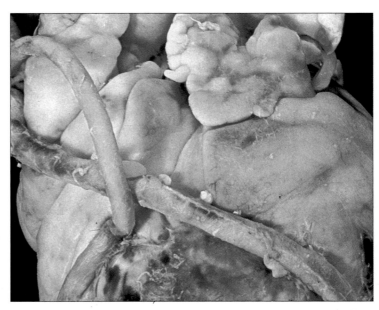

Fig. 9.83 Two venous grafts, one of which is a 'jump', being inserted side-to-side into oblique branch and side-to-end into LAD.

that the intrinsic structure of superficial veins from the legs differs along the vein. In some areas, the veins may be relatively thin walled, whereas other sites may show a thick wall with dense intimal cushions composed of fibrocellular tissues. These cushions are found particularly at the sites of venous valves. The pathologist should be aware of these variations when asked to judge whether or not an implanted vein has an intrinsic stenosis because of intramural fibrosis (phlebosclerosis). Obstruction occurs in approximately 20% of grafts inserted, the majority occluding within three months following the procedure. After one year, patency remains almost constant. The overall patency of implants of the internal mammary artery is higher, particu-

larly when the implant is attached to small coronary arteries, but the limited use conditioned by the presence of only two arteries may occasionally be a drawback.

Obliteration of venous grafts has been attributed to a variety of causes, such as increased intraluminal pressure, ischaemia of the wall of the graft, thrombosis, or deposition of fibrin and intimal injury either because of ischaemia or trauma. The main cause of occlusion of grafts, nonetheless, whether early or late, probably relates to technical facets of the procedure. Trauma during handling of the venous graft prior to implantation, or other technical flaws, play a key role.

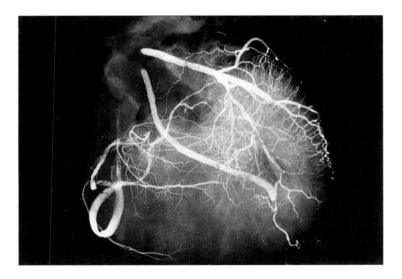

Fig. 9.84 Post-mortem angiogram of venous grafts on LAD shows poor distal run-off due to obstructive coronary disease immediately distal to site of anastomosis.

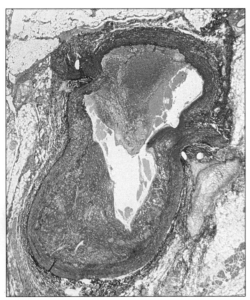

Fig. 9.85 Histological section of implanted venous graft at site of severe coronary artery obstruction; recent thrombus obliterates the lumen. E-VG stain.

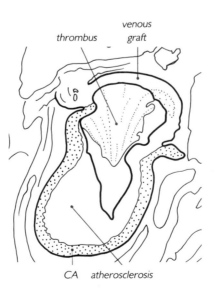

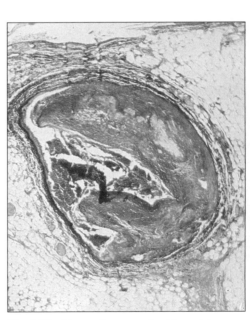

Fig. 9.86 Venous bypass graft with partial detachment of plaque and dissection of coronary artery. E-VG stain.

The eventual result of grafting is largely determined by the presence of coronary arterial stenosis distal to the site of anastomosis of the graft (Fig. 9.84). This error is often due to faulty interpretation of the coronary angiogram which, in the presence of a severe stenosis, will show a poor distal run-off. Another important technical problem is implantation at the site of another obstructive lesion. Despite the fact that, initially, the flow may be sufficiently restored through the graft, persistent obstruction may lead to thrombosis at the site of implantation (Fig. 9.85). In some instances, the atherosclerotic plaque may be partially detached, leading to localized dissection and luminal obliteration (Fig. 9.86). Once initiated, thrombosis may rapidly occlude the site of anastomosis critically and then extend into the graft (Fig. 9.87). Ultimately, the lumen may become obliterated by vascularized connective tissue, an indication of organization (Fig. 9.88).

Intimal fibrous proliferation is generally considered a late complication, being clinically apparent only after approximately one month. The injury probably occurs, however, as early as one that produces thrombotic occlusion, the main difference being that it takes more time for the proliferative response critically to stenose the lumen. The lesion is characterized by a fibrocellular proliferation which obliterates the venous lumen (Fig. 9.89).

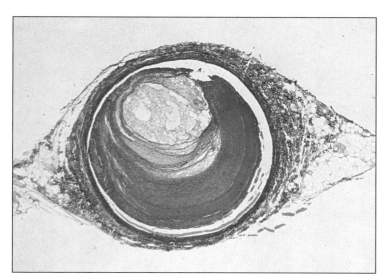

Fig. 9.87 Histological section showing recent thrombus in venous graft due to retrograde spread following implantation of graft at site of major obstruction. E-VG stain.

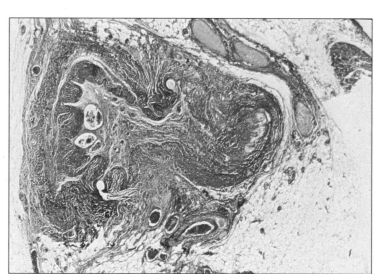

Fig. 9.88 Histological section showing graft occlusion by vascularized connective tissue at site of implantation, most likely the result of organized thrombosis. E-VG stain.

Fig. 9.89 Histological section showing fibrocellular intimal proliferation occluding lumen of venous implant. E-VG stain.

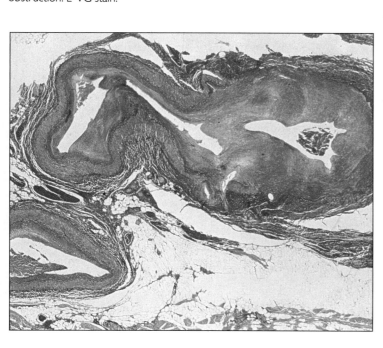

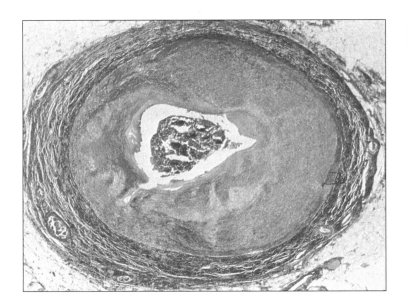

Fig. 9.90 Histological section showing fibrocellular concentric intimal proliferation obliterating lumen of venous graft. E-VG stain.

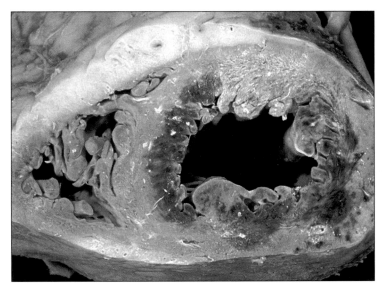

Fig. 9.91 Heart following coronary bypass surgery exhibiting almost circumferential subendocardial haemorrhages.

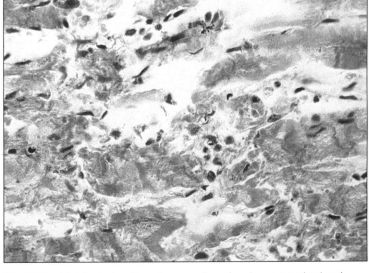

Fig. 9.92 Histological section of myocardium showing contraction band necrosis in a so-called stone heart. H&E stain.

Fig. 9.93 Post-mortem angiogram of multiple graft insertions. The jump graft on LAD does not provide peripheral filling.

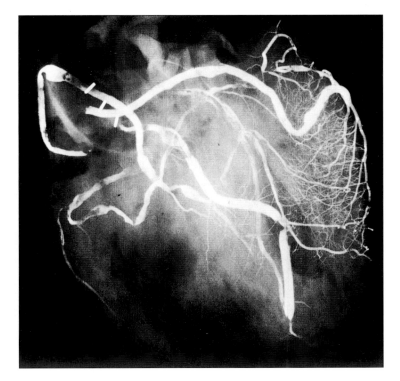

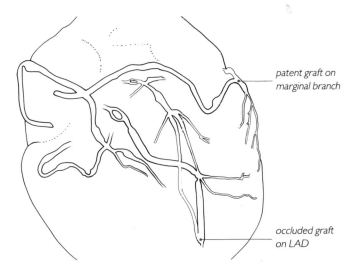

patent graft on marginal branch

occluded graft on LAD

nondiagnostic (Fig. 10.3, upper). Microscopy then reveals hypertrophy together with diffuse or patchy interstitial fibrosis (Fig. 10.3, lower). The suggestion that such changes represent the end stage of myocarditis is based largely on the presence of interstitial fibrosis as a remnant of injury and repair. Otherwise, it is made by exclusion of other possible aetiologies, rather than positive identification.

Distinguishing myocarditis from ischaemic myocardial disease can be difficult, both in the acute inflammatory stage and in the chronic stage when scar tissue prevails. Classical myocardial infarcts usually show a close correlation between obstructive coronary arterial disease and the region exhibiting an infarct, while myocarditis as a rule is more widespread. Myocardial infarcts, moreover, usually present a distinct band-like zone of infarction with central necrosis and peripheral cellular infiltration (see above). In contrast, myocarditis often shows multiple areas of myocardial necrosis and a more diffuse cellular infiltrate.

Endomyocardial biopsies

From the clinical point of view a particularly troublesome category of patients exists in which the leading feature is heart failure of unknown aetiology. An endomyocardial biopsy may be indicated under these circumstances, intended for further refinement of the final diagnosis. There are several pitfalls; as with any diagnostic procedure using biopsies, 'sampling error' plays a role. This becomes particularly important in the case of myocarditis, where the areas with myocardial necrosis and cellular infiltration may be scattered diffusely throughout the myocardium. Moreover, with elapsing time, the histopathology of the disease may change drastically. What was initially an acute inflammatory response, typified by myocyte necrosis and inflammatory cellular infiltration, can become a reparative response, characterized by fibrosis. Due to these two drawbacks, a positive diagnosis of myocarditis, using endomyocardial biopsies is relatively rare and, according to clinical experiences, even less so when more than six months have elapsed since the onset of symptoms.

Another pitfall in the context of the use of endomyocardial biopsies for the diagnosis of myocarditis is a proper definition of myocarditis in these conditions. It is presently accepted that a positive diagnosis should be based on the proper recognition of necrotic myocytes in combination with an inflammatory cellular infiltrate. The term 'borderline myocarditis' is used for specimens in which sparse cellular infiltrates are present but without distinct myocardial necrosis. In such instances, the use of immunocytochemical staining techniques may be helpful in identifying the cells present (Fig. 10.4). The use of the term 'residual myocarditis' is limited to a repeated endomyocardial biopsy required after an initial histological diagnosis of acute myocarditis, but which shows only cellular infiltration of cells without myocytic necrosis.

Despite the fact that a positive diagnosis of 'myocarditis' can be obtained only rarely, the use of endomyocardial biopsies in patients with heart failure of unknown aetiology should not be discarded, since other underlying causes such as amyloidosis may be revealed.

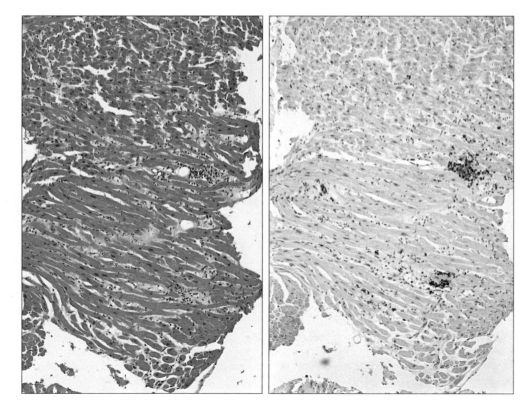

Fig. 10.4 Cells highlighted by the use of immunocytochemical staining techniques.

Infectious myocarditis

Almost any infectious disease may become complicated by myocarditis. In the Western world, viral infections are the most important, but protozoal infections may rank highest in other parts of the world. Infectious myocarditis is a common complication of opportunistic infections, such as those that occur in patients treated with cytostatic or immunosuppressive drugs.

In almost all instances, infectious myocarditis is bloodborne, septicaemia being one of the most important modes. An important condition that may underlie septic myocarditis is infectious endocarditis (see page 10.5). Infection of the aortic valve almost invariably leads to septic infestation of myocardium (Fig. 10.5).

In general, the histology of the cellular infiltrate is nonspecific. Bacterial myocarditis is often dominated by polymorphonuclear leucocytes, while viral myocarditis is dominated by lymphocytes. Cellular infiltrates with a predominance of eosinophilic cells suggest an allergic nature (Fig. 10.6). The demonstration of micro-organisms, either visualized directly or by way of *in situ* hybridization, remains the most reliable microscopical indication of an infectious myocarditis. Occasionally, bacterial toxins may play the main role in causing injury to myocardial cells; diphtheria is the best known example. A potent exotoxin inhibiting protein synthesis may directly injure myocardial cells, leading to a hyaline granular degeneration with or without a conspicuous cellular response (Fig. 10.7). Diphtheria has a marked affinity for the atrioventricular conduction tissues, with partial or complete heart block as a hazardous complication.

Viral myocarditis

A wide range of viruses can affect the myocardium, Coxsackie B viruses probably being the most common. They may play a role in the myocarditis acquired during fetal life. Infections with the Coxsackievirus often take a subclinical course and only a minority of cases results in overt cardiac disease. The signs and symptoms may be those of pericarditis, myocardial infarction, or progressive heart failure (see Chapter 9). There is evidence that idiopathic congestive cardiomyopathy may be due to infection with the virus in a good proportion of patients. A reliable diagnosis, however, is extremely difficult. It can only be made on the combined finding of rising serological titres and the demonstration of virus within samples of heart muscle.

Coxsackie viruses tend to affect both myocardium and pericardium. Pericarditis with marked exudation is a frequent finding (see Chapter 14). A mononuclear cellular infiltrate usually dominates the histological picture, varying in degree from massive infiltration with extensive myocardial necrosis (Fig. 10.8) to discrete interstitial infiltrates with only sparse foci of necrosis.

Other viruses that should be considered as potentially important are ECHO viruses, the group of psittacosis viruses, and influenza. Poliomyelitis viruses may cause myocarditis, although this complication is probably of minor significance. Infectious mononucleosis is often accompanied by electrocardiographic abnormalities that suggest myocarditis, but fatal cases are extremely rare. Almost all the viruses producing diseases of common childhood may also produce myocarditis. The actual incidence is very low given the high overall incidence of these diseases in the general population.

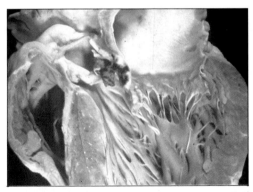
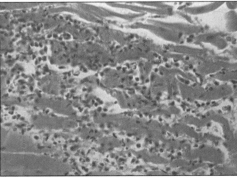

Fig. 10.5 (Upper) Longitudinal section with active bacterial endocarditis of aortic valve extending onto anterior mitral valve leaflet; (lower) focal septic myocarditis secondary to aortic valve infection. H&E stain.

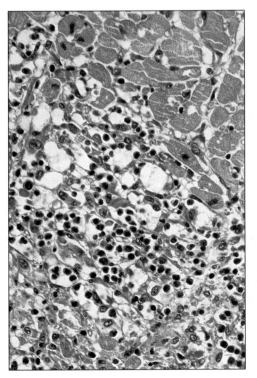

Fig. 10.6 Histological section of myocardium showing mixed zonular infiltrate with abundant eosinophilic cells suggesting allergic myocarditis. H&E stain.

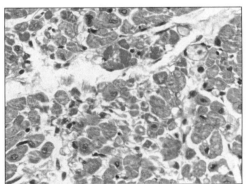
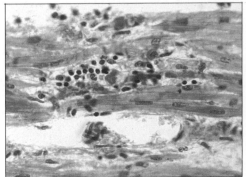

Fig. 10.7 Histology of diphtheria: (upper) spotty hyaline degeneration of myocardial cells occasionally accompanied by scant cellular infiltrate (lower), H&E stains.

Bacterial myocarditis

Bacterial myocarditis is due most commonly to infection with either staphylococci, streptococci, pneumococci, or meningococci. A suppurative response prevails and microabscesses are common (Fig. 10.9).

Tuberculosis is, in the Western world at present, an infrequent cause of myocarditis but by no means eradicated. It may occur as a tuberculoma (Fig. 10.10); as miliary granulomatous lesions, with or without caseous necrosis (Fig. 10.11); or as a diffuse (histologically nonspecific) cellular infiltration. Identification of the bacillus is necessary, giant cells and a granulomatous reaction in themselves being insufficient for diagnosis (see below). Haemorrhagic pericarditis is often the leading sign when the heart is afflicted.

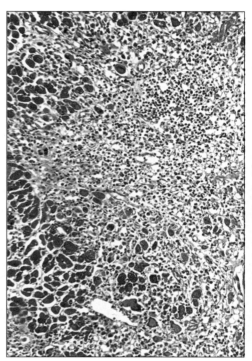

Fig. 10.8 Histology of viral myocarditis: massive mononuclear cellular infiltrate with extensive myocardial necrosis. H&E stain.

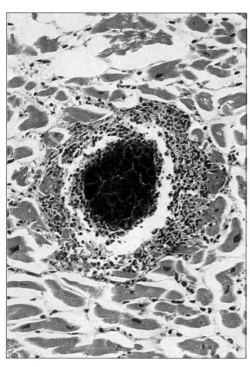

Fig. 10.9 Histology of bacterial myocarditis: microabscesses containing vast colony of staphylococci. H&E stain.

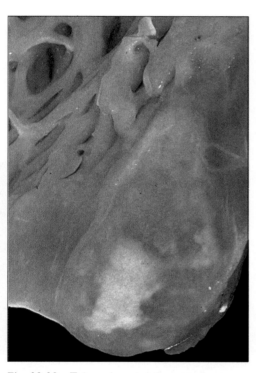

Fig. 10.10 Tuberculoma in left ventricular myocardium.

Fig. 10.11 Histology of tuberculosis: tuberculous granulomatous reaction with necrosis and epitheloid giant cells. H&E stain.

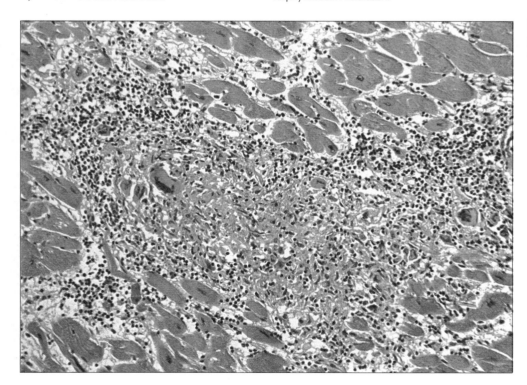

Syphilitic myocarditis can occur either in congenital syphilis as a diffuse interstitial inflammatory, or as a gummatous lesion (Fig. 10.12) when there are late manifestations in adults. A dense, predominantly mononuclear infiltrate accompanied by multinucleated giant cells together with necrosis complete the histological picture (Fig. 10.13).

Leptospirosis (Weil's disease) may seriously injure the myocardium. The histology is nonspecific in that focal necrosis occurs with a mainly mononuclear cellular infiltrate.

Lyme disease, caused by *Borellia burgdorferi*, is now recognized as being of increasing significance in patients with myocarditis (Fig. 10.14).

Whipple's disease may be accompanied by myocarditis, characterized by the presence of PAS- (periodic acid-Schiff) positive macrophages such as those seen in intestinal pathology (see p.11.6)

Fungal myocarditis

In the Western world, fungal myocarditis is almost always limited to patients with immunological deficiencies, whether as part of their principal disease or as a manifestation of therapy. Septic involvement is a common finding under these circumstances. Histological sections often reveal inflammatory foci with a non-specific cellular infiltrate (Fig. 10.15, upper), and special stains may show the organism involved (Fig. 10.15, lower). The most common agent is *Candida*. The lesions may show as yellowish nodules randomly distributed in the myocardium or they may be detected only at microscopical level. Other infections may occur, such as blastomycosis, cryptococcosis, aspergillosis, histoplasmosis, and actinomycosis, often in combination when found in an immunologically compromised heart.

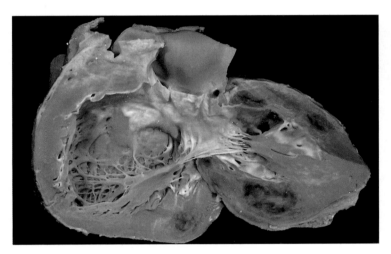

Fig. 10.12 Syphilis: gummatous lesion in left ventricular wall.

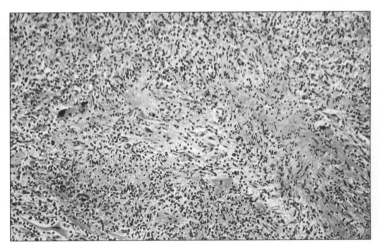

Fig. 10.13 Histology of syphilitic myocarditis; mononuclear infiltrate with giant cells and myocardial necrosis. H&E stain.

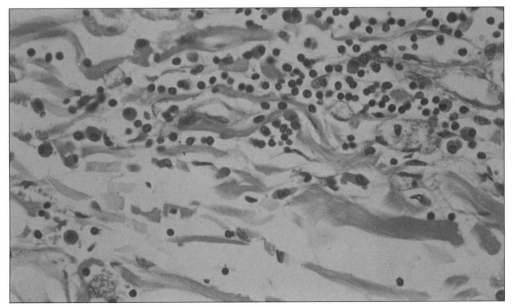

Fig. 10.14 Myocardial histology in case of Lyme disease showing a mononuclear cellular infiltrate. By courtesy of Dr. J. de Konning.

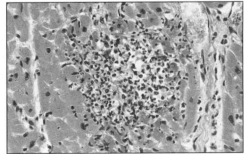

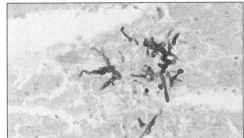

Fig. 10.15 Fungal myocarditis in immunologically-compromised patient: (upper) inflammatory focus (H&E stain); (lower) fungi shown by Grocott's stain.

Protozoal myocarditis

Protozoal myocarditis is a variant that is particularly common in South America, Chagas' disease being the major problem. The disease is due to an autoimmune reaction elicited by cross-reacting antigens of *Trypanosoma cruzi* (the causative agent) and muscle. Tissue cells, including heart-muscle cells are invaded by the organisms, where they produce pseudocysts (Fig. 10.16). In the acute stage of the disease, the heart is often dilated. Histologically, a dense inflammatory infiltrate may occur, albeit that pseudocysts in the myocardium can be found with only a scant cellular response or none at all. Polymorphonuclear leucocytes initially dominate the picture, but these cells become replaced by mononuclear cells when the disease moves into its chronic phase. Fibrous tissue then replaces the necrotic myocardial cells (Fig. 10.17). The cellular infiltrate will eventually disappear, leaving the myocardium thinned, often with attenuated myocardial fibres and varying amounts of interstitial fibrosis. The histological changes relate to the clinical findings. In the acute stage, the cardiac symptoms are dominated by electrical disturbances, whereas the later stages are dominated by cardiomegaly as a feature of progressive congestive heart failure.

Toxoplasmosis may also be complicated by myocarditis, although such a complication is relatively rare. The infection may appear at any age. It may even affect the fetus, most likely due to transplacental passage of organisms. The heart, when diseased, may contain a histologically nonspecific mixed cellular infiltrate and intracellular pseudocysts containing parasites, often occurring in the absence of inflammation (Fig. 10.18).

Other protozoal diseases, such as African trypanosomiasis, malaria, and amoebiasis, may cause myocarditis but this plays a minor role in the clinical setting of these diseases.

Drug-related myocarditis

Drugs causing myocarditis have engendered much interest of late, not least since the number of chemicals presently known to carry the risk of inducing this complication is rapidly growing. Two main categories are recognized: firstly, drugs that cause myocarditis as a result of a direct toxic effect on the myocardium and, secondly, drugs that trigger an allergic reaction.

Drug-related toxic myocarditis

Drugs included in this category are manifold. Well-known examples are emetine, lithium, phenothiazine, barbiturates, theophylline, paraquat, amphetamine, antihypertensive drugs, and a number of immunosuppressive agents.

The myocardial effects are usually dose dependent and cumulative. The histology is dominated by myocardial necrosis, albeit of variable degree and extent, accompanied by a cellular infiltrate that is initially composed mainly of polymorphonuclear leucocytes. Eosinophils are scant or absent and there are usually no giant cells. In due time, a lymphocytic response that is mainly nongranulomatous may replace the acute reaction. In other instances, the toxic effect may particularly affect the vessels and lead to necrotizing vasculitis, the myocardium then being jeopardized by ischaemia.

A particular type of drug-induced toxic myocarditis is that produced by catecholamines, particularly norepinephrine. The main myocardial lesion is contraction band necrosis (see Fig. 9.23) accompanied by a cellular reaction of mixed composition (Fig. 10.19). Known causes are phaechromocytoma, conditions accompanied by stress such as acute intracranial disease processes, and other conditions in which catecholamines are

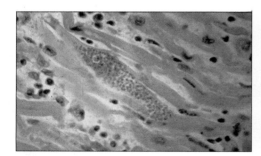

Fig. 10.16 Histology of Chagas' disease with pseudocyst in myocardium. H&E stain. By courtesy of Dr L. Becu.

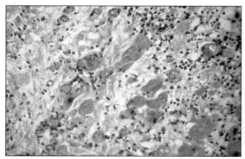

Fig. 10.17 Chronic stage, with interstitial fibrosis. H&E stain. By courtesy of Dr L. Becu.

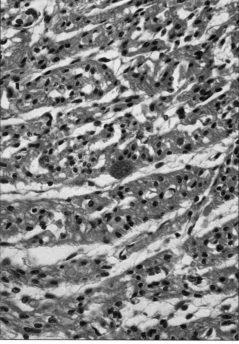

Fig. 10.18 Histology of toxoplasmosis in neonate: pseudocyst in heart muscle cell. H&E stain.

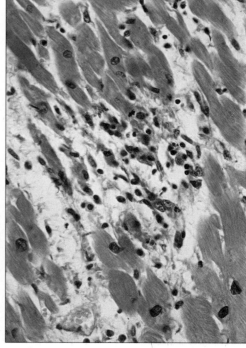

Fig. 10.19 Histological section showing catecholamine-induced myocarditis with mixed cellular infiltrate. H&E stain.

administered. The precise cellular mechanisms involved remain controversial.

Toxic myocarditis eventually leads to multifocal scarring (Fig. 10.20). In cases of repetitious injury, both acute and chronic stages can be present, randomly distributed within the same tissue section.

Drug-related allergic myocarditis

Various drugs are known to cause a side effect in the sense of an allergic myocarditis. Immune-conveyed drug myocarditis is not dose dependent. It may occur at any time and usually regresses when administration of the drug is discontinued. Many drugs are known to cause this reaction. Sulphonamides are the best known, but others such as penicillin, streptomycin, tetracycline, phenylbutazone, and methyldopa have been incriminated.

The presence of eosinophils (Fig. 10.21) and a granulomatous reaction may focus attention on the allergic nature of the disease, usually in a sensitized person. It should be emphasized, however, that the histology in itself is nonspecific.

Immune-mediated myocarditis of uncertain aetiology

Immune-mediated myocarditis of uncertain aetiology is in itself a heterogenous group of diseases. Some of the generalized auto-allergic diseases may cause myocarditis that is clinically important. Active myocarditis is usually of a temporary nature but may occasionally have a profound effect on the clinical profile of the disease.

In systemic lupus erythematosus, the myocardial lesions consist mainly of fibrinoid changes in the connective tissue, together with a cellular reaction (Fig. 10.22). The lesions are often paravascular. Valvar lesions are discussed elsewhere (see Chapter 11).

In rheumatoid arthritis, a diffuse cellular reaction can occur with massive myocardial necrosis. Most commonly, small interstitial aggregates of mononuclear cells are present which in themselves are nondiagnostic. Rheumatoid granulomas are seen in a small proportion of cases, which consist of a central zone of fibrinoid necrosis surrounded by pallisading histiocytes and fibroblasts with an outer zone of lymphocytes (Fig. 10.23). Giant cells may also be found.

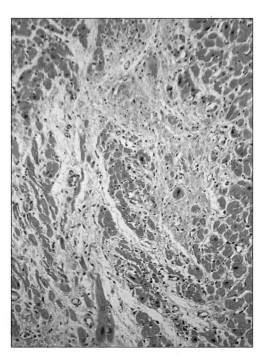

Fig. 10.20 Histological section showing focal scarring. The end result of toxic myocarditis. (H&E stain.)

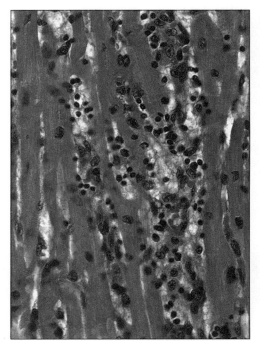

Fig. 10.21 Histological section showing allergic myocarditis, suggested by abundancy of eosinophils. H&E stain.

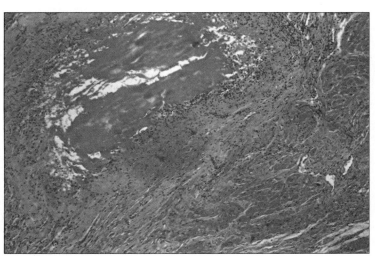

Fig. 10.22 Histology of systemic lupus erythematosus showing fibrinoid interstitial necrosis with histiocyte reaction. H&E stain.

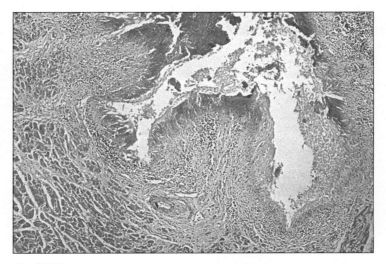

Fig. 10.23 Histological section of myocardium with rheumatoid nodule. H&E stain. By courtesy of Dr F. Eulderink.

In some diseases the outstanding pathology is formed by an allergic vasculitis, usually considered the result of depositions of circulating immune complexes. A variety of conditions is grouped together under this heading. Poly(peri)arteritis nodosa (Fig. 10.24) and Wegener's granulomatosis (Fig. 10.25) are probably the conditions that most commonly affect the heart, albeit rarely. In each, the disease is characterized by necrotizing vasculitis, which may subsequently lead to extensive ischaemic myocardial necrosis. Extensive myocarditis may also ensue in Wegener's granulomatosis. Involvement of the atrioventricular conduction tissues has been documented (Fig. 10.26).

Kawasaki's disease (mucocutaneous lymph node syndrome) most likely also belongs to the category of auto-allergic diseases. Initially considered a Japanese entity that particularly affected infants, it is now clear that the disease occurs in other parts of the world. The mortality rate varies between 2 and 8%. The most common cause of death is coronary arterial disease, with or without myocarditis. The pathology in these instances is similar to that seen in infantile periarteritis nodosa. Necrotizing arteritis of the coronary arteries with thrombosis, formation of aneurysms, and rupture leading to cardiac tamponade are the most common findings (Fig. 10.27), with myocarditis frequently present in the acute stage (Fig. 10.28).

Rheumatic fever must be considered at least briefly in terms of myocarditis although the more significant valvar pathology is discussed in detail elsewhere (see Chapter 13). Rheumatic fever is considered an auto-allergic disease following an infection with group A haemolytic streptococci. The pathologic changes are induced by cross-reactivity between some antigenic determinants of the micro-organism and certain antigens that occur in the sarcolemma and sarcoplasm of myocytes and the connective tissues. In the acute stage, this may lead to myocarditis. It is likely that, through a process of complement activation, a pattern of reaction is initiated which may result in the formation of the

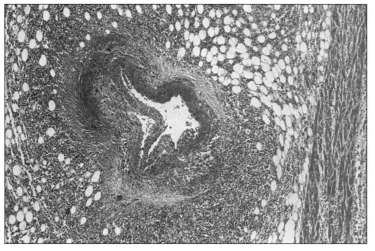

Fig. 10.24 Histology of poly(peri)arteritis nodosa showing massive necrosis of arterial wall with inflammatory reaction. H&E stain.

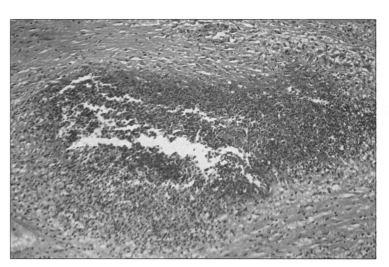

Fig. 10.25 Histological section showing necrotizing inflammatory focus in Wegener's granulomatosis. H&E stain.

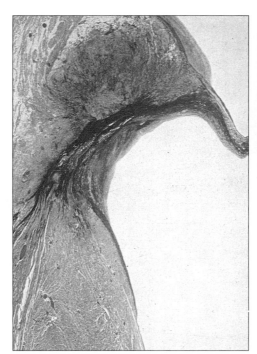

Fig. 10.26 Histology of Wegener's granulomatosis: massive necrotizing inflammation destroying atrioventricular node. E-VG stain.

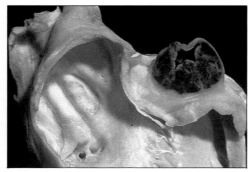

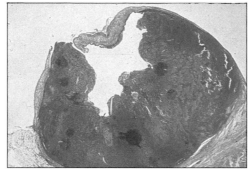

Fig. 10.27 Kawasaki's disease: (upper) ruptured aneurysm of right coronary artery; (lower) histology. E-VG stain.

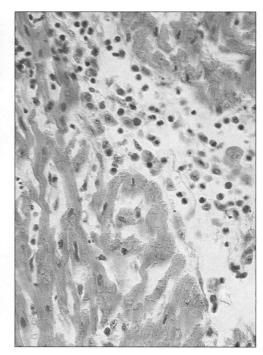

Fig. 10.28 Histology of Kawasaki's disease showing interstitial myocarditis in acute phase. H&E stain. By courtesy of Dr N Tanaka.

well-known Aschoff nodules (Fig. 10.29). The extent to which the acute inflammatory response will eventually result in scarring and interstitial fibrosis of clinical significance remains controversial. Nevertheless, there is an increased amount of interstitial fibrous tissue in the hearts of patients with valvar disease occurring secondary to rheumatic fever.

The production of auto-antibodies against the heart may also be triggered by minor changes in the structure of the pre-existent tissue antigens as a consequence of ischaemic necrosis, infections, or trauma. The postmyocardial infarction syndrome (Dressler's syndrome) and the postpericardiotomy syndrome are examples of these mechanisms although their incidence and clinical relevance remain controversial.

Acute rejection of cardiac allografts is probably best discussed under the heading of 'immune-related myocarditis'. The principal histological feature is myocarditis with a cellular infiltrate predominated by T-lymphocytes (Fig. 10.30). Endomyocardial biopsies play an important role in clinical management, providing an objective histological index of the immune response of the host to the allograft. These then allow direct assessment of the response to immunosuppressive therapy.

Miscellaneous lesions

The literature on myocarditis contains a number of so-called entities than need clarification and comment.

Granulomatous myocarditis

The term granulomatous myocarditis is purely descriptive and is based on the presence of a granulomatous reaction in the myocardium. Granulomas most likely represent a cell-mediated immunological reaction in an individual who is already sensitized. The nature of the injurious agent, nonetheless, is by no means specified and may be quite diverse. Conditions such as sarcoidosis (Fig. 10.31) and tuberculosis (see page 10.4) should always be considered. Myocardial involvement in sarcoidosis is a serious complication, involving the occurrence of disturbances of conduction and rhythm. Sudden death under these circumstances is by no means uncommon. In general, the aetiology of a granulomatous myocarditis often remains uncertain.

Giant-cell myocarditis

Giant-cell myocarditis is characterized by an inflammatory response that contains multinucleated giant cells and almost always accompanies a granulomatous reaction. The term is purely descriptive and does not allow classification according to aetiology. Indeed, giant cells may accompany various types of infectious diseases and systemic disorders. Occasionally, giant-cell myocarditis may be an incidental finding at autopsy. The adjective 'idiopathic' is often used; this is important since the term 'idiopathic giant-cell myocarditis' has also been promoted as a distinct clinicopathological entity, characterized by a rapid course and histologically by extensive serpiginous myocardial necrosis (Fig. 10.32, left) with giant-cell reaction at its margins (Fig. 10.32, right). An altered immunologic response triggered by an infection has been suggested as the most likely cause. As

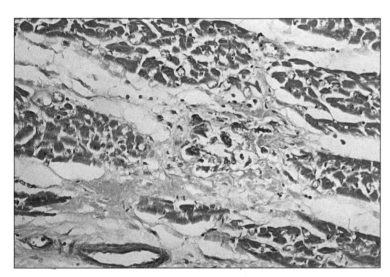

Fig. 10.29 Histology of Aschoff nodule within myocardium. H&E stain.

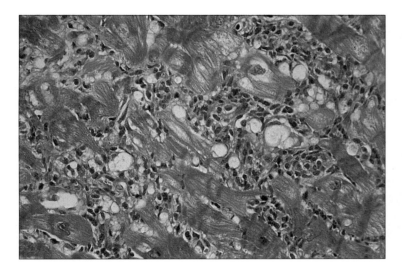

Fig. 10.30 Histological section showing myocarditis composed of lymphocytes in acute cardiac allograph rejection. H&E stain. By courtesy of Dr M.E. Billingham.

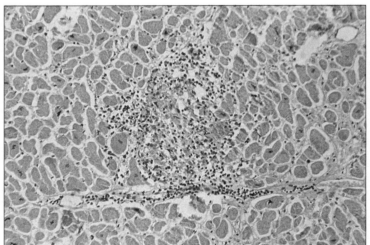

Fig. 10.31 Histological section showing granulomatous myocarditis in sarcoidosis. H&E stain.

suggested above, however, use of the term 'idiopathic giant-cell myocarditis' will inevitably promote confusion if used for the description of a discrete entity.

Fiedler's myocarditis

Patients initially described under this heading had acute myocarditis of unknown aetiology and without more widespread inflammation elsewhere in the body. In some of these cases, histology of the myocardium revealed a giant-cell reaction. In others, no giant cells were observed. Clinicians presently tend to use the term to describe an acute myocarditis of unknown aetiology. Pathologists are inclined to associate the term with the presence of giant cells or with a pronounced mixed cellular infiltrate, among which eosinophils and giant cells predominate. The term is confusing and, hence, in our opinion, should be discarded.

TOXIC CARDIOMYOPATHIES

Various drugs can injure myocardial cells without producing an inflammatory response. Within our definitions, these diseases are not classified as myocarditis. Instead, they are described as toxic cardiomyopathies.

General aspects

The main clinical feature of toxic cardiomyopathies is that of heart failure. The onset of cardiotoxicity is usually insidious and, as experience has shown, myocardial degeneration can be present long before clinical signs and symptoms become apparent. Heart failure may suddenly ensue and, at this stage, myocardial damage is usually irreversible.

It is significant that some of the drugs that produce toxic cardiomyopathy have a potentiating effect when used in combination with other drugs that may cause drug-induced myocarditis

(see above). Similarly, radiation may enhance their toxic effects and vice versa.

At autopsy, the heart usually exhibits marked dilatation of all chambers with thinning of their walls. Fibrosis is not apparent macroscopically, although microscopic sections may reveal patchy or diffuse interstitial fibrosis of limited extent. Intracavitary thrombosis is a frequent finding.

The most important cardiotoxic chemicals are antineoplastic drugs and alcohol.

Antineoplastic drugs

Cardiotoxic effects are particularly well recognized for the anthracycline antibiotics such as adriamycin (toxorubicin), adriamycin-DNA (daunorubicin), rubidazone, carminomycin, and AD32. A distinction is made between acute and chronic cardiotoxic effects: acute effects are seen during or soon after the administration of the drug and usually consist of nonspecific electrocardiographic changes; chronic effects, on the other hand, are far more serious. Two basic types of injury to myocardial cells occur. These changes are usually not readily apparent with light microscopy (Fig. 10.33) unless carefully sought. At ultrastructural level, however, the changes are most conspicuous.

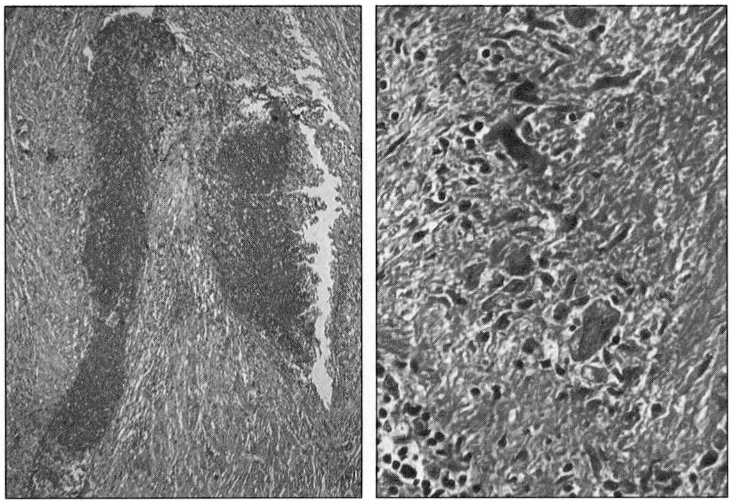

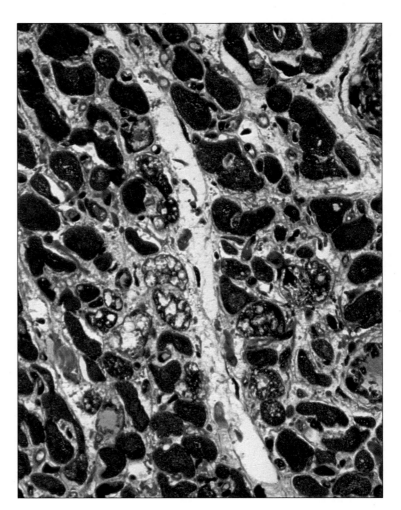

Fig. 10.33 Histological section of myocardium in adriamycin toxicity. Vacuolated myocytes indicate injury. PTAH stain. By courtesy of Dr M.E. Billingham.

Fig. 10.32 Histology of giant cell myocarditis with extensive myocardial necrosis (left) and giant cells at its margin (right) in addition to mixed cellular infiltrate. H&E stains.

One type is characterized by loss of myofibrils (Fig. 10.34); the loss is partial at first, but the degenerative process progresses gradually so that, eventually, only remnants of the Z-band may remain. Vacuolar degeneration of myocytes is the second basic feature (Fig. 10.34). Distension of the sarcotubular system is the earliest manifestation. Eventually, large membrane-bound clear spaces may form in the cytoplasm. The nucleus and the mitochondria may be unaffected by either of these changes. The myocytes thus affected usually cluster to form foci that are diffusely distributed through the myocardium. A slight increase of interstitial connective tissue may accompany the degenerative process, but inflammatory infiltrates are not a feature. Eventually, both types of myocytic degeneration lead to overt death of cells.

Since the cardiotoxic effects are present prior to clinical signs and symptoms, endomyocardial biopsies may have a role in guiding administration of drugs. In this particular clinical setting, the histological changes are typical and useful as a marker. They are not, however, specific since similar changes can occur in end-stage cardiomyopathies due to other causes.

Alcoholic cardiomyopathy

Alcohol may cause toxic damage to myocardial cells in addition to its well-known toxic effects on the nervous system, liver, and pancreas. Hence, cardiac toxicity consequent to chronic alcoholism may be produced along two pathways (Fig. 10.35). An indirect pathway may be found due to injury of the liver and the pancreas. This produces malabsorption of nutrients and, eventually, functional derangement of heart-muscle cells. On the other hand, alcohol may directly inhibit mitochondrial function. This affects the biochemical activity of myocytes through the reduced activity of oxidative enzymes, an inhibition in the uptake of calcium ions, an increase of intracellular triglycerides, and an inhibition of oxidation of fatty acids.

Disease of the heart muscle produced by alcohol does not clinically differ much from other types of congestive cardiomyopathy. No specific signs or symptoms exist. The diagnosis is usually based on circumstantial evidence. The heart usually shows dilatation of all chambers with variable degrees of fibrosis. Using light microscopy, the overall picture is again nondiagnostic. Ultrastructural studies show myofibrillar disruption, mitochondrial swelling with disruption of cristae, accumulation of lipids, and intramitochondrial inclusions of crystalline debris. These changes indicate damage to the myocardial cells but they are not specific for alcoholic cardiomyopathy.

The outbreak of rapidly progressive congestive cardiomyopathy among heavy beer drinkers in Quebec has led to the identification of cobalt as a potent cardiotoxic chemical. Thus, in the strict sense, 'beer-drinker's cardiomyopathy' is not an alcoholic disease, but rather a cobalt cardiomyopathy.

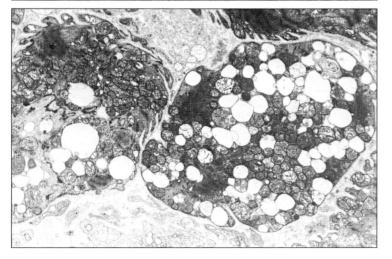

Fig. 10.34 Two types of cellular change induced by adriamycin: (upper) loss of myofilaments and (lower) extensive vacuolization. EM, × 2700 (upper), × 3600 (lower). By courtesy of Dr M.E. Billingham.

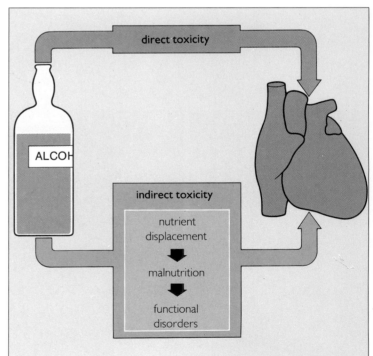

Fig. 10.35 The two main pathways in alcohol toxicity.

INFILTRATION AND STORAGE DISEASES

In this section, we describe a group of heterogeneous diseases that are linked together by an abnormal accumulation of substances within the myocardium, this having a negative effect on myocardial contractility. Only the more common forms are discussed.

Fatty change

Intracellular accumulation of fat can be caused by a variety of conditions that affect cell metabolism. Those which particularly affect the heart include carbon-monoxide poisoning, nutritional deficiencies, thyrotoxicosis, toxaemia of pregnancy, diabetes mellitus, and various toxic causes such as poisoning with chloroform and phosphorus, alcoholic intoxication and, in general, septicaemia. In childhood, the association of an acute encephalopathy and fatty degeneration of the organs, including the myocardium, is known as Reye's syndrome. The aetiology and pathogenesis remain as yet undetermined.

The heart may show endocardial striations that are known as the 'tabbycat' appearance. Microscopic sections show excessive intracellular accumulation of fat (Fig. 11.1). Since it is always possible to demonstrate a minimal amount of finely distributed fat, even in the normal heart, presence of normal amounts of fat must be differentiated from the pathological conditions discussed above.

Fatty intracellular change of myocytes should also be distinguished from fatty infiltration of the myocardium. Also known as lipomatosis cordis, this condition is usually associated with generalized obesity, although it may occasionally occur in isolation. Fat is widely dispersed throughout the myocardium, particularly in the right ventricular free wall (Fig. 11.2, left). Microscopically, islands of myocytes are seen in an ocean of adipose tissue (Fig. 11.2, right). Occasionally, no myocardial cells can be found. These changes are similar to those described in so-called arrhythmogenic right ventricular dysplasia (see Chapter 12). The condition should be distinguished from Uhl's malformation, which is congenital absence of myocardium (see Chapter 7).

In otherwise normal hearts, adipose tissue may accompany the larger intramural vascular strands and may occasionally be found subendocardially. This is relevant in the interpretation of endomyocardial biopsies, since adipose tissue in such sections is not necessarily derived from the epicardium.

Amyloidosis

Amyloidosis is encountered in two main forms: in primary amyloidosis, there appears to be no relation to an underlying disease, while secondary amyloidosis occurs in association with chronic inflammatory diseases such as rheumatoid arthritis. Cardiac amyloidosis is often seen in the primary form. In the

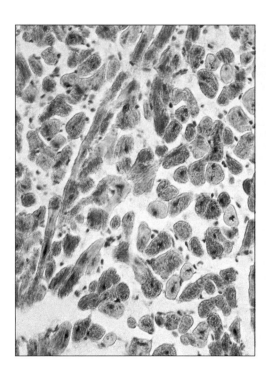

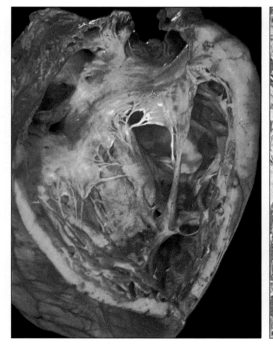

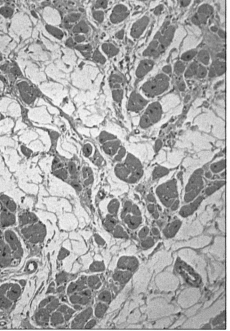

Fig. 11.1 Histological section of myocardium showing fatty change: accumulation of intracellular fat globules of different sizes. Sudan III stain.

Fig. 11.2 Fatty infiltration of myocardium: (left) outflow part is parchment-like; (right) histology. There are islands of myocardial cells amidst adipose tissue. H&E stain.

elderly, depositions of amyloid in the heart are common, often without appreciable depositions in other organs. The precise frequency cannot be given, but there is no doubt that, from 70 years of age onwards, the incidence rises sharply. At least half of all individuals over 90 will have amyloid deposited in the heart. This particular type of amyloidosis, therefore, is also known as 'senile cardiac amyloidosis'.

The pathogenesis of deposition of amyloid is not uniform. In patients with primary amyloidosis and plasma cell dyscrasias, the amyloid is derived from immunoglobulins and composed of light-chain proteins. This type of amyloid is also known as AL-protein. In other patients, in contrast, particularly in those with

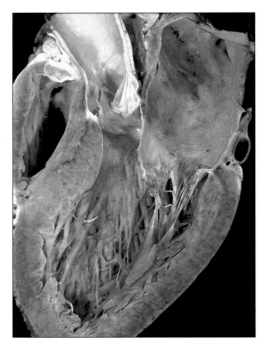

Fig. 11.3 Cardiac amyloidosis, long-axis section. The left ventricle is dilated. Note the sandy appearance of left atrial and left ventricular endocardium.

secondary amyloidosis, the protein component of amyloid is known as 'amyloid of unknown origin' or AA-protein. The latter appears to be the most important protein that can be isolated from amyloid in these cases. It shows a close relation in its sequence of amino acids and antigen determinants to SAA (amyloid-associated serum component), a precursor which normally occurs in the serum in very low concentrations. The content in the serum, however, rises markedly with increasing age, particularly over 70 years, thus suggesting a relation to so-called senile cardiac amyloidosis. Cardiac deposition of amyloid can also have an endocrine origin, with the APUD system being incriminated. Various types of phagocytic cells play a role in the deposition of the typical amyloid fibrils from the precursor substances, but the precise mechanisms are unclear.

The heart is enlarged and heavy. The myocardium, when freshly cut, maintains its shape. The chambers are usually somewhat dilated (Fig. 11.3). These pathological observations correlate well with the reduced contractility that can be demonstrated clinically. Amyloidosis is the classical example of a restrictive cardiomyopathy (see Chapter 12). It also explains why cardiac amyloidosis may present clinically with signs and symptoms resembling constrictive pericarditis (see Chapter 14).

Deposits of amyloid may produce a finely granular endo-cardial surface to the chambers and on the valves (Fig. 11.4), giving a 'sandy' sensation when palpated. This feature is particularly apparent in the left atrium following formalin fixation.

Microscopically, amyloid is found either diffusely distributed between myocardial cells (Fig. 11.5) or in the form of nodular and laminated deposits (Fig. 11.6), often related to intramural blood vessels. The reduced myocardial contractility relates directly to these features. Deposits of amyloid in the valves are frequent and usually present as nodular aggregates. In clinical terms, however, valvar pathology is of limited significance. Deposits within either intra- or extramural blood vessels are common

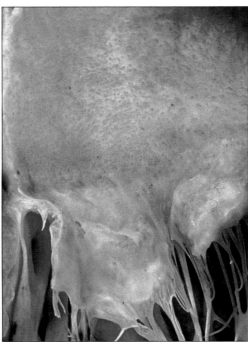
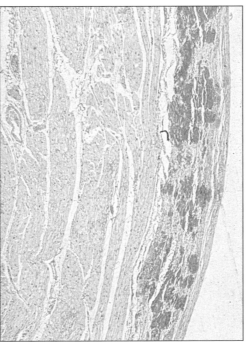

Fig. 11.4 Cardiac amyloidosis: (left) granular appearance of left atrial endocardium extending onto mitral valve; (right) subendocardial amyloid depositions. Congo red stain.

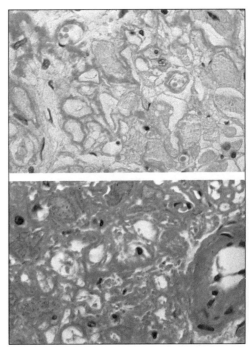

Fig. 11.5 Histology of cardiac amyloidosis: myocardial cells degenerate following extracellular deposition of amorphous eosinophilic substance enclosing the cells. (Upper) H&E, (lower) positive staining with Congo red.

(Fig. 11.7). The pericardial fat is often heavily infiltrated, and the conduction system is frequently involved. Disturbances of atrioventricular conduction are a known clinical manifestation.

Histological techniques, such as the Congo red stain (crossed polaroids result in a light-green colour) and the thioflavin-T technique (ultravoilet light results in a yellow-green fluorescence), are usually sufficient to confirm the presence of amyloid. Ultrastructurally, the typical fibrillar arrangement is the leading feature (Fig. 11.8).

Calcinosis

The most common form of deposition of calcium within the heart is dystrophic calcification, in which the calcium is deposited in degenerated cells or tissues. Dystrophic calcification appears much more readily in neonates and infants than in adults. This feature may relate to the stage of active growth and (re)modelling of bones. It is not unusual to find calcific deposits complicating myocardial infarction, even in stillborns (Fig. 11.9).

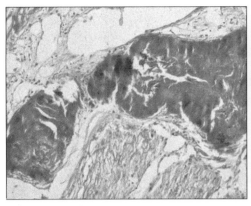
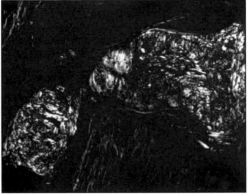

Fig. 11.6 Histology of cardiac amyloidosis: large nodular deposit in myocardium stains positive in Congo red (left) and has bright greenish birefringence with polarization (right).

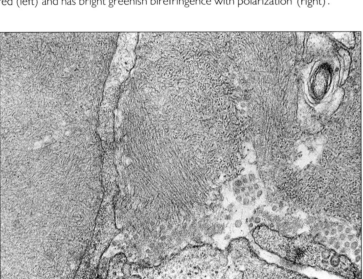

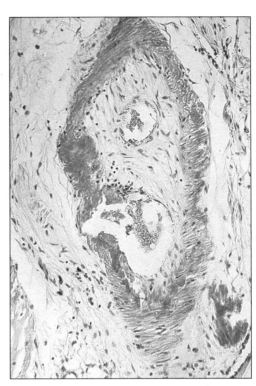

Fig. 11.7 Histological section showing amyloidosis of wall of intramyocardial coronary artery; the lumen is almost obliterated by organized thrombus (barium contrast in vascular channels). Congo red stain.

fibroblast

amyloid

collagen

Fig. 11.8 Typical fibrillar appearance of amyloid. EM, × 34,000.

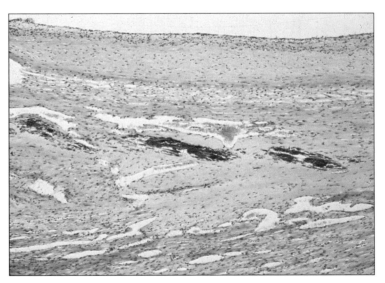

Fig. 11.9 Histological section showing scar with calcific deposits in heart of neonate. H&E stain.

Dystrophic calcification contrasts with metastatic calcification. In the latter, calcium is deposited in normal cells and tissues, usually because of an increased availability of calcium ions. Hence, metastatic calcification may accompany diseases that lead to decalcification of bones, such as leukaemia and metastatic bone disease, as well as diseases that more directly influence calcium metabolism, such as hyperparathyroidism, hypervitaminosis D, and chronic renal disease. Uraemia and chronic haemodialysis are often accompanied by severe myocardial calcification. The deposits are present in the wall of the blood vessels and within myocardial cells (Fig. 11.10).

Deposition of iron

Accumulation of iron in the myocardium may be part of an inborn error of metabolism (haemochromatosis) or may result from an excessive availability of iron, for example in cases of

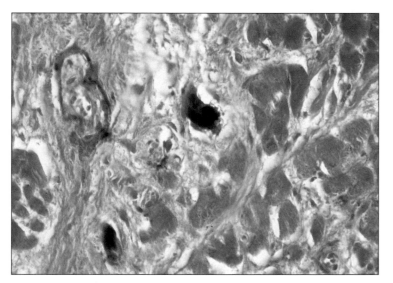

Fig. 11.10 Histological section showing calcium deposits (black) in wall of intramyocardial vessel and in myocytes, in patient with uraemia. Von Kossa's stain.

long-term haemodialysis or repeated blood transfusion (haemosiderosis). Heart failure in these conditions is usually of the congested type. Rarely, the signs and symptoms may be those of a restrictive cardiomyopathy. The heart is enlarged, often hypertrophied, and the myocardium may show a brown pigmentation. Microscopically, the iron is deposited mainly within the myocytes where it initially accumulates at the poles of the nuclei (Fig. 11.11). In advanced stages, the deposits may extend further peripherally within the cells, replacing myofibrils. Secondary degenerative changes may ensue, such as vascular degeneration and interstitial fibrosis. All contribute to the development of heart failure.

Oxalosis

The deposition of calcium oxalate in the tissues may be primary or secondary. Primary oxalosis is a genetically determined inborn error of metabolism in which large amounts of oxalate are excreted in the urine. The usual cause of death is uraemia secondary to nephrocalcinosis. Patients with longstanding renal failure may develop extensive deposits in the kidneys and the myocardium. Sections of the heart reveal the oxalate deposits as birefringent crystals (Fig. 11.12). Heart block can occur.

Glycogen storage disease

Of the different types of glycogenosis, only type II glycogen storage disease (Pompe's disease) has cardiac manifestations as a constant and leading feature. The heart may be affected in other forms, but only rarely will the cardiac abnormality become manifest. The condition is due to deficiency of the enzyme, acid maltase, which leads to an accumulation of intracellular glycogen thereby distorting normal cellular function. The heart is enlarged and the myocardium is pale-staining. Microscopically, sections stained routinely with haematoxylin and eosin exhibit extensive vacuolization of myocytes (Fig. 11.13, left). When the tissues are processed to preserve glycogen, massive accumulation of intracellular glycogen is seen (Fig. 11.13, right). Ultrastruc-

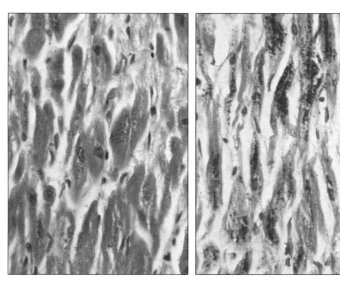

Fig. 11.11 Histology of haemosiderosis of heart showing iron deposition within cardiocytes, accumulating at nuclear poles. Iron is brown with H&E (left); blue with Perls' stain (right).

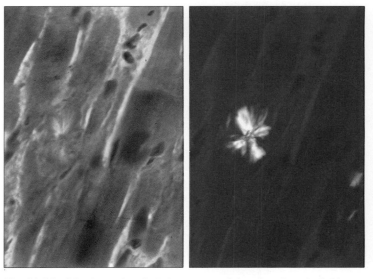

Fig. 11.12 Histology of oxalosis: intramyocardial oxalate deposits (left) show up as birefringent crystals under polarization (right). H&E stain.

CARDIOMYOPATHIES

Initially, the term cardiomyopathy was applied to any disorder affecting heart muscle. In 1980, a task force of the World Health Organisation and the International Society of Federations of Cardiology suggested that a distinction should be made between disorders of myocardium having a known cause or those associated with systemic disease, and those with an unknown cause. The former were grouped together as 'specific heart-muscle diseases'. Thus, conditions such as glycogen storage disease and amyloidosis fall in the group of specific diseases (see above). The latter group has been termed 'cardiomyopathy'. A division has since been made: this includes dilated cardiomyopathy, hypertrophic cardiomyopathy, and restrictive cardiomyopathy. Since then, however, it has become apparent that this categorization in itself is less than perfect. In some instances, it may prove impossible, clinically, to distinguish between the restrictive and dilated types. In other cases, the pathology encountered in a 'typical' case of restrictive cardiomyopathy may not fit with the 'classical' concept (see below). Furthermore, the terminology chosen suggests that hypertrophy occurs only in hypertrophic cardiomyopathy, which is definitely not the case. So-called arrhythmogenic right ventricular dysplasia is also a disorder of unknown cause and, hence, should be included within the category of cardiomyopathies. The condition is discussed in this section.

Dilated cardiomyopathy

Dilated cardiomyopathy can occur at almost any age and is characterized by symptoms and signs of congestive heart failure, often rapidly progressive. Disturbances of rhythm may be a serious complication. From a pathophysiologic point of view, the disease is characterized by decreased myocardial contractility. The diagnosis is based on the exclusion of all other forms of congestive cardiomyopathies. This may pose a problem since other diseases, such as alcoholic cardiomyopathy and the vast majority of cases of myocarditis, are not readily diagnosed. Endomyocardial biopsies may be helpful (see Chapter 10).

A particular form of dilated cardiomyopathy is associated with pregnancy and is known also as postpartum (or peripartum) cardiomyopathy.

In dilated cardiomyopathy, the heart is enlarged with dilatation of all four chambers (Fig. 12.1). Such dilatation may mask the presence of hypertrophy. The gross aspect of the myocardium is usually unremarkable, and the endocardium almost always shows diffuse or patchy fibroelastosis (Fig. 12.2). Intracavitary thrombosis is common both macro- and microscopically.

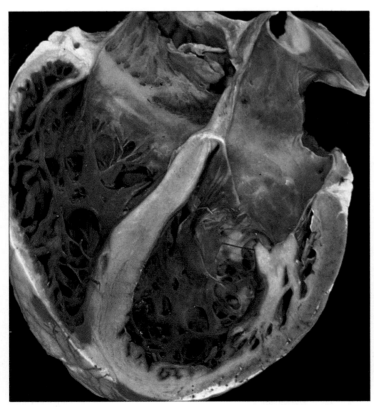

Fig. 12.1 Four-chamber section in dilated cardiomyopathy showing dilatation of both ventricles with marked wall-thinning.

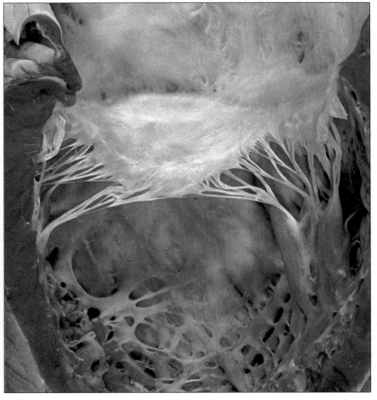

Fig. 12.2 Extensive endocardial fibroelastosis of left ventricle in dilated cardiomyopathy.

The histopathological features of the myocardium are non-specific. Endomyocardial biopsies will reveal distinct hypertrophy of myocytes (Fig. 12.3) with a varying degree of interstitial fibrosis. Occasionally, particularly in patients in whom the lapse between the onset of symptoms and the biopsy is less than six months, scant inflammatory cells, usually lymphocytes and macrophages, may be seen (Fig. 12.4). Sometimes, the endocardium present in the biopsy specimens may reveal thickening by fibroelastic tissue and the presence of smooth-muscle cells (Fig. 12.5). These observations of the myocardium in patients with dilated cardiomyopathy are often in striking contrast with the pathology seen at autopsy. In the latter instance, the myocardial cells are often excessively attenuated.

Lymphocytes may often be present in biopsy samples of the myocardium in patients with dilated cardiomyopathy. This fact, coupled with the observations made in patients affected by viral myocarditis, some of whom may develop the clinical picture of dilated cardiomyopathy without identifiable traces of a previous viral infection, have led to the assumption that, at least in some patients, dilated cardiomyopathy may be an end stage of a viral myocarditis. This is further strengthened by *in situ* hybridization of endomyocardial biopsies of patients with dilated cardiomyopathy, which occasionally demonstrate the presence of RNA sequences of Coxsackie B viruses.

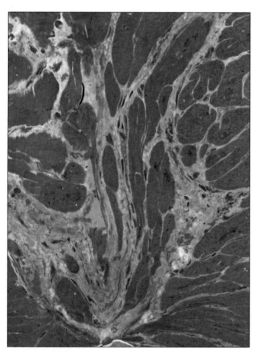

Fig. 12.3 Endomyocardial biopsy. Distinct hypertrophy of myocytes with interstitial fibrosis. (Toluidine blue stain.)

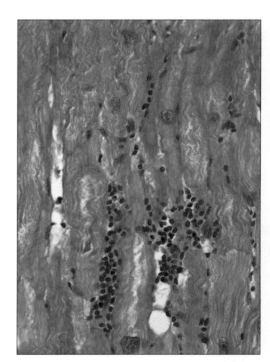

Fig. 12.4 Endomyocardial biopsy in dilated cardiomyopathy. Amidst hypertrophic myocytes scant lymphocytic infiltrates are present. (H&E stain.)

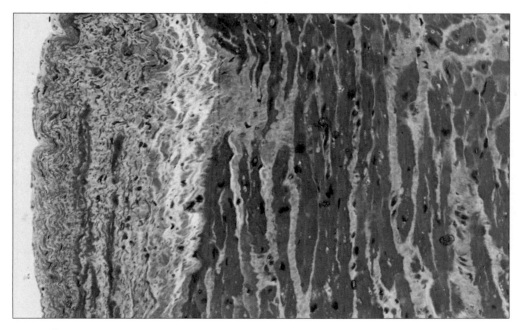

Fig. 12.5 Endomyocardial biopsy in dilated cardiomyopathy. Endocardial thickening contains smooth muscle cells. (Toluidine blue stain.)

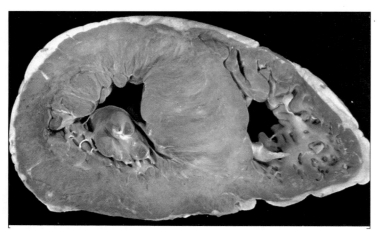

Fig. 12.6 Transverse section in hypertrophic cardiomyopathy shows asymmetric septal hypertrophy.

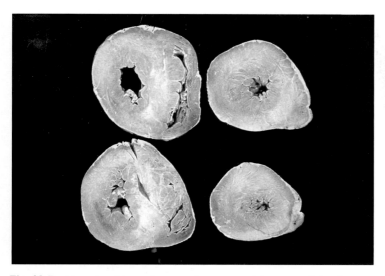

Fig. 12.7 Hypertrophic cardiomyopathy: asymmetric myocardial wall thickening extends from ventricular septum into anterior wall with almost circumferential spread in apical region. Note marked fibrosis (whitish area).

Hypertrophic cardiomyopathy

The clinical presentation of the hypertrophic form varies considerably and includes angina pectoris, syncope, cardiac failure, and sudden death. Some patients may be totally asymptomatic. The basic pathophysiologic abnormality is a decrease in diastolic myocardial distensibility.

The 'classical' pathologic feature is asymmetrical hypertrophy of the ventricular septum (Fig. 12.6). This condition should be distinguished from 'disproportionate ventricular septal thickening'. The latter may occur as a nonspecific condition in various types of congenital heart malformations, in aortic valvar stenosis, or in the adaptive left ventricular hypertrophy observed in the heart of athletes.

Many hearts with unequivocal hypertrophic cardiomyopathy do not present the classical features as outlined above. Indeed, some cases may present symmetric hypertrophy, while others may show asymmetric hypertrophy involving other areas of the left ventricle and the septum, particularly the apical region (Fig.12.7).

Even in cases with 'classical' asymmetric hypertrophy, the ventricular abnormality usually extends into the anterior left ventricular free wall. In case of septal asymmetry, the left ventricular endocardial surface shows a fibrous thickening, almost like an imprint of the overlying aortic leaflet of the mitral valve, most likely due to the impact of the leaflet during diastole (Fig. 12.8). The mere observation of this endocardial thickening on the septum may suggest the presence of hypertrophic cardiomyopathy. This may then be significant in evaluating the cause of death in young individuals dying in a sudden and unexpected fashion.

The cut surface of the abnormal thickened areas of myocardium often reveals an unusual texture of the myocardium, frequently accompanied by fibrosis (Fig. 12.9). The histological appearance of the areas of myocardium affected grossly in this fashion is that of a marked disorganization of the myofibrils

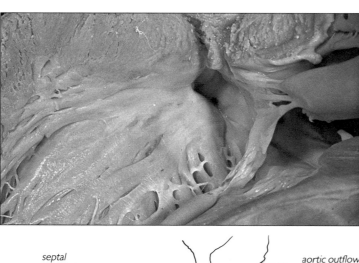

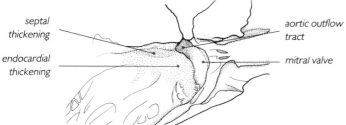

septal thickening

aortic outflow tract

endocardial thickening

mitral valve

Fig. 12.8 Hypertrophic cardiomyopathy showing narrowed left ventricular outflow tract and endocardial thickening of septum.

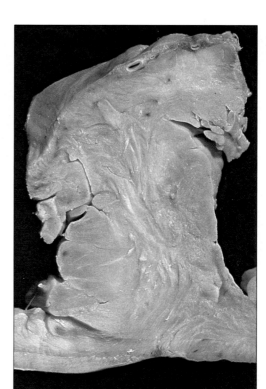

Fig. 12.9 Transverse section through ventricular septum in hypertrophic cardiomyopathy shows bizarre fibre arrangement.

(Fig. 12.10). The abnormally short and broad muscle fibres often run in different directions, showing complex bridging of adjacent fibres with abnormal intercellular contacts, leading to the formation of whirls. The myocytes are distinctly hypertrophic, with hyperchromatic and often bizarre nuclei (Fig. 12.11). The diameter of the individual myocytes often measures 90–100 μm, as compared with the range of 5–12 μm in normal hearts and an average diameter of cells hypertrophied due to any other cause of approximately 20–25 μm.

An increased cellular branching and extensive side-to-side intercellular junctions are also noted ultrastructurally (Fig. 12.12).

In themselves, neither the light-microscopic nor the ultrastructural changes are unique for hypertrophic cardiomyopathy. Nevertheless, the gross appearance, together with the extent of the microscopic changes will lead almost without exception to a proper diagnosis of this condition. It is important to realize, however, that 'disorganization' as such, particularly when observed in small samples, is not diagnostic for hypertrophic cardiomyopathy. This is particularly the case when evaluating endomyocardial biopsies. Naturally occurring 'disorganization' is common subendocardially on both the right and left sides of the ventricular septum.

The deranged architecture of myocardial fibres in hypertrophic cardiomyopathy is often further complicated by excessive fibrosis (Fig. 12.13) and, occasionally, by myocardial infarction. Such fibrotic changes are usually accompanied by extensive obstructive changes in intramural coronary arteries, characterized by a proliferation of longitudinally orientated smooth-muscle cells within the intimal layer (Fig. 12.14).

The aetiology and pathogenesis of hypertrophic cardiomyopathy remain as yet unknown. An autosomal dominant pattern of inheritance has now been established in familial cases and it has been shown that, in this kindred, the gene responsible is located on chromosome 14.

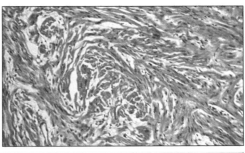
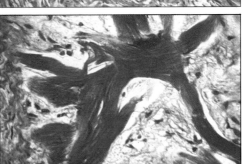

Fig. 12.10 Histology of hypertrophic cardiomyopathy: (upper) disarray in infant heart; (lower) high power bizarre perpendicular branching amidst fibrosis. E-VG (upper), Mallory's trichrome stain (lower).

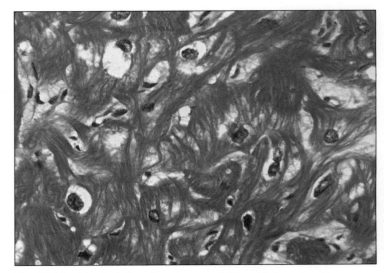

Fig. 12.11 Histological section of young adult heart in hypertrophic cardiomyopathy shows combination of unusual texture with excessive hypertrophy and intracellular abnormalities. H&E stain.

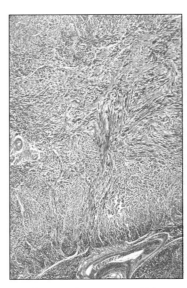

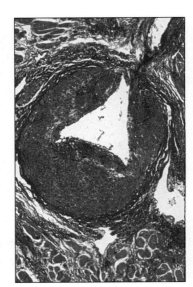

Fig. 12.12 Ultrastructural appearances of hypertrophic cardiomyopathy include disorientated myofibrils, interweaving myofilaments and irregular Z-bands. EM, × 29,400. By courtesy of Dr K.P. Dingemans.

Fig. 12.13 Marked interstitial fibrosis (blue-green). Mallory's trichrome stain.

Fig. 12.14 Histology of hypertrophic cardiomyopathy: intramural coronary artery with hypertrophic media and muscularization leading to luminal narrowing. E-VG stain.

Restrictive cardiomyopathy

This restricted form of cardiomyopathy is characterized functionally by a loss of ventricular compliance. The left ventricle is resistant to filling and demands high diastolic filling pressure. Systolic function is normal.

Cardiac amyloidosis long served as the classical example of restrictive cardiomyopathy. The current definition, however, dictates that amyloidosis is categorized as a 'specific heart-muscle disease'. Nevertheless, this disorder may be one of the most important conditions to be excluded; endomyocardial biopsies may be helpful in this respect. Furthermore, disease characterized primarily by loss of systolic force, such as dilated cardiomyopathy, may eventually be further complicated by loss of compliance, this occurring consequent to myocardial injury and interstitial fibrosis. Thus, dilated cardiomyopathy may eventually turn into a restrictive type of cardiomyopathy. This is yet another example of the deficiencies of the current classification of cardiomyopathy. Indeed, loss of compliance and systolic force may represent extremes of a spectrum of myocardial lesions. Clinical characteristics of both may occur in some patients with end-stage cardiac disease. This has been designated collectively as 'mildly dilated cardiomyopathy'.

Presently, the 'typical' example of restrictive cardiomyopathy is characterized by a heart of normal size but with ventricular cavities that are markedly obliterated by extensive endocardial thickening (Fig. 12.15). The apparatus of the atrioventricular valves is usually included in the obliterative change. Histology reveals endomyocardial fibrosis (Fig. 12.16). These changes probably represent 'end-stage' disease. At earlier stages, the disease may be characterized by an inflammatory process, with an eosinophilic cellular infiltration often accompanied by an early proliferative endocardial reaction (Fig. 12.17). These abnormalities may be revealed in endomyocardial biopsies.

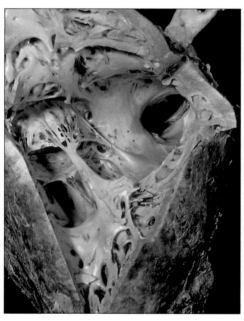

Fig. 12.15 Opened right ventricular outflow tract in a heart with restrictive cardiomyopathy caused by endomyocardial fibrosis. There is endocardial thickening with partial obliteration of the right ventricular apex.

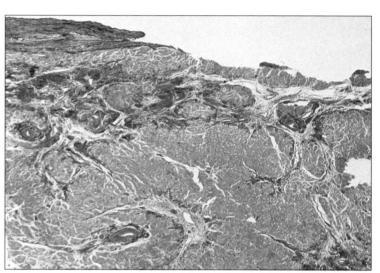

Fig. 12.16 Histological section of left ventricular wall in endomyocardial fibrosis showing fibroelastic thickening of endocardium and fibrosis extending into myocardium. E-VG stain.

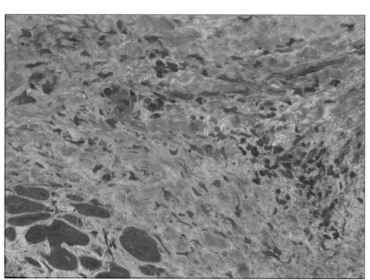

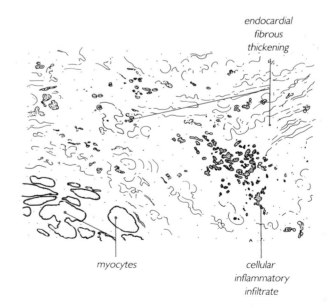

endocardial fibrous thickening

myocytes

cellular inflammatory infiltrate

Fig. 12.17 Endomyocardial biopsy in restrictive cardiomyography. There is endomyocardial thickening which contains an inflammatory cellular infiltrate.

Apart from this 'classical' histopathological picture, |cases do occur with none of these features; instead, the pathology is dominated by extensive interstitial fibrosis (Fig. 12.18). Such examples may reflect end-stage disease of a disorder which, initially, may have presented as heart failure of unknown cause.

Arrhythmogenic right ventricular dysplasia

Arrhythmogenic right ventricular dysplasia is characterized by excessive fatty infiltration of the myocardium, particularly in the right ventricle. Sites of predilection occur in the right ventricular inflow, particularly in its inferior border, in the apex of the right ventricle, and in the anterior wall of the right ventricular infundibulum. The condition is important because of its association with ventricular arrhythmias and sudden death.

The gross appearance of the heart is that of fatty replacement of the myocardium (Fig. 12.19). Microscopical studies will reveal that the myocardium has been extensively replaced by fat (Fig. 12.20). The disease is not restricted to the right ventricle, but may also extend into the left ventricle (Fig. 12.21). The aetiology and pathogenesis of this condition remain as yet unclear (see Fig. 11.1).

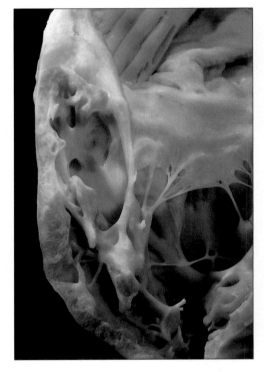

Fig. 12.19
Arrhythmogenic right ventricular dysplasia. Inferior wall of right ventricle showing almost total replacement of myocardium by adipose tissue.

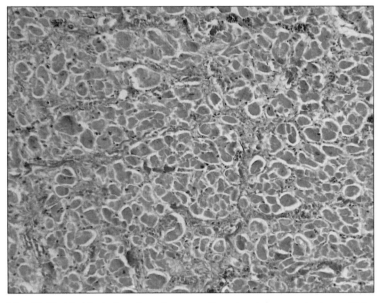

Fig. 12.18 Histological section of myocardium showing extensive interstitial fibrosis. The patient presented the clinical picture of 'restrictive cardiomyopathy'. (EVG stain.)

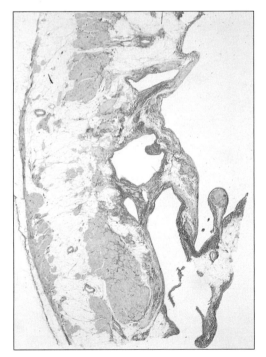

Fig. 12.20
Histological aspect of ventricular wall in arrhythmogenic right ventricular dysplasia. Islands of myocardium are still present amidst fat tissue. (EVG stain.)

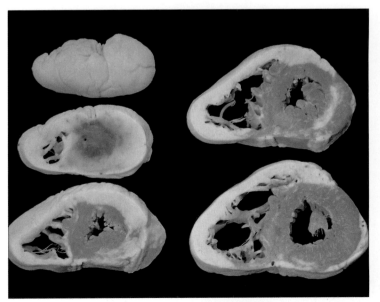

Fig. 12.21 Arrhythmogenic right ventricular dysplasia. Cross sections of heart show extension of fatty tissue into left ventricular myocardium, apart from extensive right ventricular involvement.

The affect of pressure/ volume load

ACQUIRED CONDITIONS PRIMARILY
AFFECTING PRESSURE/VOLUME LOAD

13 ACQUIRED CONDITIONS PRIMARILY AFFECTING PRESSURE/VOLUME LOAD

Among the cardiac conditions that primarily affect the pressure or volume load of the heart, valvar pathology ranks highest. In general terms of functional pathology, a valve can either be stenotic or insufficient, although a combination of the two is common. Valvar pathology on the left side of the heart may have a profound effect on the pulmonary vascular bed as well as affecting the right side of the heart (see Section 3). Abnormalities of the valves of the right heart may also affect the left heart, but usually to a lesser extent.

The types of prevailing valvar abnormalities differ from one part of the world to another and even within the West important shifts in prevalence have occurred over the past decades. Rheumatic valvar disease, for instance, has become less of a problem, whereas conditions such as prolapse of the mitral valve and age-related valvar diseases (see also Chapter 15) have gained in significance. Infective endocarditis, in previous decades a disease of young people with pre-existing cardiac pathology, has veered markedly towards the elderly patient without a history of heart disease. Iatrogenic cardiac disease, moreover, can no longer be considered a bagatelle.

IMMUNE-RELATED VALVAR HEART DISEASE

Under this heading we will discuss auto-allergic diseases such as systemic lupus erythematosus, rheumatoid arthritis and rheumatic fever. The pathology that results from the latter is collectively known as rheumatic valvar disease.

Rheumatic valvar disease

In the Western part of the world the significance of rheumatic disease is declining thanks to early prevention, although in many other parts of the world rheumatic fever remains prevalent and is still a major disabling condition. Among the auto-allergic diseases rheumatic fever is the most important as far as the heart is concerned. It is generally considered that, following an infection of the throat, auto-allergy is elicited by cross-reactivity between the membrane antigen determinants of ß-haemolytic streptococci, and certain proteins present in the heart. Recurrent attacks may thus produce repeated episodes of injury and repair. When located in the valves, these eventually result in scar formation and functional impairment. Interstitial myocardial fibrosis is of less clinical significance than the valvar malformations that eventually ensue.

In the acute stage, the injury causes an inflammatory reaction dominated by oedema. Fibrinoid necrosis of connective tissues and a cellular reaction may occur. The valvitis leads to verrucous deposits of fibrin along the line of closure of the leaflets (Fig. 13.1), indicating a process of traumatic injury secondary to forceful closure. This observation is relevant since the deformities that eventually lead to cardiac disability show preference for those valves that sustain the highest pressures. The frequency with which the different valves are said to be involved depends upon the type of investigation. Pathological studies usually report a higher incidence than do clinical reports. Nevertheless, the mitral valve is by far the most commonly affected, although the combined involvement of mitral and aortic valves is the most frequent.

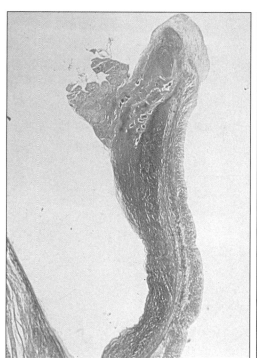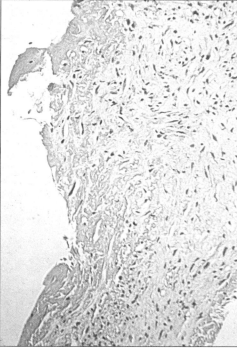

Fig. 13.1 Histology of the aortic valve in acute rheumatic fever: (left) verrucous fibrin depositions at site of closure; (right) fibrinoid necrosis with cellular reaction. E-VG (left), H&E (right) stains. By courtesy of Dr C.C. Lenox.

The healed stage of rheumatic valvar disease (often referred to as 'chronic') is characterized by deformities representing a longstanding and continuous process of injury and repair.

The mitral valvar apparatus is usually seriously affected by fibrosis of the leaflets, fusion of commissures and fibrosis of cords with obliteration of the intercordal spaces (Fig. 13.2). As a consequence, the normally high mobile valve is transformed into a rigid, irregularly thickened and funnel-like structure. The principal orifice is narrowed and displaced into the left ventricular cavity. These features are well demonstrated in a long-axis section (Fig. 13.3).

The degree and extent of the changes varies from one individual to another. Cases can occur with retraction of the leaflets as the dominant pathology (Fig. 13.4) and insufficiency as the main clinical feature, whilst in other cases, commissural and cordal fusion dominate the pathology (Fig. 13.5), with stenosis the prevailing clinical consequence. In advanced cases with extreme commissural fusion and funnel-like adherence of leaflets and cords, particularly when further aggravated by valvar calcifications, simple commissurotomy brings little relief. The same applies to the long term effects of balloon valvoplasty, which basically can be considered to represent commissurotomy.

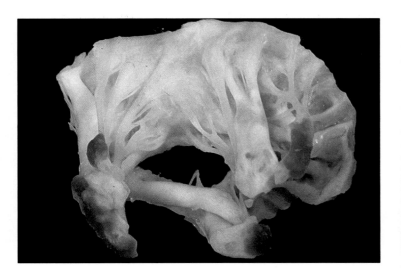

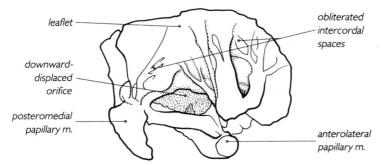

leaflet

downward-displaced orifice

posteromedial papillary m.

obliterated intercordal spaces

anterolateral papillary m.

Fig. 13.2 Resected and stenotic valve in chronic rheumatic valve disease showing fibrosis of leaflets and cords and fusion of commissures.

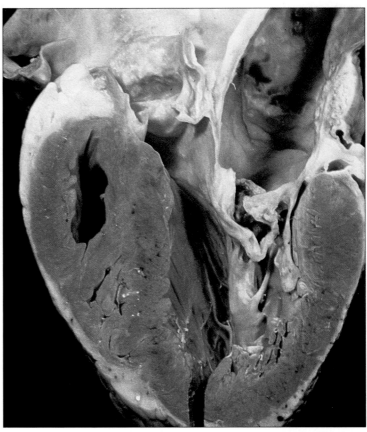

Fig. 13.3 Long-axis section showing funnel-shaped stenosis of a rheumatic mitral valve.

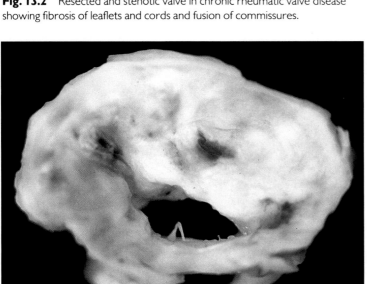

Fig. 13.4 Atrial view of resected rheumatic mitral valve showing retraction of the mural leaflet as the dominating feature producing insufficiency.

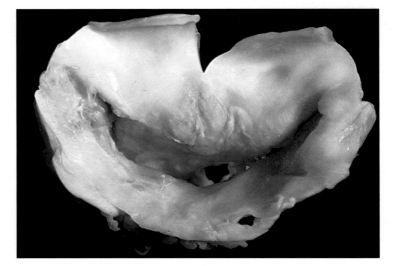

Fig. 13.5 Atrial view of resected rheumatic mitral valve showing commissural and cordal fusion as the dominating pathology producing stenosis.

In many instances, the basal part of the leaflet adjoining the aortic root is less affected and still pliable and transparent (Fig. 13.6). This part of the leaflet may thus produce a convexity towards the left atrium and, for a long time, ensure efficient closure of the valve despite advanced rheumatic involvement

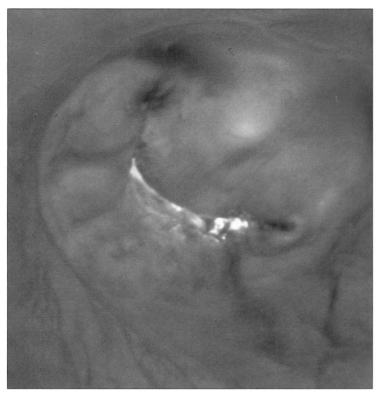

Fig. 13.6 Atrial view of rheumatic mitral valve showing its crescent-shaped orifice. Transillumination from the ventricular side shows the preserved transparency of the basal aspect of the aortic leaflet.

with retraction of the leaflets. The corvexity should not be confused with prolapse (see below). Even in the presence of severe disease the shape of the aortic leaflet is essentially preserved, whereas the usual scalloping of the mural leaflet tends to disappear, leaving a semicircular fibrous shelf (Fig. 13.6). The growth of relatively large-calibre vessels into the leaflet illustrates the inflammatory nature of the valvar deformity (Fig. 13.7). Contrary to common belief, however, this feature is not diagnostic of rheumatic disease.

Clinical rheumatic disease of the mitral valve, itself produced over a long period of time, is usually associated with an enlarged left atrium. In cases of longstanding insufficiency the left atrium can be huge. The endocardium is often corrugated and calcifications are common (Fig. 13.8). The deformed valve may show dystrophic calcifications with a preference for the commissural sites, in particular the posteromedial commissure. The calcific deposits may invade the junctional attachment of the leaflets and the adjacent myocardium, and a calcified rheumatic valve may coexist with so-called calcified mitral ring (see Chapter 15). The calcific deposits occur predominantly on the ventricular side of the valve, but occasionally they erode the atrial surface (Fig. 13.9). Thrombosis adherent to such exposed calcifications is common and may be a source of thromboembolism. Restenosis following commissurotomy carries a high incidence of dystrophic calcification as a late complication. Calcific embolization can also occur, although rarely with mitral valve disease. The dilated left atrium can be largely filled with mural thrombosis but the pulmonary venous channels are usually preserved (Fig. 13.10). Massive left atrial thrombosis occurs more frequently with mitral stenosis than with mitral insufficiency. Thrombus of the left atrial appendage is almost always present when rheumatic mitral disease is complicated by atrial fibrillation. Thromboembolism may then become a serious complication.

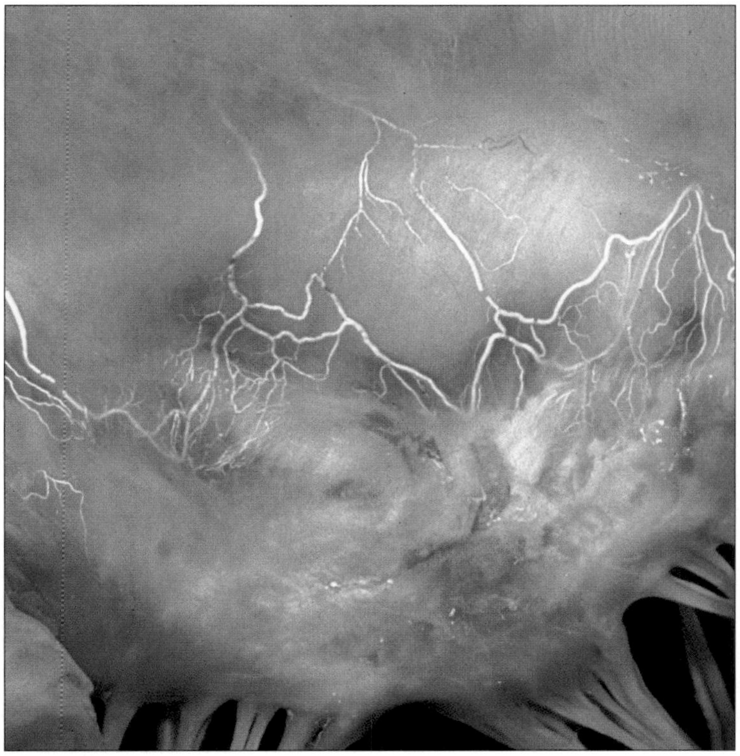

Fig. 13.7 Rheumatic mitral valve with extensive vascularity. The vessels have been injected with barium.

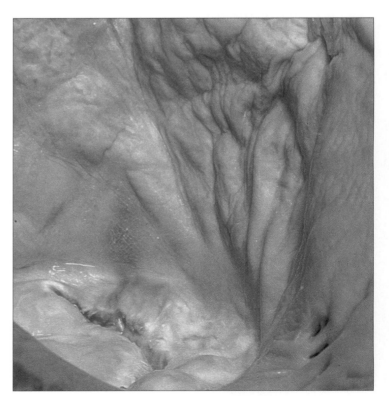

Fig. 13.8 Rheumatic stenosis of the mitral valve and huge dilatation of the left atrium with corrugated endocardium containing calcifications.

Right ventricular hypertrophy is a common cardiac consequence, being particularly outspoken in hearts with pure mitral stenosis. In such cases the marked right ventricular hypertrophy contrasts strikingly with the non-hypertrophied left ventricle (Fig. 13.11) and is followed by right atrial dilatation. Atrial fibrillation is a common, though non-specific, clinical finding.

The aortic valve exhibits similar changes to those in the mitral valve. The pathology is dominated by fibrosis and commissural fusion, often eccentric in nature (Fig. 13.12) and calcification may accompany these changes. Eccentric commissural fusion may mimic a congenitally bicuspid aortic valve with a raphé in the conjoined leaflet. However, close inspection will usually

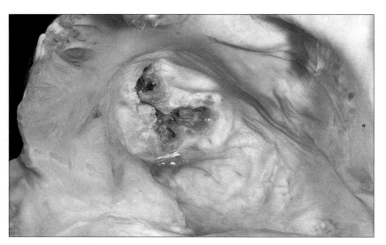

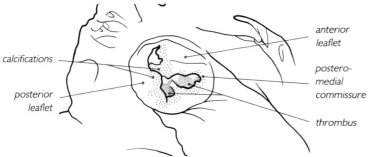

Fig. 13.9 Rheumatic mitral valve showing gross calcifications extending onto adjacent leaflets. There is adherent thrombosis.

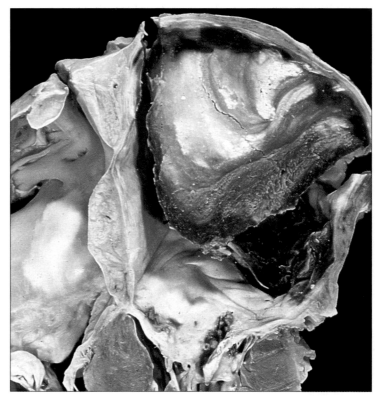

Fig. 13.10 Four-chamber section showing dilated left atrium largely filled with mural thrombosis. The pulmonary venous channels were preserved.

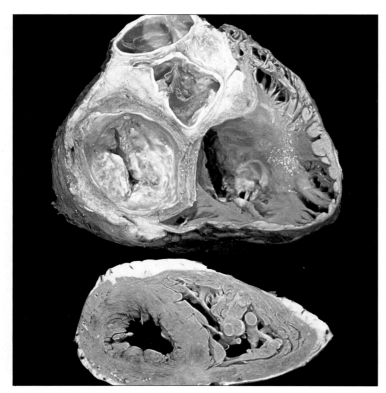

Fig. 13.11 Isolated rheumatic stenosis of the mitral valve and marked hypertrophy of the right ventricle contrasts with non-hypertrophied left ventricular wall.

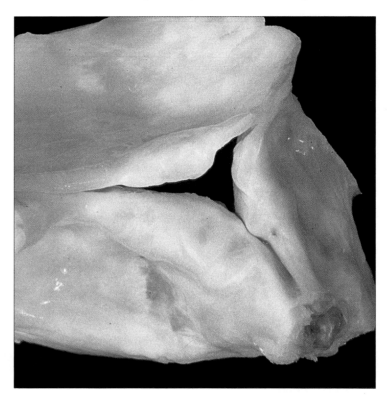

Fig. 13.12 Aortic aspect of resected aortic valve with fibrosis of the leaflets and eccentric commissural fusion with calcifications – signs of rheumatic disease.

reveal the two leaflets to be 'glued' together (Fig. 13.13). Histological sections of the commissural site show extensive fibrosis as the 'glue' (Fig. 13.14). The nature of these changes is as in the apparatus of the mitral valve, with friction between different components playing an important role.

In longstanding cases the aortic valve becomes more heavily calcified (Fig. 13.15), often with a corrugated surface and adherent thrombosis. The gross aspect of this end-stage pathology is non-specific. So-called isolated calcific aortic stenosis occurring on the basis of degenerative diseases may have a similar appearance.

The tricuspid valve, when affected, shows fibrosis of the leaflets and fusion of commissures (Fig. 13.16) very similar to rheumatic lesions affecting the mitral valve. Cordal fusion, however, is not a striking feature and calcification is exceptional. In the Western world, tricuspid stenosis is exceptionally rare as the dominating clinical feature. Tricuspid insufficiency, on the other hand, is much more common. The combination of leaflet retraction in the setting of a hypertrophied and dilated right ventricle consequent to left-sided valvar pathology may underlie this particular complication.

The pulmonary valve is only rarely involved. In the event that it is, the changes are similar to those seen in the aortic valve. The incidence of pulmonary valvar disease is probably greatly influenced by the pressure of sustained pulmonary hypertension consequent to left heart disease.

Fig. 13.13 Aortic aspect of rheumatic aortic valve showing eccentric commissural fusion. The two leaflets can still be identified.

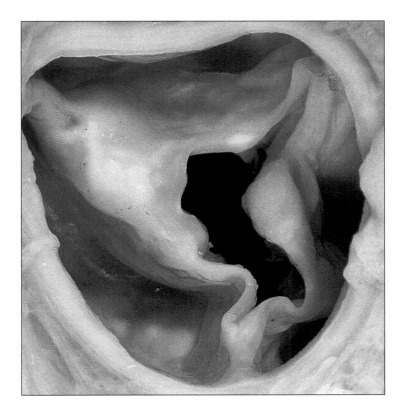

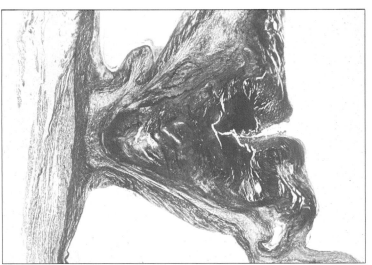

Fig. 13.14 Histological section through affected commissure showing dense fibrous tissue interposed between two leaflets at the site of commissural fusion. E-VG stain.

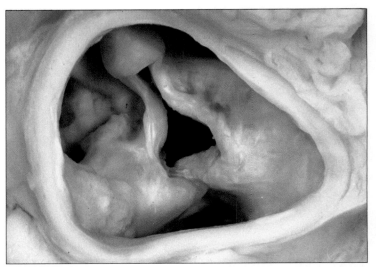

Fig. 13.15 Rheumatic aortic valve with involvement of all three commissures and more extensive calcifications affecting commissural sites as well as extending onto the leaflets.

Rheumatoid arthritis

This disease also belongs to the category of auto-allergic diseases and is characterized by the occurrence of antibodies against altered IgG. The aetiology is unknown. Like other generalized auto-allergic diseases, different organs may be involved, usually via an immune complex vasculitis, although whether this mechanism is involved in the pathogenesis of rheumatoid valvar disease remains unclear. Rheumatoid valvar disease most commonly affects the mitral valve. Involvement of the aortic valve is the next most common, followed by combined involvement of the aortic and mitral valves. Lesions of the tricuspid valve, or involvement of all four valves, are exceedingly rare. The valvar lesions are largely confined to the fibrous layers and consist either of small granulomatous lesions or areas of fibrinoid necrosis with a granulomatous marginal zone (Fig. 13.17). Fibrosis could ensue in these patients, particularly following sustained treatment with steroids.

Ankylosing spondylitis, considered a variant of rheumatoid arthritis, leads to dilatation of the aortic root and, hence, to aortic regurgitation. The valvar lesions are usually secondary to the altered haemodynamics.

Systemic lupus erythematosus

Systemic lupus erythematosus is a generalized auto-allergic disease, characterized by the occurrence of antibodies directed against a variety of auto-antigens, such as DNA, RNA, lymphocytes, complement factors and intracellular organelles. The aetiology is unknown. Pathology is induced mainly by depositions of immune complexes, and many organ systems may be involved, including the heart. One of the most important cardiac effects is acute pericarditis (see Chapter 14), but myocardial lesions also occur (see Section 5).

The pathology is dominated by a distinctive type of valvar and mural endocarditis, so-called Libman–Sacks endocarditis. This is characterized by the presence of verrucous greyish lesions along the closure line of the valves, as well as being draped along the undersurface and extending onto the mural endocardium. The lesions are composed of aggregates of fibrin and platelets. The mitral valve is most frequently affected, with the tricuspid valve a close second. Despite the fact that valvar involvement is common, haemodynamically significant lesions are rare. When reported, however, aortic and mitral insufficiency is the dominant feature. Mitral stenosis can occur, while haemodynamically

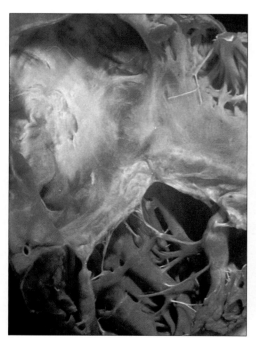

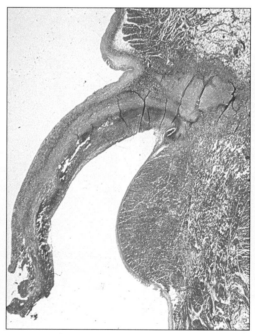

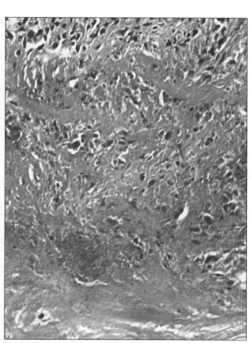

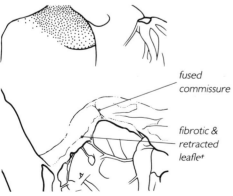

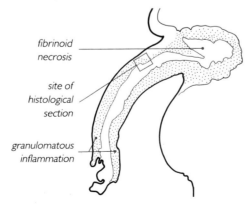

Fig. 13.16 Rheumatic involvement of the tricuspid valve includes fibrosis and retraction of leaflets together with commissural fusion. The cordal abnormalities are less striking.

Fig. 13.17 Histology of mitral valve in rheumatoid arthritis (left), fibrinoid necrosis of the fibrous layer with granulomatous marginal zone seen in detail (right). H&E stain. By courtesy of Dr F. Eulderink.

significant aortic stenosis, due to extensive thrombotic vegetations, has been described. Bacterial endocarditis may complicate the valvar lesions and spontaneous valve perforation can occur (Fig. 13.18).

The histology is characterized by fibrinoid degeneration of collagen with a marginal cellular reaction composed mainly of mononuclear inflammatory cells and fibroblasts. In itself, this is a non-specific reaction, and beyond the active stage the lesions may heal leaving fibrous scars. Treatment with steroids may change the pathologic spectrum of the cardiac lesions. Healed lesions characterized by fibrosis would dominate the picture instead of the classically described exuberant multivalvar vegetations.

FLOPPY MITRAL VALVE

In the West the waning clinical relevance of rheumatic valve disease as a cause of mitral insufficiency has led to waxing interest in an anomaly best designated as 'floppy mitral valve'. The lesion is known by a variety of names such as myxomatous mitral valve, ballooning or billowing mitral valve, prolapse of the mitral valve, mitral valve click syndrome and Barlow's syndrome.

Inaccurate definitions have led to much confusion, particularly since prolapse of the mitral valve leaflets can occur in a variety of conditions, such as ischaemic heart disease and hypertrophic cardiomyopathy. The terms 'idiopathic' and 'primary versus

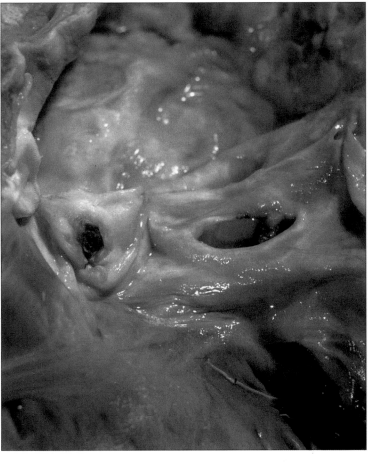

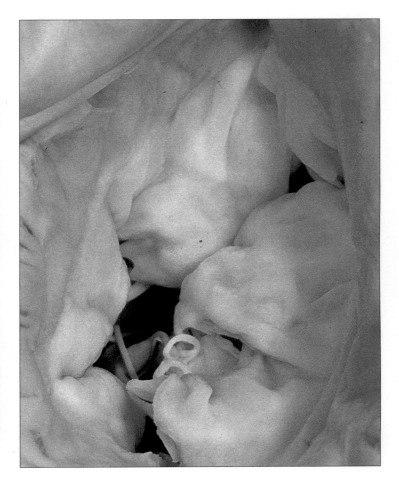

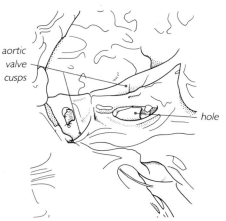

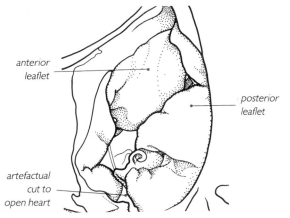

Fig. 13.18 Gross aspect of the aortic valve in a patient who had suffered systemic lupus erythematosus. The cusps show 'punched out' holes; infectious endocarditis was ruled out.

Fig. 13.19 Left atrial view of floppy mitral valve.

secondary' have been introduced to distinguish between these various forms of prolapse.

In the present context, the term 'floppy mitral valve' is used for an abnormality in the absence of a clearly identifiable aetiology. In general terms, the mitral valve shows redundant leaflets with domes projecting towards the left atrial cavity (Fig. 13.19). The domes may show a distinct overshoot producing an anatomical substrate for mitral insufficiency (Fig. 13.20). Not all mitral valves designated as floppy by the pathologist will necessarily have been insufficient during life (Fig. 13.21). Almost any part of the leaflets may be affected, although the lesion tends to concentrate around the posteromedial commissure, leaving the

anterolateral commissure and its bordering leaflets less affected (Fig. 13.21). The deformities are usually most pronounced in the mural leaflet (Fig. 13.22). The dome-shaped deformities should not be confused with the 'hoods' that occur naturally as atrial convexities of the leaflets between the sites of cordal anchorage.

The cords supporting the floppy leaflets are often attenuated, although in some areas the cords may be thickened. An abnormal lacework of cords is often present at the site of anchorage, leaving large areas of leaflet devoid of proper cordal insertions (Fig. 13.23), with cordal rupture the most common complication

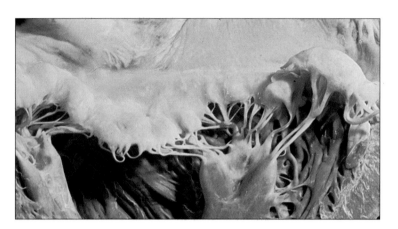

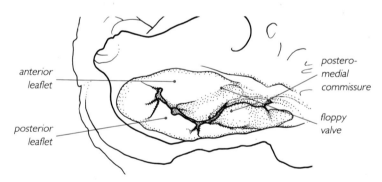

Fig. 13.20 Floppy mitral valve with overshoot of the middle scallop of the posterior leaflet unequivocally producing insufficiency.

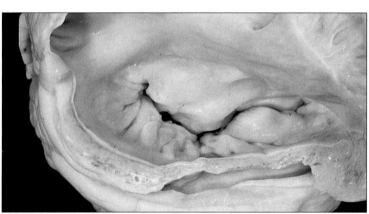

Fig. 13.21 Floppy leaflets located around the posteromedial commissure of the mitral valve but without overshoot.

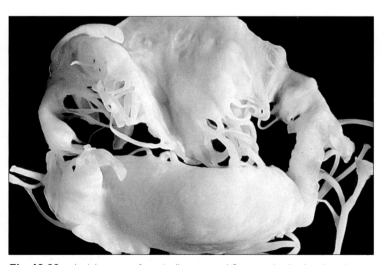

Fig. 13.22 Atrial aspect of surgically resected floppy mitral valve showing gross prolapse of middle scallop.

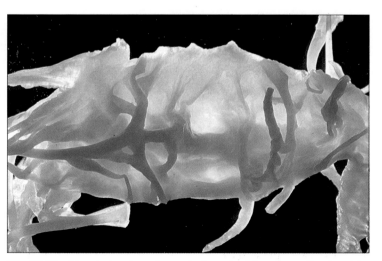

Fig. 13.23 Ventricular view of a surgically excised floppy mural leaflet of the mitral valve showing abnormally textured cords.

(Fig. 13.24). The typical history in such cases is that of a patient known for some time to have signs of a floppy mitral valve in whom a sudden onset of aggravation of mitral insufficiency occurs in the absence of signs of infectious disease. Depending upon the overall nature of the deficient cordal support, rupture may lead to minor (Fig. 13.25) or major (Fig. 13.26) prolapse.

Floppy mitral valve has been described as the underlying disease in patients with transient ischaemic cerebral attacks, although the mechanism involved remains unclear. It has also been associated with angina pectoris in the presence of normal coronary arteries with ventricular arrhythmias and sudden death.

Another association that cannot be accounted for by chance is the combination of floppy mitral valve and large atrial septal defects within the oval fossa. The abnormality of the valve tends to be confined to the area of the posteromedial commissure, suggesting lack of support as the underlying mechanism. Floppy mitral valve is also a common finding in patients with Marfan's syndrome (Fig. 13.27).

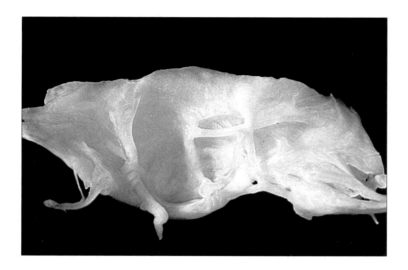

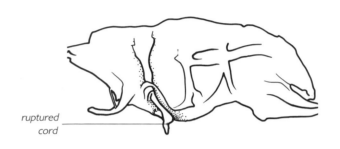

Fig. 13.24 Ventricular view of a surgically excised mural leaflet from a floppy mitral valve showing cordal rupture.

ruptured cord

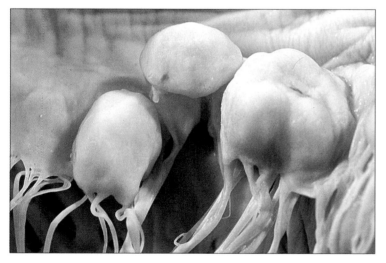

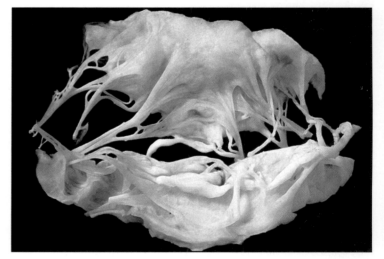

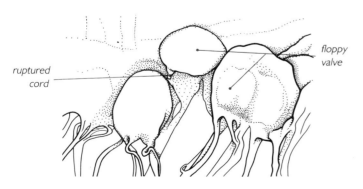

ruptured cord

floppy valve

Fig. 13.25 Cordal rupture in a floppy mitral valve showing minor prolapse.

prolapse of mural leaflet

ruptured cordae

Fig. 13.26 Left ventricular aspect of surgically excised specimen of floppy mitral valve with cordal rupture and major prolapse of the mural leaflet.

The aetiology and pathogenesis of floppy mitral valve remain controversial. Valves thus affected show an excessive accumulation of glycosaminoglycans (Fig. 13.28). The atrial aspect, moreover, may show a thickening composed of layers of collagen fibres (Fig. 13.29) secondary to regurgitant flow and abnormal friction. Different opinions emerge regarding the interpretation of these findings. Most investigators take the myxomatous change as the primary underlying cause of idiopathic mitral valve prolapse. In this respect, Marfan's syndrome serves as the paradigm.

The myxoid change observed histologically, however, could also represent an expression of a secondary event, such as prolonged or undue stress on the valvar apparatus causing accelerated collagen degradation. The observation of a wide spectrum of cordal arrangements in normal hearts, rendering parts of the leaflets less well supported than others, together with the observation that resected specimens of floppy mitral valve exhibit abnormalities in cordal anchorage, endorse the concept of a secondary mechanism as at least one of the possibilities (Fig. 13.30).

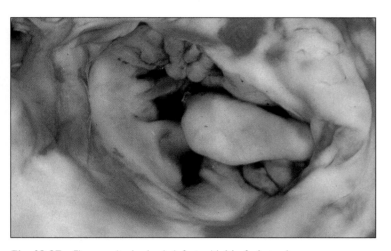

Fig. 13.27 Floppy mitral valve in infant with Marfan's syndrome.

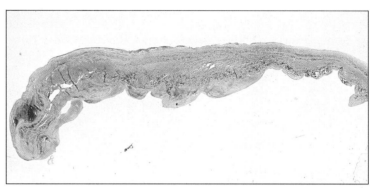

Fig. 13.28 Histological section of floppy leaflet showing excessive accumulation of glycosaminoglycans.

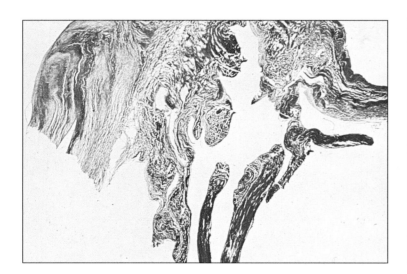

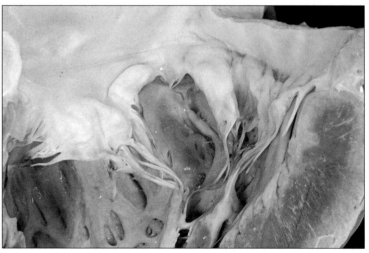

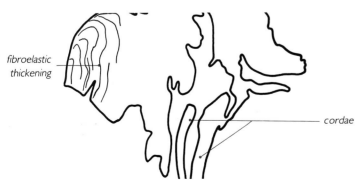

fibroelastic thickening

cordae

Fig. 13.29 Histological section of prolapsed leaflet of the mitral valve showing excessive fibroelastic tissue at atrial aspect. E-VG stain.

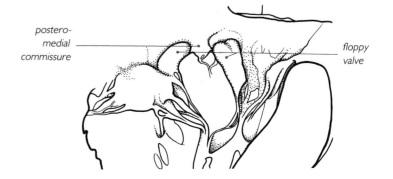

postero-medial commissure

floppy valve

Fig. 13.30 Floppy mitral valve in which the affected segment, centring around the posteromedial commissure, has almost no cordal support.

INFECTIVE ENDOCARDITIS

The term 'infective' is preferred over 'bacterial' endocarditis since it is well acknowledged that a wide variety of organisms may cause this disease. An important shift has taken place in recent years regarding the type of patient involved. In the 'old' days, infective endocarditis particularly affected patients with rheumatic valvar or congenital heart disease. Presently, the average age of the patient has markedly risen and, usually, there is no past history of heart disease. Instead, degenerative valvar changes play an important role in elderly patients, not only in cases with overt changes such as calcific aortic valvar disease or calcified mitral ring (see below), but also in patients with apparently no valvar abnormalities. The process of 'wear and tear' that affects the tissues of valves over the years may render them susceptible to infection, particularly when organisms invade the elderly patient with an altered immune-defense capacity. In valves showing such 'wear and tear' changes, the endothelial surface of the valves is altered and the line of closure

often accentuated (Fig. 13.31). More detailed histological studies often reveal adherent aggregates of fibrin and platelets. Such lesions may thus form a nidus for circulating microorganisms and form the foundation for infective endocarditis in an apparently normal valve (see also Chapter 15). At present, it is also important to consider iatrogenic causes for infective endocarditis. The number of patients with intracardiac pacemaker electrodes and prosthetic valves (see below) is ever increasing. Furthermore, since the longevity of patients with congenital heart disease has improved considerably, thanks to corrective and palliative cardiac surgery, the risk of acquiring infective endocarditis is a constant threat in this set of patients. The problem of the increasing number of drug addicts in whom infective endocarditis is a common and often fatal complication must also be faced. Whatever the background, the source of infection is not always clear. Dental and gingival infections, infections of the respiratory and urinary tracts, as well as skin infections, are still the most important primary sites. The list of micro-organisms able to produce endocarditis is enormous. For

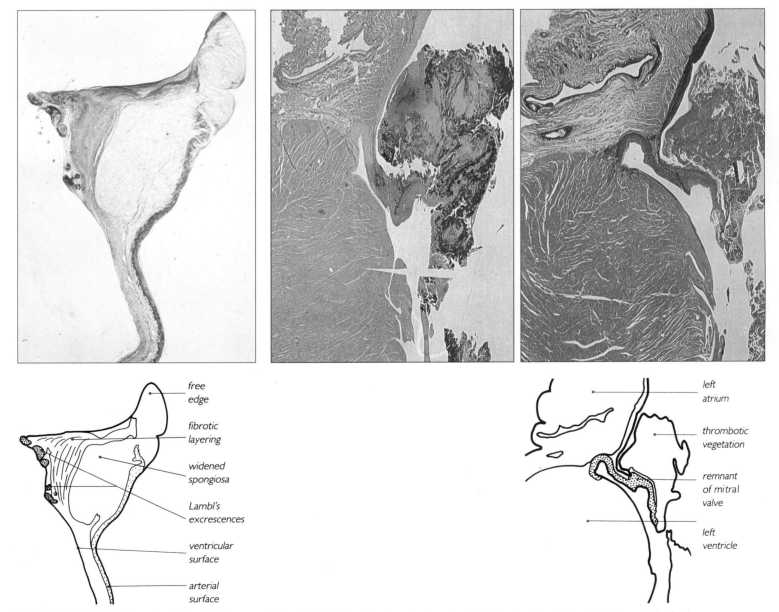

Fig. 13.31 Histological section of a leaflet from the aortic valve showing surface alterations at the site of closure. E-VG stain.

free edge
fibrotic layering
widened spongiosa
Lambl's excrescences
ventricular surface
arterial surface

Fig. 13.32 Histological section showing virtual destruction of a leaflet of the mitral valve by staphylococci. (Left) Gram stain; (right) E-VG stain.

left atrium
thrombotic vegetation
remnant of mitral valve
left ventricle

practical purposes every micro-organism (including viruses), thus far reported has the potential to produce endocarditis.

Infective endocarditis predominantly affects the valves. Mural endocarditis usually occurs as an extension from a diseased valve. Pre-existent mural endocardial changes, such as those evoked by jet or cordal friction, may occasionally underlie a primary endocarditic lesion. The left side of the heart is most commonly affected, the mitral valve having a slightly higher incidence of primary infection than the aortic valve. Tricuspid involvement is infrequent and infection of the pulmonary valve is extremely rare.

Basically, infective endocarditis is a disease that destroys the valve (Fig. 13.32). The type of micro-organisms involved, the immune state of the host, and the speed with which the disease is properly diagnosed and treated all determine the clinical course and outcome. For these reasons, a division into acute and sub-acute endocarditis is nowadays of less significance. If left un-treated, the prognosis is largely determined by the damage present when the disease is controlled. The complications of infective endocarditis can thus be classified into destructive

effects on the valve, invasive effects onto neighbouring cardiac structures and septic embolic effects. A late consequence of infective endocarditis occurs when the immune complexes evoked produce generalized vasculitis, with renal involvement then being a particular threat.

Infective endocarditis of the mitral valve tends to occur at its atrial surface, initially at the site of coaptation of the leaflets (Fig. 13.33). This is also the natural site for age-related changes. A thrombotic mass usually adheres to the site of infection and often contains vast colonies of micro-organisms (Fig. 13.32). This is one of the reasons why high doses of intravenous anti-biotics are mandatory if they are to be effective at those sites. The infection may easily spread onto adjacent parts of the leaflet (Fig. 13.34) as well as onto the cords. Cordal destruction can then lead to prolapse of the affected leaflet and massive mitral insufficiency (Fig. 13.34). Eventually, the central part of the leaflet may be completely destroyed, leaving a hole amidst infected tissue (Fig. 13.35). When cured at this stage, subsequent valve replacement is almost always necessary (Fig. 13.36).

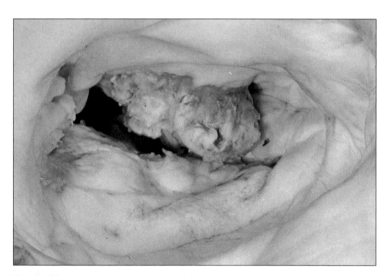

Fig. 13.33 Infective endocarditis of the mitral valve showing destruction of atrial aspect, predominantly on the aortic leaflet, with adherent thrombosis.

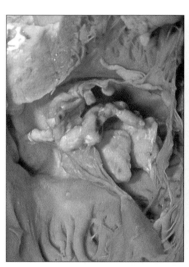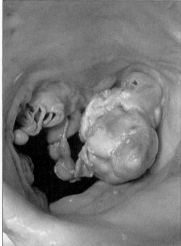

Fig. 13.34 Infective endocarditis of the mitral valve with cordal rupture: (left) left ventricular view; (right) left atrial aspect with prolapsing leaflets at the posteromedial commissure.

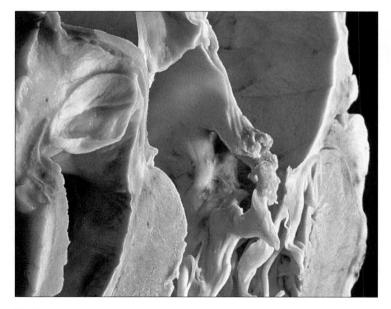

Fig. 13.35 Infective endocarditis: destruction of a leaflet of the mitral valve in active stage with defect amidst infected tissue.

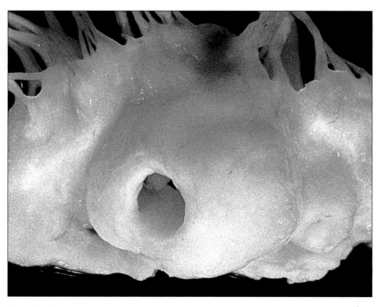

Fig. 13.36 Infective endocarditis of the mitral valve: surgically resected aortic leaflet with 'healed' lesion.

Calcific mitral ring is notably prone to infection (see also Chapter 15). The abnormal morphology and function renders the valve vulnerable to infection, for instance along its free edge and atrial surface (Fig. 13.37). The undersurface of the valve, which contains the degenerative calcific process (see Chapter 15), is also in jeopardy (Fig. 13.38). An infection at the annulus carries a poor prognosis since it may easily lead to the formation of an abscess (Fig. 13.39) which is often difficult to diagnose and treat. Pericarditis and death readily ensue. The development of pericarditis in any patient with clinical signs of an infectious disease of unknown nature should always raise the possibility of infective endocarditis.

Infective endocarditis of the aortic valve tends to occur on the ventricular aspect, again with the line of closure as the usual site (Figs 13.31, 13.40). For full understanding of the ensuing complications, it is necessary to have a complete knowledge of the topography of the aortic root (see also Chapter 1). The infection may spread anteriorly into the epicardium in the angle

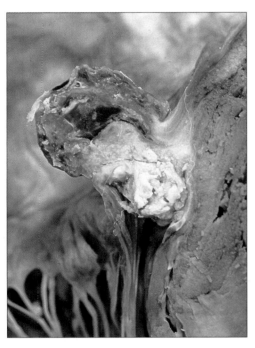

Fig. 13.37 Infective endocarditis on atrial aspect of the mural leaflet of the mitral valve complicating calcification of the ring.

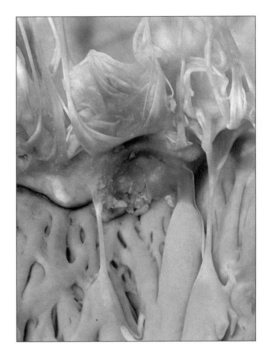

Fig. 13.38 Infective endocarditis at the site of calcification of the ring of the mitral valve showing the infected angle between the leaflet and the ventricular wall.

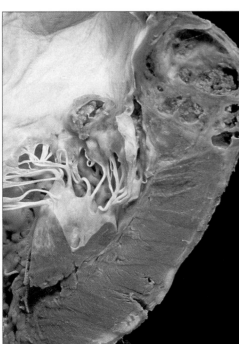

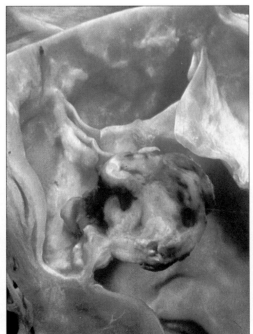

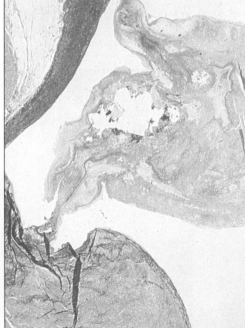

Fig. 13.39 Infective endocarditis: ring abscess of the mitral valve extending into epicardial fat tissue. The atrial aspect of the valve is eroded.

Fig. 13.40 Infective endocarditis of the aortic valve: (left) leaflet with thrombotic vegetation; (right) histology revealing destruction of the leaflet. E-VG stain.

between the right ventricular outflow tract and the zone of aortic–mitral valvar fibrous continuity (Fig. 13.41). It may give rise to an epicardial abscess in this location, with consequences as described for an abscess of the mitral ring. The infection may also spread into the right ventricular outflow tract (Fig. 13.42) as well as to the right (Fig. 13.43), and left atrial walls. The axis of atrioventricular conduction tissue may become involved, with production of heart block. The infection may then spread directly onto the ventricular surface of the adjoining mitral valvar leaflets (Fig. 13.44). Infective endocarditis of the aortic valve may thus result in infective mitral valvar disease. The occurrence of mitral insufficiency in the clinical setting of aortic valvar endocarditis is difficult to evaluate, even with sophisticated echocardiographic techniques, because aortic valvar endocarditis in itself can produce mitral insufficiency as a consequence of left ventricular dilatation and papillary muscle dysfunction.

The regurgitant and infected flow through a damaged aortic valve can lead to infection of the mitral valve at more remote sites (Fig. 13.45). Moreover, superficial spread on the left ventricular septal surface may lead to selective damage of the left

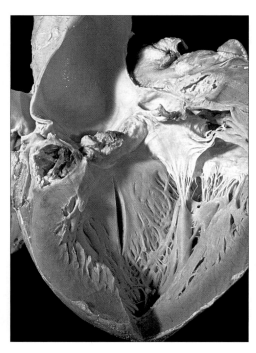

Fig. 13.41 Infective endocarditis of aortic valve leading to an abscess in the aortic root.

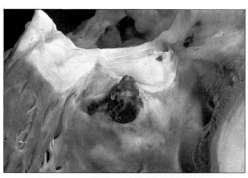

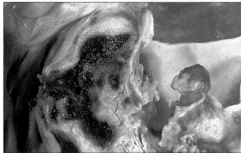

Fig. 13.42 Infective endocarditis of the aortic valve, which has perforated into the outflow tract of the right ventricle (upper); section showing root of spread (lower).

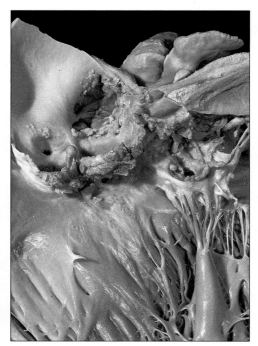

Fig. 13.43 Extension of infective endocarditis from the aortic valve into the right atrium.

Fig. 13.44 Direct spread of infective endocarditis from the aortic onto the mitral valve.

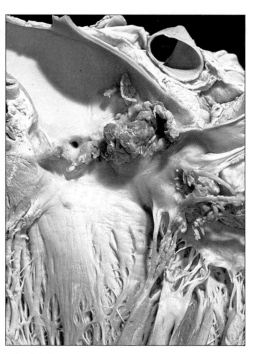

Fig. 13.45 Infective endocarditis: distant involvement of the aortic leaflet of the mitral valve and its cords. Note the unaffected segment of leaflet beneath the infected aortic valve.

bundle branches and, hence, to partial or complete left bundle branch block (Fig. 13.46). As with infective endocarditis of the mitral valve, the infection may have destroyed the valve so extensively prior to cure that replacement becomes necessary. In some patients, the disease may take a fulminant course resistant to medical treatment which necessitates surgical replacement of the valve in the acute stage (Fig. 13.47). As previously stated, septic emboli are a frequent complication. In our autopsy series all patients who died in the setting of aortic valve infection had septic myocarditis (see also Section 5). This is particularly relevant when instituting appropriate treatment during life.

Infective endocarditis of the tricuspid valve is increasingly seen as a complication of drug addicts (Fig. 13.48). It is a misconception to think that other valves are not, or only rarely, affected in such individuals. Infection of the septal leaflet, which is located close to the membranous septum, may easily spread to the atrioventricular node and penetrating atrioventricular bundle. Disturbances of atrioventricular conduction may thus appear as an early complication. The signs and symptoms of infection of the tricuspid valve are different from those that occur with left-sided endocarditis. Septic embolization into the lungs cause recurrent pulmonary infections and should alert to infection of the tricuspid valve, particularly in young individuals.

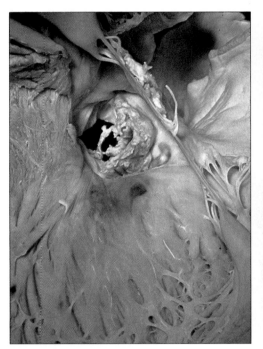

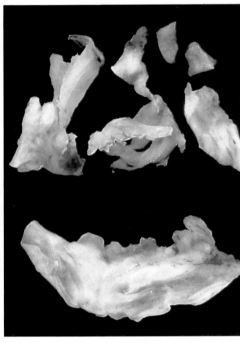

Fig. 13.47 Surgically removed aortic valve showing acute phase of bacterial endocarditis.

Fig. 13.46 Infective endocarditis of the aortic valve spreading onto the left ventricular surface and producing left bundle branch block. Note involvement of the mitral valve.

Fig. 13.48 Infective endocarditis of tricuspid valve in a known heroin addict.

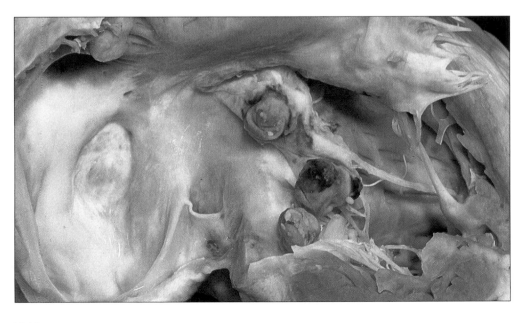

DEGENERATIVE PATHOLOGY OF THE AORTIC VALVE

Degenerative disease of the aortic valve is of major clinical importance. The lesions found are almost always heavily calcified (Fig. 13.49), hence the often used term 'isolated calcific aortic valvar' disease. In approximately half of the patients, the aortic valve is congenitally malformed, either bicuspid or (rarely) unicuspid in nature, while the remainder show a normal aortic valve with three leaflets. The common denominator in each category is degeneration of tissues as part of a process of wear and tear (see below). Dystrophic calcification occurs as a secondary effect (Fig. 13.50).

The unicuspid aortic valve is usually intrinsically stenotic and is one of the common forms of aortic stenosis in the very young (see also Section 4). Nevertheless, isolated stenosis of this type may occur in adult patients, the average age at which symptoms occur being approximately 40 years. The oldest patient we have seen with stenosis of a unicuspid valve was 69 years old.

Congenitally bicuspid aortic valves are not usually intrinsically stenotic. The vast majority of such valves encountered in adults and first recognized at autopsy contain gross calcific deposits.

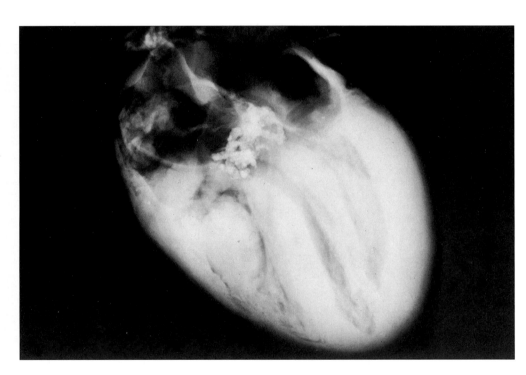

Fig. 13.49 Postmortem radiograph showing isolated pathology of the aortic valve.

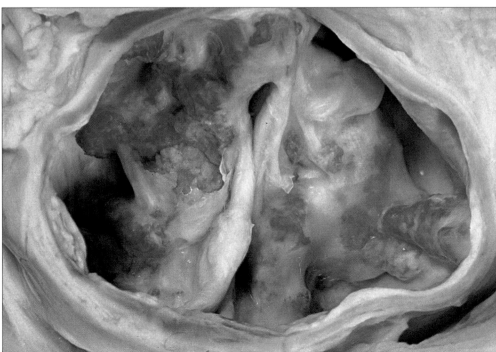

Fig. 13.50 Calcific stenosis due to a congenitally unicommissural and unicuspid valve in a male patient 69 years of age.

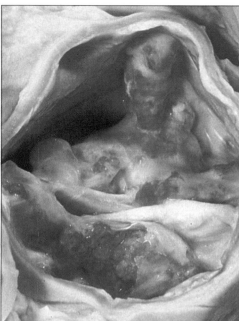

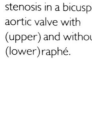

Fig. 13.51 Calcific stenosis in a bicuspid aortic valve with (upper) and without (lower) raphé.

These valves are rigid and non-pliable, irrespective of whether or not there is a conjoined leaflet with a raphé (Fig. 13.51).

As previously indicated, isolated pathology of the aortic valve also occurs in the aortic valve with three leaflets (Fig. 13.52), usually in patients over 65 years of age. The underlying degenerative changes in these valves again relate to a process of wear and tear. In the congenitally unicuspid and bicuspid aortic valves, enhanced degeneration is caused by the excess in pressure load on a single leaflet. In aortic valves with three leaflets, variations in size of the individual leaflets occur as a rule (Fig.

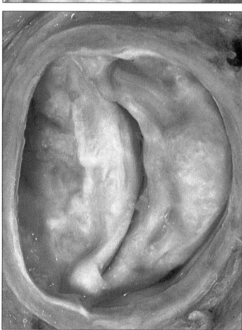

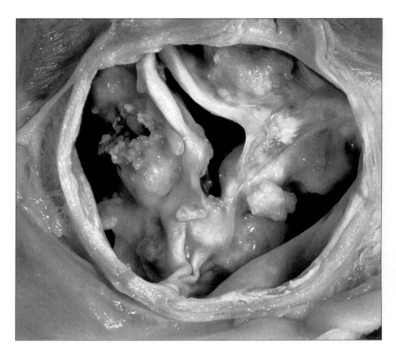

Fig. 13.52 Isolated calcific stenosis of the aortic valve in which the basically trifoliate nature is still recognizable; calcifications on the aortic sides of the leaflets are typical of age-related valvar pathology.

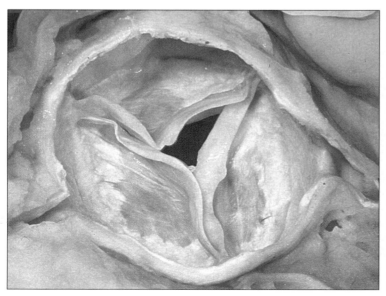

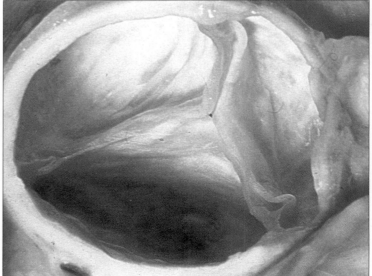

Fig. 13.53 Non-stenotic aortic valves: (left) three leaflets of almost equal sizes; (right) marked differences in sizes of the leaflets, the left coronary leaflet being tiny.

13.53). Hence, there is an unequal distribution of forces exerted on the leaflets both in diastole and systole. This fact provides the anatomical basis for enhanced 'wear and tear'.

Degenerative disease of the aortic valve usually results in stenosis and sudden death is well-known when the stenosis is severe. Death may be unexpected, particularly in the elderly patient, because the valvar pathology had passed unnoticed, once more emphasizing the enormous capacity of the myocardium for adaption (see also Chapter 3). Indeed, colossal left ventricular hypertrophy is always present, but usually it is accompanied by signs of ischaemic myocardial damage (Fig. 13.54), thus providing a basis for sudden death.

Occasionally, signs of valvar insufficiency can be found in the presence of a heavily fibrotic and calcified valve (Fig. 13.55). Nonetheless, the incidence of valvar insufficiency as the dominant feature of degenerative disease of the aortic valve in elderly patients is low. Infective endocarditis, on the other hand, is by no means an infrequent complication (Fig. 13.56).

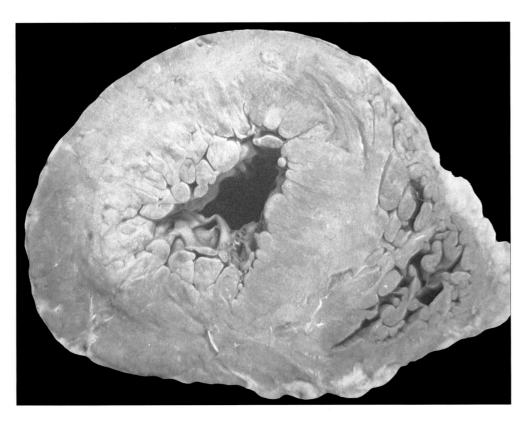

Fig. 13.54 Left ventricular hypertrophy in isolated calcific stenosis of the aortic valve exhibiting ischaemic changes confined mainly to the subendocardial zone.

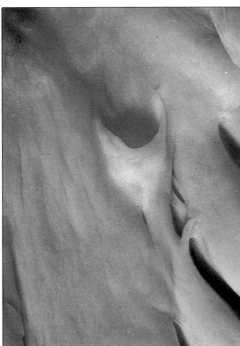

Fig. 13.55 Discrete endocardial fibrous pocket on the left ventricular aspect of the septum indicating insufficiency of the aortic valve.

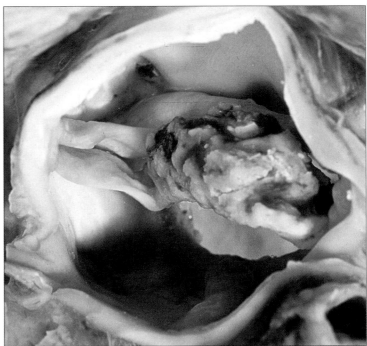

Fig. 13.56 Infective endocarditis of a congenitally bicuspid aortic valve with destruction of the base of the anterior leaflet. Calcifications are absent.

VALVAR AND ENDOCARDIAL PATHOLOGY: MISCELLANEOUS LESIONS

Acquired abnormalities of the cardiac valves and mural endocardium occur with a variety of diseases. It is beyond our scope to attempt a full account of all such abnormalities. Disease of the aortic valve producing significant symptoms may occur in patients suffering from such diverse diseases as syphilis, ankylosing spondylitis, Ehlers–Danlos syndrome or idiopathic and non-inflammatory dilatation of the aortic root. The common denominator in all these conditions is a widening of the aortic outflow tract at the level of attachment of the leaflets. Depending on the underlying disease, the leaflets themselves may either be transparent and non-pliable or somewhat fibrosed, but, in almost all instances, the free edges of the leaflets are rolled.

Syphilis

In the West, the chronic stage of syphilistic aortitis is of minor clinical significance at present. The disease is characterized by fibrosis and retraction of the leaflets with the commissures being slightly opened (Fig. 13.57, left). The aortic side of the commissure may be compromised by a prominent hyaline plaque (Fig. 13.57, right). Occasionally, these plaques fuse in circular fashion.

Non-inflammatory dilatation of the aortic root

The largest single cause of clinically significant aortic regurgitation is idiopathic and non-inflammatory dilatation of the aortic root. The disease is characterized by an increase in the diameter of the aortic root at the level of the peripheral attachments of the commissures (Fig. 13.58). The immediate cause of insufficiency in these instances is prolapse of the leaflets which, in time, leads to fibrous thickening of their free edges (Fig. 13.59). Dilatation of the ascending aorta a few centimetres above this level is a common feature in the elderly and has no effect on the function of the aortic valve.

The pathogenesis of this important disease remains, as yet, enigmatic. The similarities with classical Marfan's disease has led to the supposition that non-inflammatory dilatation is a *formes fruste* of Marfan's syndrome. There is no firm scientific basis for this concept, despite the fact that isolated dilatation of the aortic

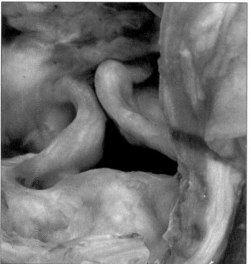
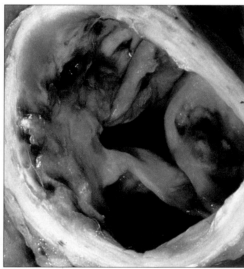
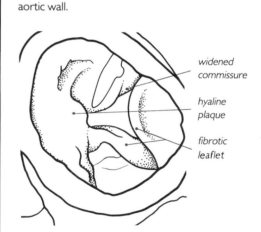

Fig. 13.57 Aortic root in syphilis: (left) typically widened commissures; (right) hyaline plaque on aortic wall.

widened commissure

hyaline plaque

fibrotic leaflet

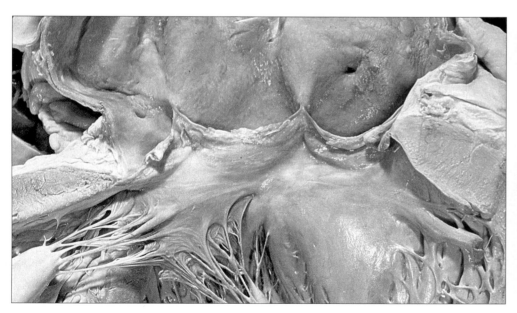

Fig. 13.58 Dilatation of the aortic root.

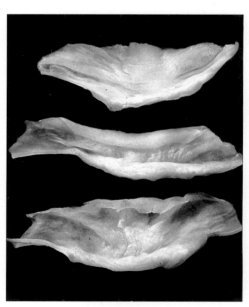

Fig. 13.59 Surgically excised leaflets of the aortic leaflets showing rolled free edges.

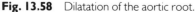

root may occur among relatives of patients with classical Marfan's disease. The histological findings in the aortic root show various degrees of fragmentation of elastic and collagen fibres, with accumulation of glycoaminoglycans. Such changes, from a histological point of view, indicate a process of injury and response of the aortic wall rather than being specific for any particular disease such as Marfan's syndrome. Since the disease shows a positive correlation with age, it is tempting to speculate that haemodynamic factors, associated with the altered geometry of the left ventricular outflow tract in the elderly, play a role in causing early degeneration of the supporting tissues.

Aortic valvar insufficiency may appear as a complicating feature in patients suffering from mitral insufficiency of various causes. Surgically excised valves from such cases show no appreciable pathology other than the changes mentioned above. A chronic and undue pull on the leaflets of the aortic valve via the aortic leaflet of the mitral valve in a dilated left ventricle may be the underlying pathogenetic mechanism.

Marfan's syndrome

Marfan's syndrome requires a full discussion because valvar pathology is one of its major manifestations. The disease is characterized by the production of an abnormally structured collagen-like protein and, hence, affects the integrity of the supportive tissues. These features play an important role in the pathogenesis of all its cardiovascular complications. Dissecting aneurysm of the aorta, dilatation of the aortic root and excessive laxity of the valvar leaflets leading to insufficiency are the most common abnormalities which affect the heart. Indeed, Marfan's syndrome is the classical example of prolapse of the leaflets of the mitral valve consequent to a floppy change (see Fig. 13.27). Usually, in addition to the floppy leaflets, the orifice of the mitral valve is markedly dilated. Aortic valvar insufficiency in these patients is then due to prolapse of the leaflets and dilatation of the aortic root, the leaflets showing extreme laxity (Fig. 13.60). Dissecting aneurysm of the ascending aorta may cause or aggravate aortic valvar insufficiency as a direct consequence (Fig. 13.61). Rupture of a dissecting aortic aneurysm into the pericardial cavity leads to cardiac tamponade. It is the second most frequent form of acute haemorrhagic pericardial effusion and death, following rupture of the free wall of the left ventricle (see Section 5). The dissecting haematoma may also cause narrowing of the orifices of the coronary arteries, particularly the right, with myocardial ischaemia and infarction as a result. This feature may compromise the clinical differentiation between dissecting aneurysm and acute myocardial infarction.

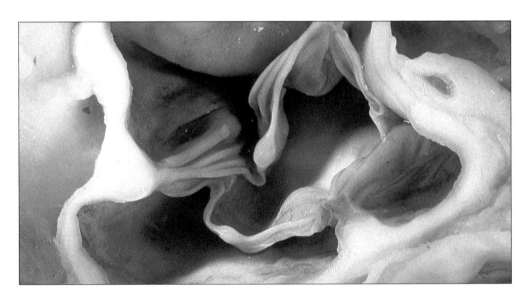

Fig. 13.60 Dilatation of the aortic root with floppy leaflets in Marfan's syndrome.

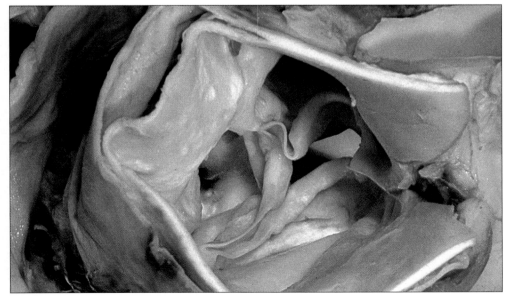

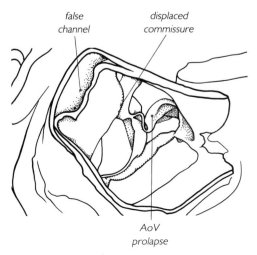

Fig. 13.61 Aortic dissection; an intramural haematoma has displaced the commissure leading to prolapse of leaflets and valvar insufficiency.

false channel   *displaced commissure*

AoV prolapse

Thrombotic endocarditis

Non-bacterial thrombotic endocarditis is another example of pathology afflicting the valves that may accompany a variety of diseases. The condition is known under various names of which 'non-bacterial thrombotic endocarditis' and 'marantic endocarditis' are the most widely used. The entity is characterized by verrucous and thrombotic vegetations adherent to the site of the closure of the valvar leaflets (Fig. 13.62). The mitral valve is most commonly affected, followed by the aortic valve and combined lesions involving the aortic and mitral valves. The tricuspid and pulmonary valves are rarely involved. The condition may easily be mistaken for infective endocarditis. Close observation, nonetheless, will show that the leaflets themselves are unaffected (Fig. 13.62) apart from alterations to their surface that occur with advanced age (see Chapter 15). Non-bacterial thrombotic endocarditis, however, may form the nidus for infection in the presence of circulating micro-organisms and when the immune status of the patient is compromised. The size and extent of the vegetations varies considerably. In some cases, the thrombotic mass may cover the full circumference of the line

of closure, giving the impression of functional stenosis (Fig. 13.63).

Non-bacterial thrombotic endocarditis occurs predominantly in patients with a malignant disease. Tumours of the prostate, ovaries, pancreas, stomach and testis appear especially prone to producing these lesions, although they may coexist with any other tumour, as well as with non-tumorous diseases. As a rule, non-bacterial thrombotic endocarditis does not lead to clinical symptomatology. Its presence is usually an incidental autopsy finding. Thromboembolic complications, particularly in the cerebral vessels, can be the first sign of its presence. Similarly, thrombotic occlusions of the coronary arteries, both epicardial and intramural, may occur. Myocardial infarction is then a complication.

Non-bacterial thrombotic endocarditis is considered part of a more generalized 'pre-thrombotic state' of the blood, typified by a chronic form of intravascular clotting. The relation between hypercoagulability and malignancy is well founded. As a consequence, thrombotic arterial occlusions in these patients may be part of 'spontaneous' thrombosis rather than embolism, with the lesions on the valves as the prime source.

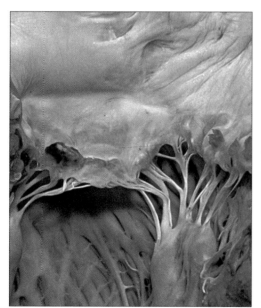
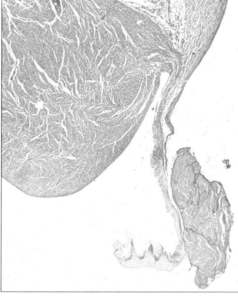

Fig. 13.62 Non-bacterial thrombotic endocarditis on the mitral valve: (left) thrombotic vegetations located along the line of closure; (right) histology shows thrombus adherent to an intact leaflet. E-VG stain.

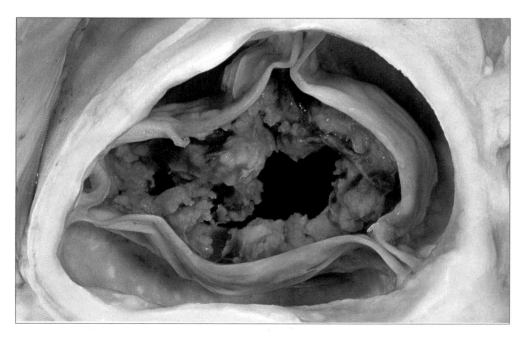

Fig. 13.63 Extensive non-bacterial thrombotic endocarditis narrowing the orifice of the aortic valve.

Carcinoid heart disease

The heart is involved in approximately half the patients who have a carcinoid tumour with metastatic spread. The right side of the heart is predominantly affected, although the mitral valve is involved occasionally. Carcinoid involvement of all four heart valves has been described in association with deficiency of the oval fossa. Carcinoid lesions appear as white plaques that cover the valves or the mural endocardium. The leaflets of the tricuspid (Fig. 13.64, left) and the pulmonary (Fig. 13.64, right) valves thus become markedly thickened, often with retraction and muscular ingrowth. The lesions are not usually confined to the leaflets but extend onto the tendinous cords and the mural endocardium related to the valves. Tricuspid insufficiency and pulmonary stenosis are common clinical findings.

Histologically, the carcinoid lesions are composed of relatively acellular 'young' fibrous tissue, sharply delineated from the underlying endocardium. The endocardium and valvar leaflets themselves are normal. The lesions are characteristically superimposed on the ventricular aspect of the atrioventricular valves and the pulmonary side of the arterial valve (Fig. 13.65). The composition of the lesions may differ slightly from one case to another, varying from an acellular ground substance with a few spindle-shaped cells as the dominant feature to a predominantly collagenous aggregation, thus reflecting the age of the proliferative lesion. Ultrastructurally, the proliferating cells are shown to be smooth muscle-like cells or myofibroblasts. The pathogenesis of the carcinoid lesions remains unclear as yet.

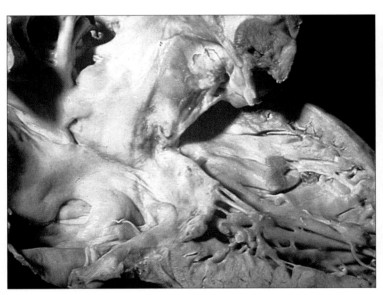

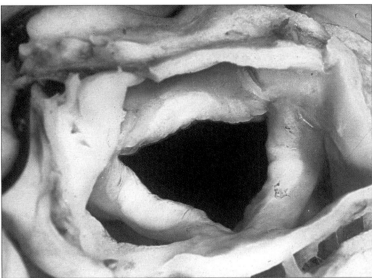

Fig. 13.64 Carcinoid heart disease: marked thickening of the leaflets of the tricuspid (left) and pulmonary valves (right).

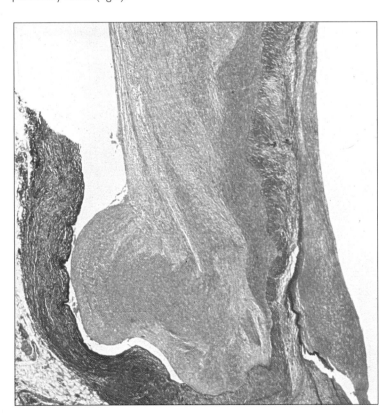

Fig. 13.65 Histological section of a leaflet from the pulmonary valve in carcinoid heart disease showing deposition of fibrous tissue, mainly localized in the sinus; the leaflet is basically normal. E-VG stain.

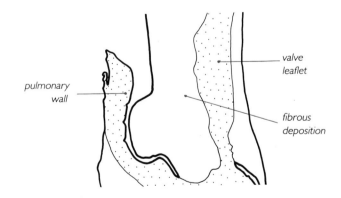

PATHOLOGY OF PROSTHETIC VALVES

The success of replacement of cardiac valves is greatly influenced by pre-existent pathology. Conditions such as a heavily calcified valve with extensive myocardial involvement, or massive myocardial hypertrophy with a small ventricle, may necessitate adjustments of technique during surgery. The preoperative state of the heart, and optimalization of myocardial preservation during the procedure, are widely accepted as key factors determining the outcome. Clinicians and pathologists alike should be aware of the complexity of the issue when confronted with pathology afflicting prosthetic valves.

Valvar dysfunction

Dysfunction can be due to a variety of causes. In the early days, variance in the size of the ball due to absorption of lipids was a serious problem. The ball turned yellow and became pliable. Fragmentation would occur (Fig. 13.66) with peripheral emboli-zation of fragments or, occasionally, of the ball itself (Fig. 13.67). The incidence of these complications has drastically fallen with improvements in the manufacturing process of the occluders and poppets. Local problems, nonetheless, such as calcific deposits at the base of the valve or formation of rings of fibrous tissue (Fig. 13.68) still pose a problem and, on occasion, cause postoperative prosthetic valvar dysfunction.

Ventricular geometry plays an important role, particularly since the indications for replacement of a valve are no longer dependent upon age. The geometry of the left ventricle, particularly the shape of its outlet, changes with age. Indeed, important moulding occurs within the outflow tract. A subaortic septal bulge is almost invariably present in the elderly person (Fig. 13.69). In addition, the angle between the planes of the orifices of the mitral and aortic valves is less obtuse than in the young. These features together create a setting in which the orifice of the mitral valve tends to face the ventricular septum rather than the apex. This alteration may jeopardize the success of valvar replacement. Use of caged-ball prostheses in the mitral position

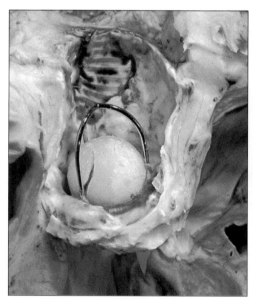
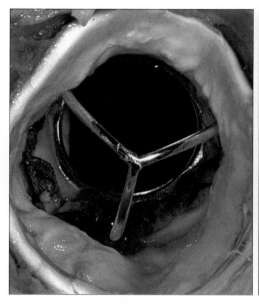

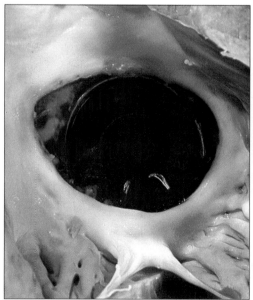

Fig. 13.66 Surgically inserted ball valve. The fragmented ball is yellow because of infiltration of lipids.

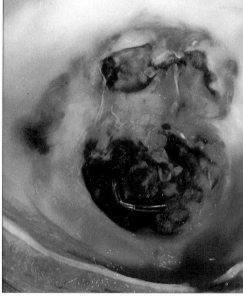

Fig. 13.67 Embolism from a caged-ball valve prosthesis: (left) empty cage; (right) ball lodged in abdominal aorta at the iliac bifurcation.

Fig. 13.68 Valvar dysfunction: (left) fibrous ring underneath disc hampering its proper function; (right) atrial aspect of the same prosthetic valve covered by organized thrombus.

has long been known to involve the risk of obstruction to the outflow tract (Fig. 13.70), while septal friction can lead to endocardial fibrosis and, occasionally, septal laceration. The alterations in geometry may also affect the use of other types of artificial valves (Fig. 13.71). Even disc valves may show dysfunction because of an intimate relation between the disc and septum (Fig. 13.72). Prosthetic valvar dysfunction may then trigger the onset of thrombosis, particularly when the dysfunctioning valve is in mitral position (Fig. 13.73). Eventually, the valve may become virtually immobilized by organized thrombus covering its atrial aspect (Fig. 13.68, right). Thrombosis of a prosthetic valve, however, can also occur as a late phenomenon in the agonal state, and is not necessarily related to the principal cause of cardiac deterioration. It is important, therefore, to distinguish these processes.

The main concern regarding the use of bioprostheses is their durability. Dysfunction due to calcification of the leaflets is well documented. This phenomenon is particularly likely to occur in young patients. Biochemical changes of collagen, in part induced by the pretreatment with glutaraldehyde together with deposition of thrombi, play a major role in the pathogenesis of calcification. The precise mechanisms, however, remain controversial.

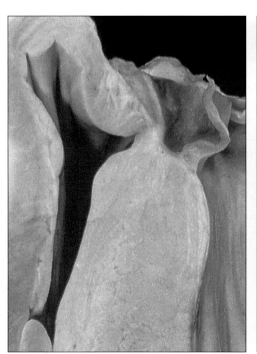

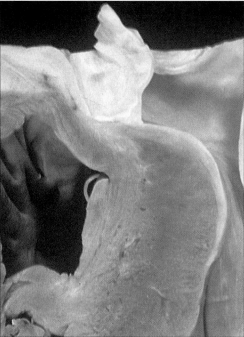

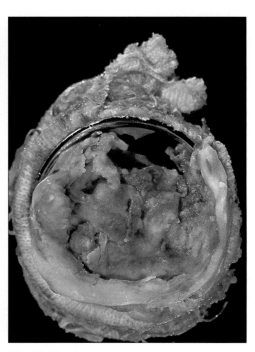

Fig. 13.69 The outflow tract from the left ventricle is almost straight in the young (left) but shows subvalvar bulging in the elderly (right).

Fig. 13.70 Caged-ball prostheses in both aortic and mitral positions. The mitral prosthesis obstructs the outlet from the left ventricle.

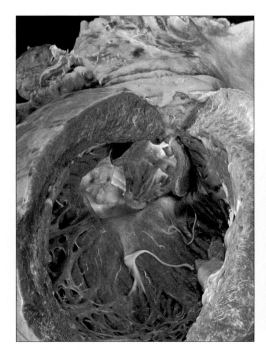

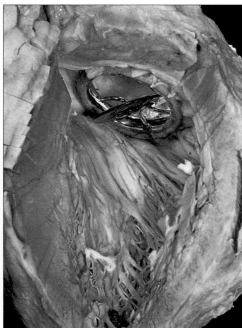

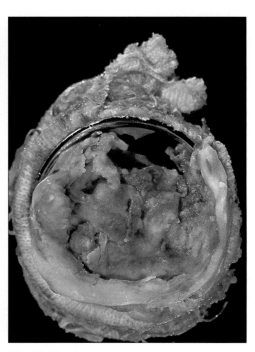

Fig. 13.71 Bioprosthesis in mitral position obstructing the outlet from the left ventricle.

Fig. 13.72 Disc valve in mitral position showing intimate contact between the disc and the ventricular septum leading to valvar dysfunction.

Fig. 13.73 Surgically excised prosthetic mitral valve almost completely covered by thrombus.

Injury and laceration

In the early period of closed commissurotomy for rheumatic stenosis of the mitral valve, the aortic or mural leaflets were sometimes split instead of the commissure (Fig. 13.74). Even when properly executed, insufficiency following commissurotomy was a problem. Restenosis was largely determined by the pre-existent valvar pathology. These complications have subsided since the introduction of open heart procedures.

Insertion of a prosthetic valve may induce myocardial laceration. Injuries to the atrioventricular junction are more likely in hearts with calcifications that extend into the myocardium or, in cases of pathology involving the aortic or mitral valve, onto its neighbouring valve. Removal of excess tissue to permit implantation of the prosthesis may lead to separation of the left atrium from the left ventricle, or of the aortic root from the base of the heart. Hence, false aneurysms develop at these sites. The close relation between the aortic valve and the atrioventricular conduction tissues is well recognized, and heart block following surgery on the aortic valve is extremely rare. Transverse ventricular disruption is an important, though often concealed, complication (Fig. 13.75). Hearts with chronic rheumatic disease of the mitral valve are prone to this form of injury. Direct surgical trauma is unlikely. The pathogenetic mechanism promoted is that of disruption of an important functional longitudinal binder by detachment of the papillary muscles from the mitral valve, thus permitting stretch damage to the myocardium.

A particular type of injury is the occurrence of perioperative myocardial infarction. Improved techniques for myocardial preservation have minimized this risk. Direct injury to coronary arteries can occur, but this complication is extremely rare. The circumflex artery is especially at risk when replacing a diseased mitral valve with extensive calcification of the atrioventricular junction (Fig. 13.76).

Stenosis of a prosthetic valve in the aortic position is an important cause of postoperative low cardiac output (Fig. 13.77) when the diameter of the aortic root is too small for the prosthesis inserted. Undue stretch of the aortic root, moreover, transforms the orifices of the coronary arteries into narrowed slit-like structures (Fig. 13.78). Myocardial perfusion is then further jeopardized. Since preoperative assessment of the size of the aortic root may prevent this complication, and with improving experience in handling these conditions at surgery, this form of pathology is becoming less significant. In some patients, nonetheless, primarily those with prosthetic valves placed in both aortic and mitral position, the postoperative period may be complicated by progressive pump failure of the left ventricle which then leads to death. No apparent cause can be demonstrated at autopsy. It may well be that a similar, but more complex, situation is occurring in these cases. It should not be forgotten that, during the period of disease, the heart has adjusted to the gradually progressive changes in valvar pathology. The whole scene is abruptly changed when the surgeon creates unobstructed blood flow through the orifices. An unstable equilibrium built up over the years suddenly collapses, and the myocardium is unable to cope with the new situation at such short notice.

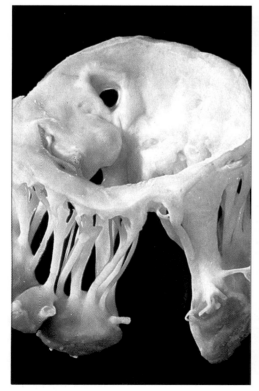

Fig. 13.74 Surgically resected rheumatic mitral valve showing a split in the aortic leaflet due to false route from previous commissurotomy.

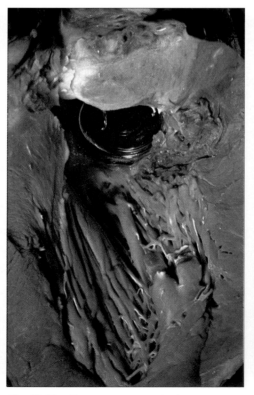

Fig. 13.75 Transverse ventricular laceration following replacement of the mitral valve.

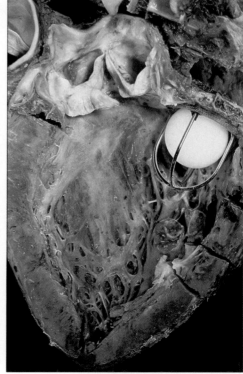

Fig. 13.76 Inferior and lateral infarction of the left ventricle produced by injury to the circumflex artery during replacement of the mitral valve.

Dehiscence of valves

Dehiscence of prosthetic valves, leading to a so-called paravalvar leak, may be an early complication. It usually results from faulty surgical technique. Small openings are mostly due to retraction of tissues from the sewing ring (Fig. 13.79). A large dehiscence almost always occurs because stitches pull apart. Pre-existent abnormalities, such as infarction or secondary infection, play an important role. In time, the edges of the paravalvar leak become smooth and lined by thickened endocardium. An endocardial jet lesion may develop secondary to the localized regurgitant flow (Fig. 13.80). Although small openings are usually considered of little clinical relevance, it is our experience that, on occasion, a small dehiscence will have important haemodynamic consequences. Thus, an annuloplasty of the tricuspid valve became forcefully disrupted when a small paravalvar leak along a prosthesis inserted in mitral position, sought but not found at operation, was left unclosed.

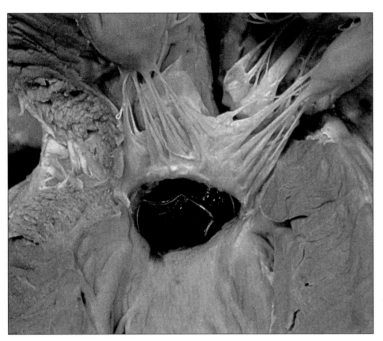

Fig. 13.77 Prosthetic valvar stenosis: a disc valve in aortic position is in excess of the diameter of the orifice.

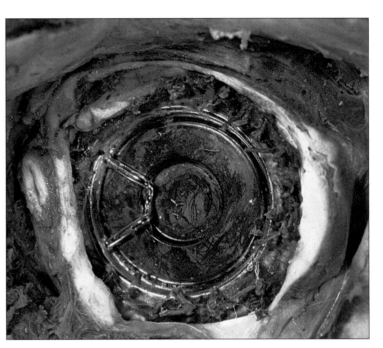

Fig. 13.78 Disproportionate prosthetic valve in aortic position leading to stretching of aortic root and slit-like transformation of the orifices of the coronary arteries.

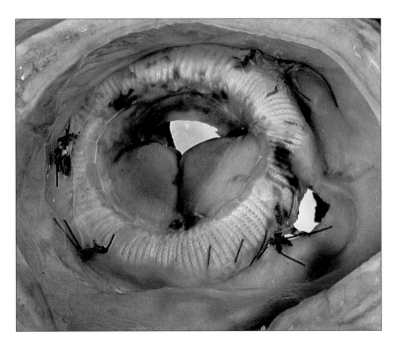

Fig. 13.79 Paravalvar leak due to dehiscence of the valvar ring.

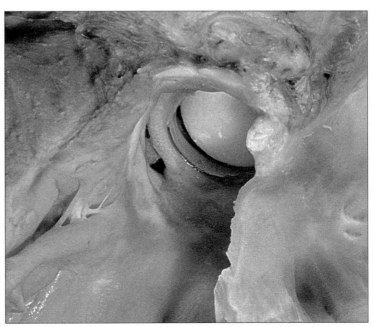

Fig. 13.80 Paravalvar leak along a mechanical valve inserted in aortic position showing an endocardial jet lesion on ventricular septum.

Infection of prosthetic valves

Any prosthetic valve is liable to endocarditis. The coating of the valve ring and sutures by platelets and fibrin serve as niduses for infection. Endocarditis of porcine xenografts almost always involves the leaflets and, most likely, develops from within the deposits of fibrin overlying their surfaces.

Hence, infection in mechanical prostheses usually leads to detachment (Fig. 13.81) and formation of abscesses in the junction, whereas disruption of leaflets is the dominating feature of infection of a bioprosthesis (Fig. 13.82).

As with infective endocarditis in general (see above), almost any organism is capable of producing prosthetic endocarditis. The infection is basically destructive in nature. The infected area is usually covered by thrombi (Fig. 13.83) which often leads to impaired function of the valve and septic thromboembolization. Mycotic aneurysms of the ascending aorta may occur, either at the site of the aortic incision or due to mechanical trauma produced by the struts of the prosthesis (Fig. 13.84). Prophylactic treatment with antibiotics is advisable in all patients who have had surgery on cardiac valves, irrespective of the type of valve inserted, whenever the patient subsequently undergoes a procedure likely to produce bacteraemia.

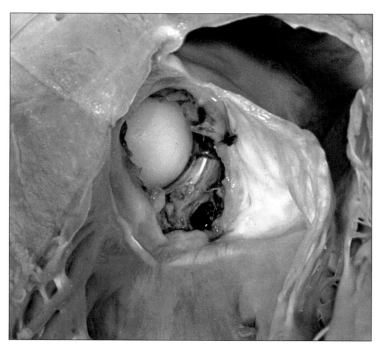

Fig. 13.81 Infection of a mechanical valve inserted in aortic position leading to dehiscence of the valve.

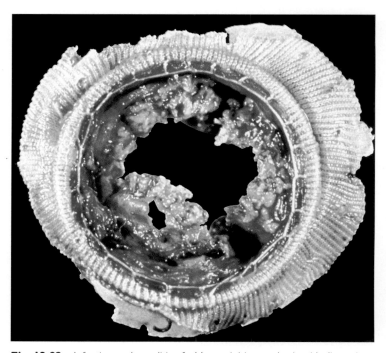

Fig. 13.82 Infective endocarditis of a Hancock bioprosthesis with disruption of the valvar tissue. By courtesy of Prof G. Thiene.

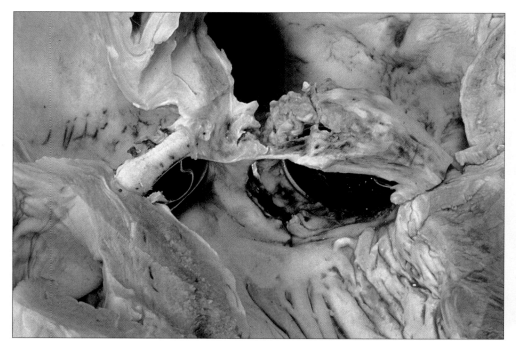

Fig. 13.83 Infection of disc valve in mitral position leading to dehiscence at the ring and excessive thrombosis covering the site of infection. Note the disc valve in aortic position.

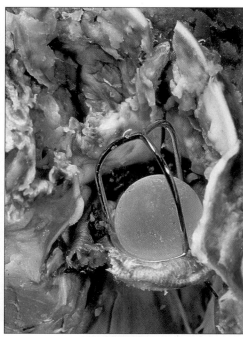

Fig. 13.84 Late infection of the ascending aorta following replacement of the aortic valve.

Miscellaneous conditions

14   PERICARDIAL HEART DISEASE

The term 'pericardial heart disease' directly associates abnormalities of the pericardium with cardiac performance. From a pathological point of view, the term 'pericarditis' is commonly used, indicating any response of the pericardium to injury, whether infectious or non-infectious.

Abnormalities of the pericardium may primarily affect either contractility or the pressure and volume load of the heart. Tumours involving the pericardium are discussed in Chapter 16.

Pericardial heart disease is commonly seen by pathologists, but the clinician is less familiar with this particular anomaly. William Osler, as early as 1892, said 'probably no serious disease is so frequently overlooked by the practitioner'. Post-mortem experience shows how often pericarditis is not recognized, or has proceeded to resolution and adhesion without having attracted notice. 'Pericardial disease', therefore, is an incidental finding, endorsing the notion that diseases of the pericardium are frequently underdiagnosed and apparently often asymptomatic.

From the viewpoint of pathology, the pericardial response to injury is limited, and is clinically dominated by the stage and extent of exudation. A fibrinous exudate is the initial reaction, although histologically non-specific. Nevertheless, it does under-lie the typical signs of pericardial friction rub. The nature and severity of the initiating injury largely determines whether the response will remain confined to the fibrinous stage, resolve completely or pass on to a more excessive stage of exudation characterized by the accumulation of fluid. In this final stage, signs and symptoms of pericardial effusion with cardiac tamponade may ensue. The nature of the disease, and the response of the host, will then determine whether there is to be complete resolution or whether a reparative response will ultimately lead to dense fibrosis with adhesion of the pericardial layers, a condition that, clinically, may result in constrictive pericarditis.

Histologically, the disease is usually non-specific and only rarely will it be possible to make a definite diagnosis regarding aetiology from a specimen of pericardial tissue. This situation is much like that found with myocarditis (see Chapter 13).

Fibrinous pericarditis

In this condition, the pericardial layers are 'glued' together by a fibrinous exudate (Fig. 14.1) which may, on occasion, totally cover the heart, giving rise to the typical 'bread and butter' appearance (Fig. 14.2).

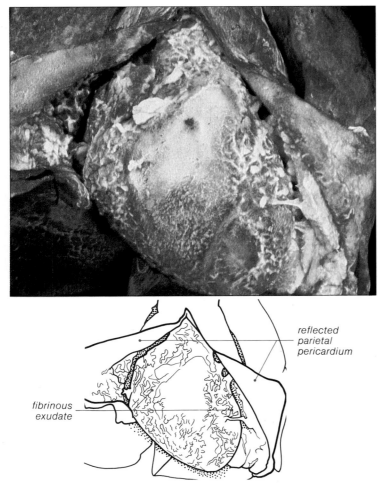

reflected
parietal
pericardium

fibrinous
exudate

Fig. 14.1   Fibrinous pericarditis.

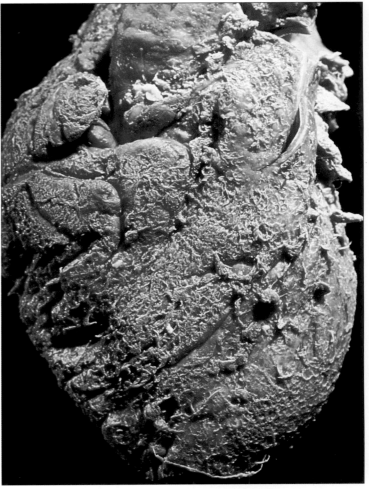

Fig. 14.2   Extensive fibrinous exudation gives rise to typical 'bread and butter' appearance.

As previously outlined, almost any pericarditis will start off with fibrinous exudation and, therefore, may be categorized under this heading at some stage. Consequently, disappearance of the friction rub may indicate that either the exudate has resolved or that it has become watery or haemorrhagic.

One of the commonest diseases underlying fibrinous pericarditis is acute myocardial infarction, and under these circumstances it is almost diagnostic for transmural infarction. In general, most diseases that cause myocarditis as the principal disorder also have the potential to evoke a pericardial response. A pericardial friction rub may, therefore, accompany almost all infectious diseases as well as most immune-related disorders that affect the heart. Consequently, the identification of fibrinous pericarditis is an important warning sign and usually indicates a more widespread cardiac involvement whilst, similarly, infective primary pericardial disease and neoplastic involvement may, in their early stages, present with the principal signs of fibrinous pericarditis (see below).

Histologically, the pericardial lesion is characterized by fibrinous deposits, often with a non-diagnostic inflammatory cellular infiltrate and prominent vascular reactivity (Fig. 14.3). It is rare to find specific signs of a particular disease at this stage.

Pericardial effusion

Any accumulation of fluid in excess of 50 ml within the pericardial cavity can be considered to represent an effusion. The amount of fluid which can lead to cardiac tamponade is largely determined by the time span in which the effusion accumulates. When accumulated rapidly, for example in cases of cardiac rupture, 250 to 300 ml are sufficient to cause fatal tamponade, although in cases of chronic pericarditis, effusions of more than one litre can occur. The nature of the effusion is important with regard to possible aetiology.

Serous fluid is characterized by its watery appearance and it is a common feature of all conditions accompanied by protracted congestive heart failure or hypoalbuminaemia. Moreover, it is the usual type of fluid encountered in patients with so-called idiopathic and recurrent benign pericarditis which is probably a disease of viral origin, with coxsackie viruses as the most likely agent. This concept is supported by the observation that a viral pericarditis with similar characteristics occurs in apes (Fig. 14.4). A particular form of serous pericarditis is so-called cholesterol pericarditis which is characterized by a high content of cholesterol in the serous fluid, and the epicardial surface may have a glistening golden appearance due to the depositions of cholesterol crystals. This form of effusion is seen in patients with hypothyroidism, rheumatoid arthritis and, occasionally, in patients with tuberculosis.

Blood as the main constituent of the pericardial effusion (Fig. 14.5) can be found with a variety of conditions and commonly dominates the pericarditis that occurs in the setting of acute

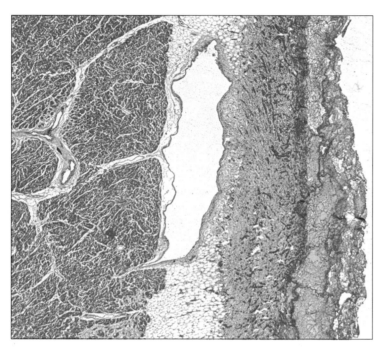

Fig. 14.3   Histology of fibrinous pericarditis showing thickened epicardium with marked vascularity and fibrinous deposition. H&E stain.

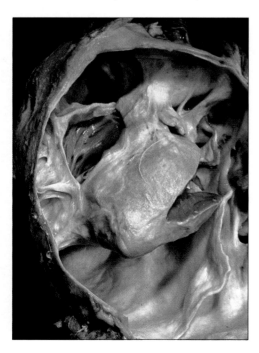

Fig. 14.4   Viral pericarditis with excessive accumulation of fluid and distension of pericardial cavity in chimpanzee.

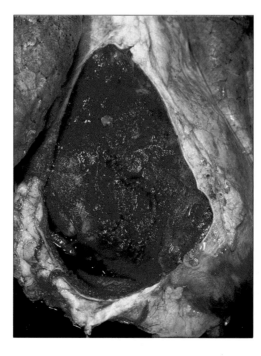

Fig. 14.5 Haemorrhagic pericarditis.

myocardial infarction, although in other settings its presence should always alert to the possibility of malignancy as the underlying disease (see Chapter 16). Tuberculous pericarditis (Fig. 14.6) and uraemia also have a high incidence of haemorrhagic effusions and, hence, should rank high in the differential diagnosis. Pericarditis may be the first sign of the underlying tuberculous infection, and proper recognition is important since the pericarditis is usually an expression of either local extension from inflamed mediastinal lymph nodes or disseminated disease. In uraemia, and particularly in patients on chronic haemodialysis, sudden haemorrhagic effusion may occur which, when accumulating rapidly, can lead to severe cardiac tamponade and, if left

untreated, to death. All diseases accompanied by clotting disorders, including iatrogenic conditions, may change a fibrinous exudate into a serosanguinous effusion.

Cardiac injury and rupture are not discussed in this section, but obviously can lead to the accumulation of pure blood.

A purulent effusion (Fig. 14.7) is an almost certain indication of infection, and in this situation micro-organisms can usually be cultured. Septicaemia, particularly in patients with deficient immunological defence, is the most common cause. Infective endocarditis may spread to involve the epicardium and is an important aetiology, at present, for purulent pericarditis (see also Chapter 13).

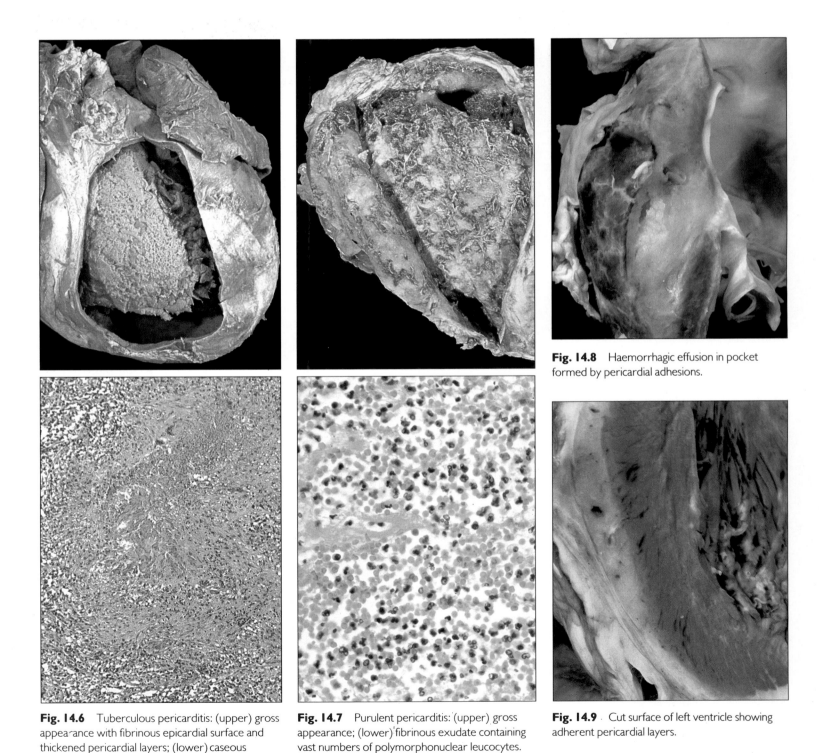

Fig. 14.6 Tuberculous pericarditis: (upper) gross appearance with fibrinous epicardial surface and thickened pericardial layers; (lower) caseous tuberculous lesion in pericardium. H&E stain.

Fig. 14.7 Purulent pericarditis: (upper) gross appearance; (lower) fibrinous exudate containing vast numbers of polymorphonuclear leucocytes. H&E stain.

Fig. 14.8 Haemorrhagic effusion in pocket formed by pericardial adhesions.

Fig. 14.9 Cut surface of left ventricle showing adherent pericardial layers.

Fibrous pericarditis

Any type of pericardial disease may eventually lead to fibrosis. This affects the epicardial and parietal layers either locally or in a diffuse manner. Of clinical importance is the situation where distinct fibrosis is associated with adhesion of the pericardial layers. This may lead to localized encapsulated areas which often contain an effusion (Fig. 14.8), and localized cardiac constriction can then occur. In other instances, large areas of the heart (Fig. 14.9), or indeed the whole heart, may become enclosed in a thick fibrous capsule. This situation has serious clinical implications.

As previously stated, constrictive pericarditis of this type can occur as a late manifestation of almost any type of pericardial disease. Clinically, the aetiology usually remains obscure, although tuberculosis and the postirradiation syndrome are particularly associated with this complication. Likewise, neoplastic involvement may lead to fibrosis of the pericardium and constriction and, in many such instances, the tumour itself encapsulates the heart (see Chapter 16). Only rarely does pericardial constriction develop as a complication of cardiac surgery, in spite of an open pericardium. Fibrosis probably results from the combined effects of trauma, haemorrhages, drying and exposure to pericardial irrigants. The postpericardiectomy syndrome (Dressler's syndrome) may also lead to constrictive pericarditis in rare cases.

Calcification may further complicate fibrous (adhesive) pericarditis. Deposition of calcium is an end-stage process and, hence, histological examination in such instances will hardly ever lead to an aetiological diagnosis, although almost any type of disease can eventually end with calcifications. The calcium deposits are sometimes spotty (Fig. 14.10), which has little clinical relevance. In other instances the calcium may encapsulate large parts of the ventricles (Fig. 14.11), and functional impairment is then the rule.

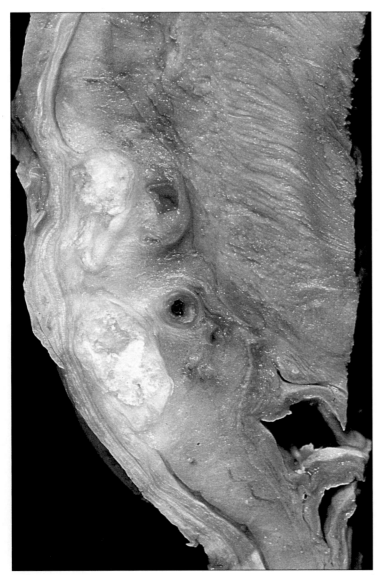

Fig. 14.10 Adhesive pericarditis with localized calcific deposits.

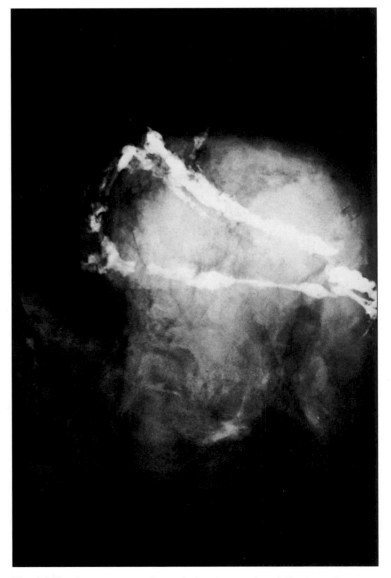

Fig. 14.11 Postmortem radiograph showing annular calcification as late result of adhesive pericarditis causing constriction.

15   THE AGEING HEART

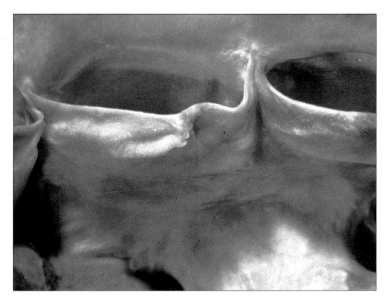

Fig. 15.1   Aortic valve of an elderly person. The line of closure is eccentrically accentuated. The leaflets are thickened due to fibrosis. Note yellowish plaques on the aortic leaflet of the mitral valve.

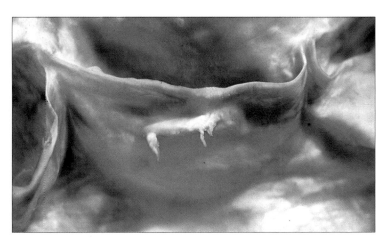

Fig. 15.2   Lambl's excrescences on the aortic valve.

In the Western world, increasing longevity has led to a corresponding waxing interest in geriatric medicine. In the heart, the most prominent ageing changes relate to the supportive tissues, that is, the fibrous skeleton and the valves.

There are many disease processes which increase in incidence with age, such as atherosclerosis, myocardial hypertrophy, interstitial myocardial fibrosis on the basis of impaired myocardial perfusion, and so-called senile cardiac amyloidosis. None of these conditions, however, can be considered an ageing process in the strict sense.

General aspects

The cardiac valves are thin and transparent at birth. With age, the atrial aspect of the atrioventricular valves and the ventricular surface of the arterial valves thicken because of fibrosis. In addition, the line of closure becomes accentuated (Fig. 15.1) with the development of so-called Lambl's excrescences (Fig. 15.2). These papillary outgrowths, composed of a fibrous core with scattered concentrically-arranged elastic fibres, are particularly prominent on the aortic and mitral valves. The tricuspid (Fig. 15.3) and the pulmonary valves are only rarely involved. These 'natural' changes have long been considered of no clinical relevance. They could, however, play a role in serving as nidi for infective endocarditis (see Section 5), and may be further aggravated by additional pathologic conditions, such as raised pressures and regurgitant flow. The development of almost tumour-like papillary lesions may occasionally happen (Fig. 15.4) and their distinction from papillary fibroelastoma (see Chapter 16) may then become almost impossible. It is extremely difficult, if not impossible, to indicate precisely, in any given individual, where the natural process of physiological ageing ends and pathology begins.

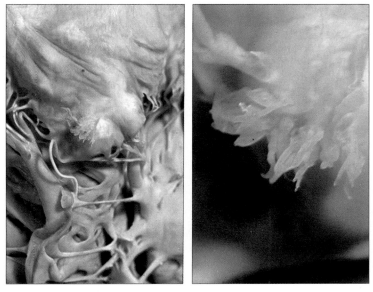

Fig. 15.3   Lambl's excrescences on the tricuspid valve: (left) general view; (right) detail.

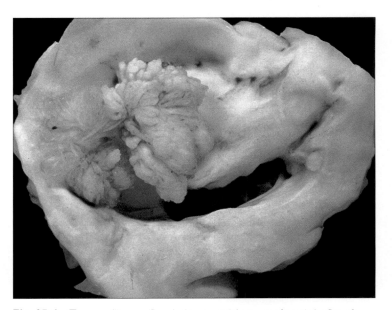

Fig. 15.4   Tumour-like papillary lesion on atrial aspect of aortic leaflet of surgically excised rheumatic mitral valve.

The aortic valve

In the elderly, valve fibrosis is often accompanied by a separation of leaflets from the aortic root along the base of their semilunar attachments. Degenerative changes occur in the supportive tissues and secondary dystrophic calcifications ensue (Fig. 15.5). This process results in spotty calcifications which are seen mainly within the sinuses, at the base and on the aortic aspect of the leaflets. The valve so affected is often described as having 'aortic valve sclerosis'. This usually has little haemodynamic consequences other than producing the harsh systolic ejection murmur which is often audible in older people. The degenerative process that causes this is generally considered to be the consequence of wear and tear and the changes are, in fact, similar to those seen in degenerative aortic valvar stenosis (see Section 5), albeit in a mitigated form. From a pathogenetic viewpoint, however, the two processes can be considered as extremes in a spectrum of ageing that affects the aortic valve and, eventually, may cause stenosis (Fig. 15.6).

The mitral valve

The mitral valve may similarly exhibit degenerative changes. These changes result in valvar fibrosis with accentuation of the line of closure (see above), but, in addition, become prominent at the 'hinge' with the ventricular wall, and at sites of insertion of tendinous cords. Lipid accumulation, often grossly visible (Fig. 15.7), is an almost constant finding at these sites in adults over 40 years of age. Histologically, moreover, marked alterations are found in the staining characteristics of the collagen (Fig. 15.8), indicating a degenerative process. This may render the tissues susceptible to calcium deposition, and the process of 'wear and tear' in the mitral valve may progress, eventually, to a stage known as calcified mitral ring. The latter condition, particularly when clinically relevant, has a distinct preference for females, although the mechanisms which underlie this increased susceptibility remain unclear.

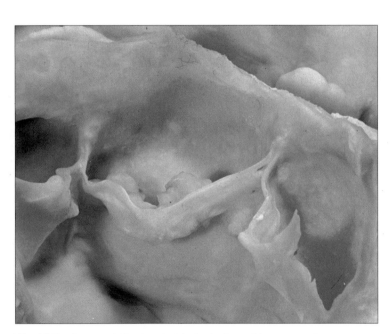

Fig. 15.5 Spotty calcifications inside the leaflets of the aortic valve cusps is a typical change in the elderly.

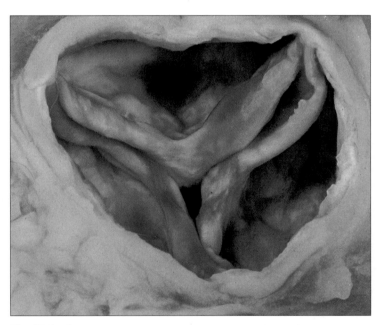

Fig. 15.6 Stenosis of the aortic valve secondary to advanced ageing changes. Note absence of commissural fusion.

Fig. 15.7 Ventricular aspect of the mitral valve at site of insertion into ventricular wall. Note spotty lipid accumulations.

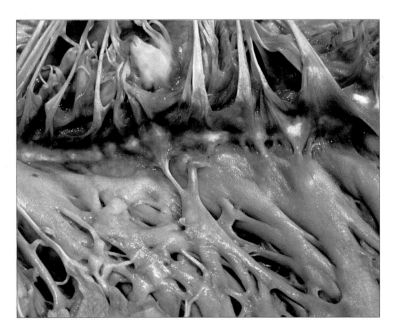

Calcification of the mitral ring in its classical form presents as a horseshoe-shaped ridge (Fig. 15.9) on the ventricular surface of the mitral valve. The calcific deposits are localized in the angle between the leaflets and the ventricular wall, and usually extend onto the valve leaflet to incorporate cordal attachments. The lesion may be confined to the middle part of the mural leaflet (Fig. 15.10) or it may extend in an almost circular fashion (Fig. 15.11). Massive calcification can occur, immobilizing the greater part of the valve leaflet (Fig. 15.12). Mitral insufficiency is the usual clinical feature under these circumstances. The calcific deposits may also extend into the myocardium of the left ventricular free wall (Fig. 15.13), and the calcified ring can show central softening, rather like a caseous abscess. It probably reflects the structural alteration in the composition of collagen, basic to the anomaly, but without much calcium deposited as yet.

Thrombosis can occur beneath the leaflets of the mitral valve, in a position which corresponds to the calcified ring (Fig. 15.14). Thrombotic deposits may eventually organize and calcify, but subvalvar thrombosis is no longer considered to be the underlying pathogenetic mechanism in the appearance of mitral calcification. The combined occurrence of calcific aortic disease and calcified mitral ring is a particularly common finding in the elderly (Fig. 15.15).

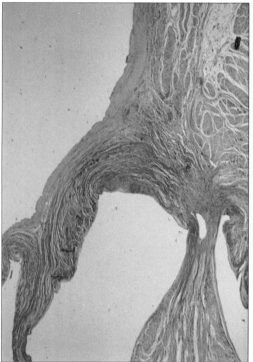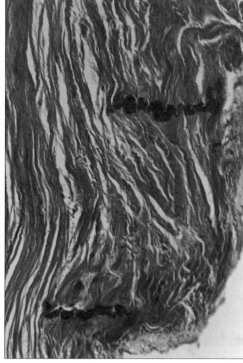

Fig. 15.8 Histological appearance of an ageing mitral valve. The left hand panel shows the valve at the atrioventricular junction. At the base of the valve leaflet, close to the insertion of a cord, irregular cross bands appear stained intensely red, as a sign of collagen degeneration. The right hand panel shows the area in more detail.

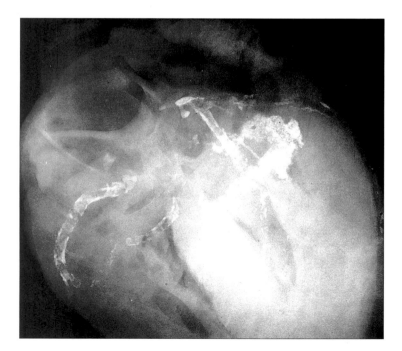

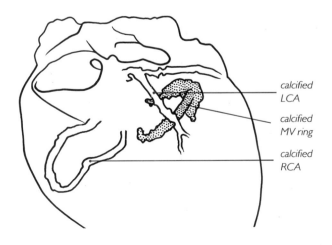

Fig. 15.9 Post-mortem radiograph showing horseshoe-shaped calcification in the mitral valve. The coronary arteries also exhibit marked calcifications of their walls.

calcified LCA

calcified MV ring

calcified RCA

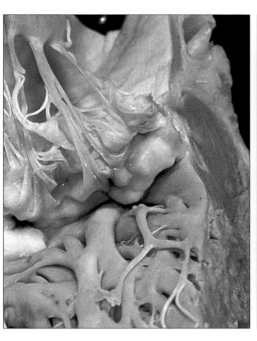

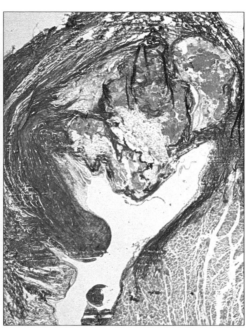

Fig. 15.10 Calcified mitral ring: (left) calcific deposits beneath the mural leaflet of the valve; (right) histology showing calcified mass in base of leaflet; note endocardial fibrosis as friction lesion. E-VG stain.

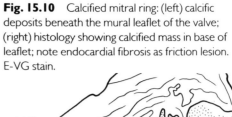

calcifica-tions

valvar leaflet

endocardial fibrosis

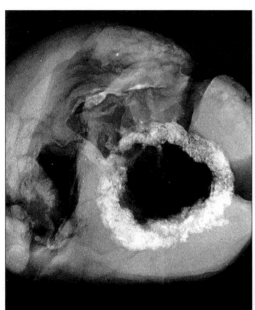

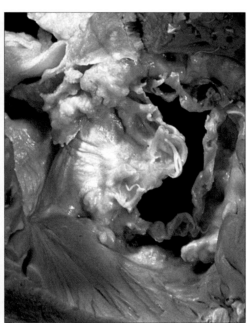

Fig. 15.11 Calcified mitral ring: (left) post-mortem radiograph, craniocaudal view, showing ring-like calcification of the valvar orifice; (right) ventricular aspect exhibiting subvalvar calcifications extending onto fibrous tissue, thus completing the 'ring'.

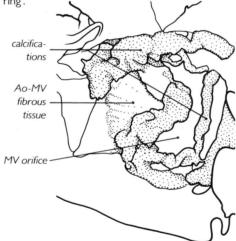

calcifica-tions

Ao-MV fibrous tissue

MV orifice

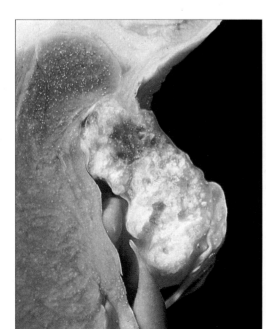

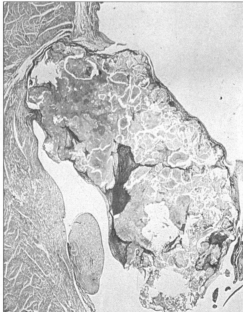

Fig. 15.12 Calcified mitral ring: (left) extensive calcification of the leaflet; only the most distal part of the leaflet is pliable; (right) histology reveals massive involvement of leaflet and its cordal attachments. E-VG stain.

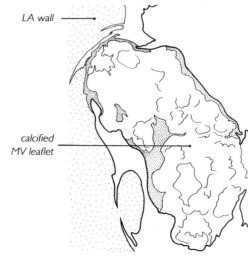

LA wall

calcified MV leaflet

Right heart valves

Ageing changes in the right heart are less outspoken than the left-sided changes, although the large anterosuperior leaflet of the tricuspid valve almost always shows fibrous thickening (Fig. 15.16). In elderly patients with pulmonary disease and right ventricular hypertrophy, the atrial surface of the leaflets may be highly irregular, with surface depositions of fibrin, resembling ulceration. The pulmonary valve shows similar fibrosis, particularly in cases with sustained pulmonary hypertension, irrespective of its cause.

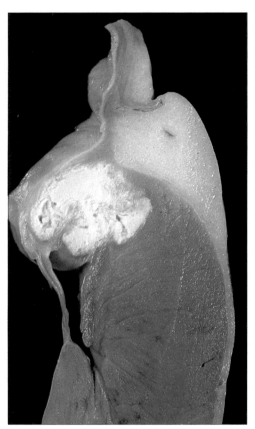

Fig. 15.13   Calcified mitral ring extending into myocardium. The central part is soft, exhibiting a superficial resemblance to caseous necrosis.

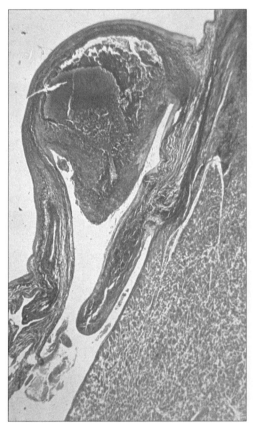

Fig. 15.14   Partially organized subvalvar thrombosis. E-VG stain.

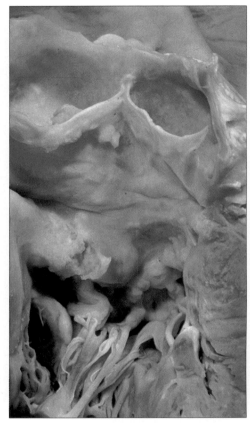

Fig. 15.15   Extensive calcific ageing changes of the apparatus of both aortic and mitral valves. Calcific deposits extend onto the ventricular septum.

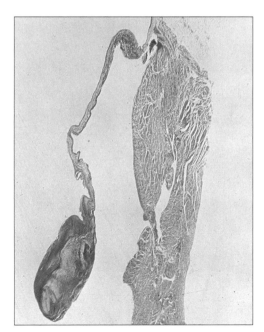

Fig. 15.16   Histology of leaflet of the tricuspid valve with marked fibrosis on atrial aspect. E-VG stain.

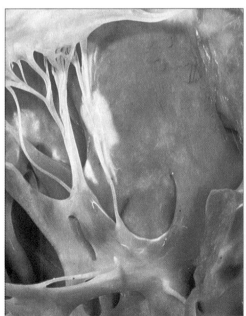

Fig. 15.17   Friction lesions of cords: fibrous lesion on right ventricular aspect of septum encapsulating cord.

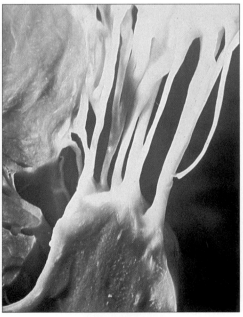

Fig. 15.18   Fibrous encasement of cords of the mitral valve.

Endocardium

Endocardial thickening frequently occurs in relation to tendinous cords. These friction, or rub, lesions are particularly prominent in hearts with ventricular hypertrophy. Septal lesions are commonly seen in association with right ventricular hypertrophy (Fig. 15.17), whereas, with left ventricular hypertrophy, lesions are often encountered in the posterobasal aspect (Fig. 15.18). These lesions may progress from small imprints of overlying cords to large fibrous encapsulations of one or several cords. The larger examples may contribute to impaired function of the valve and, occasionally, form the nidus for mural endocarditis. The incidence of endocardial friction and rub lesions increases with age, but their appearance is enhanced by other circumstances. From that point of view, therefore, these changes should not be considered ageing changes in the strict sense.

The cardiac skeleton and conduction

The process of 'wear and tear' of the cardiac skeleton probably underlies the gradual separation of the aortic root from the ventricular septum in the elderly. This contributes to the so-called sigmoid septum and the altered geometry of the left ventricular outflow tract (see also Section 5).

Calcification of the central fibrous body can also occur (Fig. 15.19, left), whereby the calcified mass may extend onto the ventricular septum and impinge on the atrioventricular bundle and bundle branches, thus producing heart block (Fig. 15.19, right). The calcific mass in these instances represents the end-stage of a process of 'wear and tear' of the central fibrous body. This is relevant since the conduction tissues have to pass through the fibrous skeleton in order to descend onto the ventricular myocardium (see also Chapter 1). Consequently, the disintegration of the cardiac skeleton may lead to attenuation and fibrosis of the conduction fibres. This degenerative process probably underlies the common finding of proximal atrioventricular dissociation, known as Lev's disease, in elderly patients. The fibrocalcific nature of this disease should be distinguished from idiopathic bundle branch fibrosis, known as Lenègre's disease, which affects the more peripheral parts of the bundle branch system.

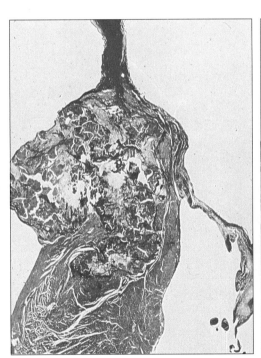
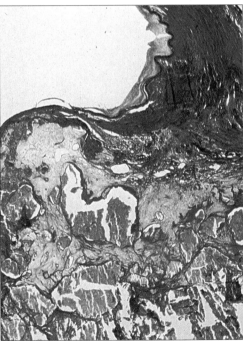
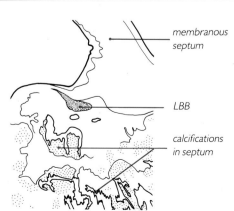

Fig. 15.19 Histological section showing extensive septal calcifications as part of age-related pathology: (left) general view; (right) detail. The left bundle is entrapped by massive calcifications. E-VG stain.

Insertion of pacemakers

In cases of heart block, the insertion of pacemakers may introduce other forms of pathology. They carry a particular risk of producing endocardial laceration and of providing nests for thrombosis and infection. The incidence of these complications is directly related to the amount of time a catheter is in place. Thrombosis rapidly develops as heat around the catheter and is particularly likely to develop at sites of endocardial laceration. The thrombotic event may give rise to further complications, such as inlet obstruction or thromboembolism. Infection is a most serious complication, albeit rare. When it does occur, the removal of the pacemaker is usually necessary for complete recovery, regardless of whether the lead is endocardial or pericardial.

In time, catheters can become partly encapsulated by fibrous tissue. These fibrous sheaths favour sites of mural contact and electrode catheters left in place for a long time may become encased within the right atrium, usually near the entrance of the superior caval vein. Such encasement also occurs at the site of contact with the tricuspid valve and within the right ventricle, usually near the apex where the catheter tip is lodged between trabeculations. However, Tricuspid insufficiency is relatively uncommon, despite fibrous encasement and secondary reactive changes. In addition, proper pacemaker function is rarely interfered with by the development of fibrous tissue at the electrode tip, although the changes which are evoked remain as possible sites for infective endocarditis.

A division is made between primary neoplasms of the heart and pericardium and metastatic tumours, the latter being by far the most frequently encountered.

PRIMARY TUMOURS

Primary tumours of the heart and pericardium are exceedingly rare. In the overall population, cardiac myxoma is by far the most common, accounting for approximately 25% of all primary cardiac neoplasms, although the most frequent tumour found in children and infants is the rhabdomyoma.

Cardiac myxoma

Myxomas arise as pedunculated tumours extending from the walls of the cardiac chamber. Approximately 95% of these tumours arise from the endocardial surface of one of the atria, the left atrium being affected in approximately 75% of cases. The remaining cardiac myxomas arise with almost equal incidence from the right or left ventricular endocardium. Multiple myxomas occur in approximately 5% of instances, with left atrial myxoma always dominating the clinical presentation. The circulatory effects of cardiac myxoma can be grouped under the heading of obstructive, embolic and constitutional features. These are largely determined by the primary site of origin, the size and mobility of the tumour and the nature of its surface. The leading signs and symptoms of right heart myxomas, apart from the constitutional aspects, are different from those caused by left-sided myxomas. Obstruction of the tricuspid orifice and pulmonary emboli predominate, and the most common site of attachment is the atrial septum, just below the region of the superior rim of the oval fossa (Fig. 16.1, left). Other atrial locations occur in approximately 10% of cases, although myxomas rarely originate from the cardiac valves. Cardiac myxomas present grossly as pedunculated masses either with a villous surface, which often harbours adherent thrombus, or with a smooth and lobulated surface. Atrial tumours frequently extend through the corresponding atrioventricular orifice (Fig. 16.1, right). The stalk is usually short but with a small diameter, which often permits marked mobility of the tumour. This feature is well demonstrated on echocardiograms. Because of this, the position of a cardiac myxoma may change. For instance, a left atrial myxoma, depending on its position, may cause obstruction of either the pulmonary venous inflow or the left ventricular inlet. In some instances, the gross appearance of a left atrial myxoma may reveal its obstructive nature, there being a sharp distinction between the whitish surface of the ventricular part, caught during systole in the mitral orifice and thus exposed to high

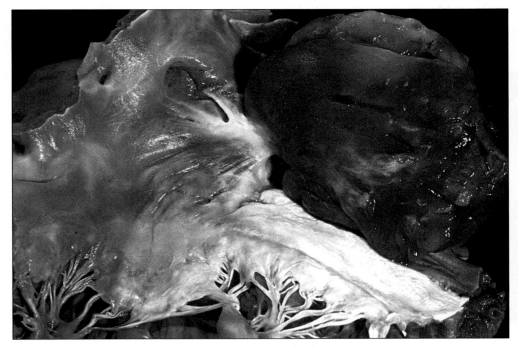
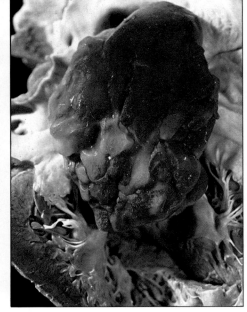

Fig. 16.1   Mobile myxoma: (left) the tumour arises from a stalk in the left atrium; (right) the myxoma in the orifice of the mitral valve.

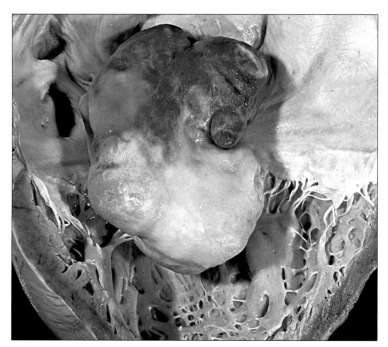

Fig. 16.2 Left atrial myxoma within the orifice of the mitral valve. Note the sharp distinction between ventricular (pale) and atrial (haemorrhagic) aspects.

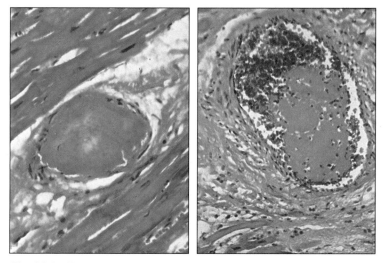

Fig. 16.4 Thromboemboli in intramural coronary arteries derived from myxoma. H&E stains.

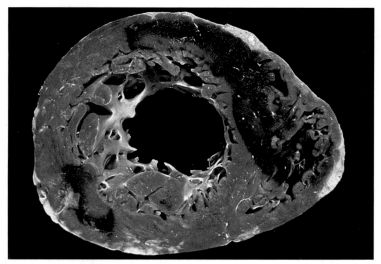

Fig. 16.5 Recent, almost circumferential, transmural myocardial infarction following massive thromboembolism from a left atrial myxoma. NBT technique (viable muscle stains dark blue).

pressures, and the haemorrhagic aspect of the low pressure atrial part (Fig. 16.2). The villous surface (Fig. 16.3) may serve as a source of thromboemboli which occasionally may obstruct coronary arteries (Fig. 16.4) and cause myocardial infarction (Fig. 16.5). On the other hand, the friable appearance of such tumours permits detachment of myxomatous fragments and results in tumour emboli (Fig. 16.6). Longstanding atrial myxomas may calcify, and occasionally it seems that the tumour might have been detected on a routine chest radiograph (Fig. 16.7). The stalk usually contains large vessels of large calibre which can

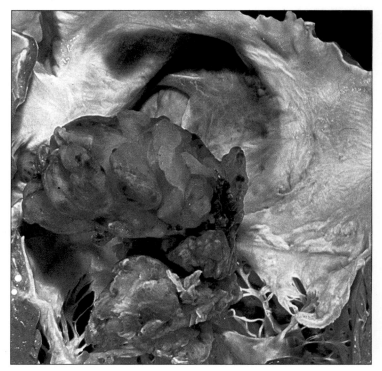

Fig. 16.3 Left atrial myxoma with friable villous surface.

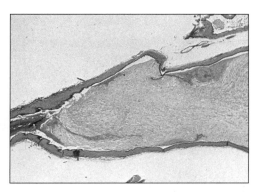

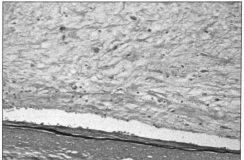

Fig. 16.6 Myxoma emboli in an artery: (upper) low power; (lower) detail. E-VG stains.

sometimes be seen on coronary angiography. The presence of a left atrial myxoma in intimate contact with the mitral valve may account for secondary pathology, and may necessitate replacement of the mitral valve. Ventricular myxomas also vary in size and gross appearance. Obstruction of the ventricular cavity is usually the main haemodynamic problem (Fig. 16.8).

Histologically the tumours are composed of polygonal cells embedded within a mucoid ground substance rich in acid glycos-aminoglycans (Fig. 16.9, upper). The cellular make-up is variable from one site to another. In some areas, scattered single cells may appear, often stellate in shape, whereas other areas may present nests of polygonal cells. Spindle-shaped cells may appear and transformation into smooth muscle cells is common (Fig. 16.9, lower). Iron pigment is widely distributed and foci of haematopoietic cells are often encountered. A fibrinoid stromal appearance is common at the periphery, giving resemblance to a softening thrombus.

Myxomas are considered as true neoplasms, originating from undifferentiated mesenchymal cells that occur naturally in the subendocardial layer.

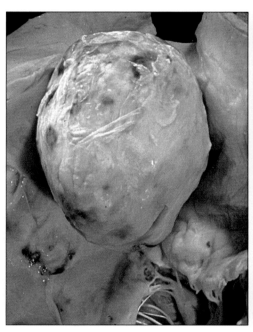
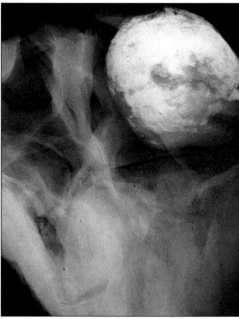

Fig. 16.7   Calcified left atrial myxoma: (left) gross appearance; (right) postmortem x-ray.

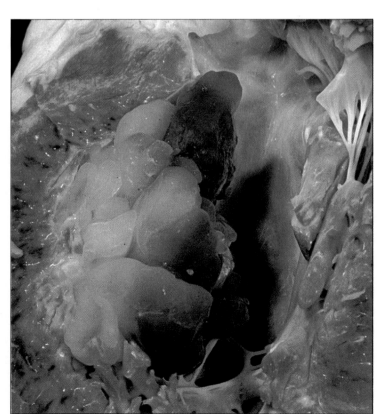

Fig. 16.8   Left ventricular myxoma obstructing cavity.

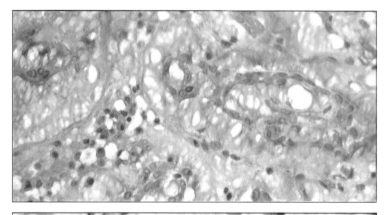
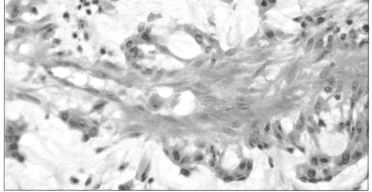

Fig. 16.9   Histology of myxoma: (upper) strands and nests of myxoma cells amidst stroma. Alcian blue stain. (Lower) transformation into spindle-shaped cells. H&E stain.

Papillary fibroelastoma

This lesion is known also as a papillary tumour of the cardiac valve or as a giant Lambl's excrescence (see chapter 15). Papillary fibroelastoma occur relatively frequently in adults but hardly ever in children and infants. Although usually found on the valves, with a preference for the aortic valve, similar lesions can originate from the mural endocardium of a cardiac chamber. In the majority of cases, the lesions are found as an incidental finding at necropsy (Fig. 16.10) or on inspection of a surgically excised valve. Clinical signs and symptoms have not been unequivocally connected with these lesions, although the association with paroxysmal angina pectoris and sudden unexpected death has been reported. The gross appearance resembles that of a sea anemone, with a bouquet of filiform threads attached to the endocardium by a short pedicle. Histologically, the threads consist of a central core of dense collagen surrounded by a loose matrix of connective tissue (Fig. 16.10), and elastic fibres are often present in abundance. The pathogenesis of these lesions is controversial. Thrombosis, friction and true neoplasia have all been proposed, whilst the resemblance with Lambl's excrescences is striking (see also Figs 11.3 & 11.4). We wonder, therefore, whether the origin of the papillary fibroelastoma should not be considered along the same line as that for the excrescence.

Rhabdomyoma

These tumours occur almost exclusively in infancy, with more than half of all primary heart tumours found in patients of one year of age or younger being rhabdomyomas. Two main categories exist – those presenting as the direct cause of morbidity (or mortality), and those found incidentally at autopsy. In the latter group, it is signs and symptoms of tuberous sclerosis which have usually dominated the clinical profile. It has been argued that rhabdomyomas are always accompanied by tuberous sclerosis of the brain, whether or not the latter condition is clinically manifest.

In patients in whom the rhabdomyoma is clinically manifest, two further groups are distinguished. In some patients, the cardiac lesion has led to either stillbirth or death within a few days following birth. In the remaining patients, cardiomegaly with congestive heart failure with, or without, cardiac arrhythmias predominate. Sudden and unexpected death may be caused by an otherwise clinically silent rhabdomyoma. On the other hand, there is evidence that some rhabdomyomas may regress spontaneously.

The clinical significance of cardiac rhabdomyomas is largely determined by their size (Fig. 16.11), by whether they occur as solitary or multiple lesions, and by whether or not they extend into a cavity (Fig. 16.12). Intracavitary extension is particularly frequent in those patients who have functional impairment. The demonstration of an intracardiac mass in a symptomatic child under five years of age is strongly suggestive of this diagnosis. Almost all instances of rhabdomyomas appear to be multifocal, even though multiplicity can, in some instances, only be detected with the aid of the microscope.

Histologically, the tumour is composed of swollen myocytes, which have an almost empty cytoplasm traversed by tiny strands of cellular matrix which may exhibit cross-striations (Fig. 16.13, upper). The nucleus may thus appear suspended within the cell, hence the term 'spider cell' (Fig. 16.13, lower). The glycogen content of these cells is best demonstrated on fresh-frozen sections. The distinction from glycogen storage disease should be no problem since, in the latter, the myocardial histology is monotonous and does not show grotesquely swollen myocytes typical for rhabdomyoma (see Fig. 11.13). At present rhabdomyomas are considered to represent hamartomas.

Teratoma

These tumours are relatively rare in adults and children, but are the second most frequent tumour encountered in infants. By definition, they contain elements derived from all three germ layers. Most teratomas are extracardiac, albeit intrapericardial, with their usual position being at the base of the heart, attached to the root of the arterial pedicle. Intrapericardial teratomas in young infants may hamper cardiac function due to pericardial effusion, whilst in older infants the first indication is the compression of airways.

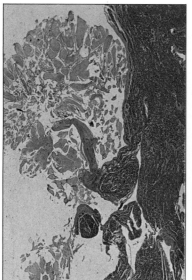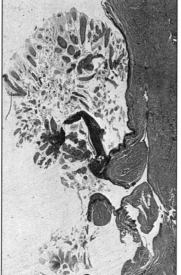

Fig. 16.10 Fibroelastoma of mural endocardium of left ventricle: (left) H&E, (right) E-VG stains.

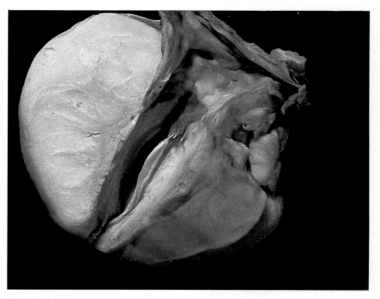

Fig. 16.11 Cardiac rhabdomyoma which takes up almost all of the wall of the left ventricle, reducing the cavity to a virtual slit.

Fibroma

Fibroma is the second most commonly encountered neoplastic lesion in children and ranks third in infants, although it is rare in adults. The clinical signs and symptoms are largely dependent on its location, with a distinct tendency for fibromas to occur in the ventricular septum. This may relate to the high frequency of sudden and unexpected death among those cases. Compression of the atrioventricular conduction system may occur in such instances. Fibromas may grow to a large size (Fig. 16.14) and usually present as circumscript, solid, firm and whitish lesions with a distinct fibromatous architecture.

Histologically, the lesions are composed of interweaving bundles of collagen fibres intermingling with elastin fibres, the latter fibres often appearing fragmented. Islands of haemato-poietic cells can be encountered, and smooth muscle cells may be present (Fig. 16.15).

In practical terms, cardiac fibromas should be considered as slow-growing and potentially aggressive lesions which, when suspected on clinical grounds, may be surgically excised. The resemblance to soft tissue fibromatosis, in both natural history and light and electronmicroscopic characteristics, has led to the suggestion that the two are identical diseases. Because of this, the term 'cardiac fibromatosis' has been advocated.

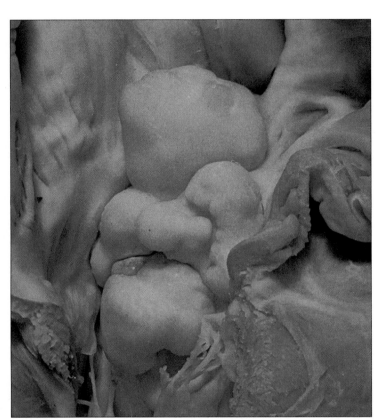

Fig. 16.12 Intracavitary extension of rhabdomyoma from the right atrium through the orifice of the tricuspid valve into the right ventricle.

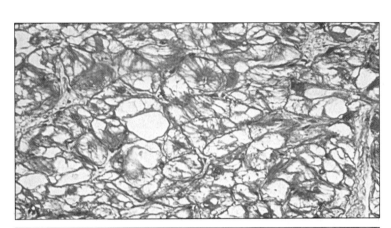

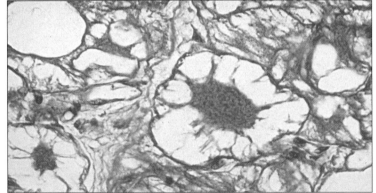

Fig. 16.13 Histology of rhabdomyoma showing bizarre vacuolated cells: (upper) low power; (lower) detail of spider cell. Mallory's phosphotungstic acid-haemotoxylin stains.

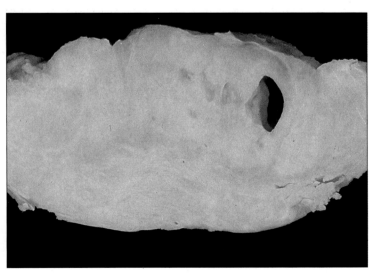

Fig. 16.14 Surgically excised cardiac fibroma from a three-week-old baby: the cut surface shows the fibrous nature of the lesion.

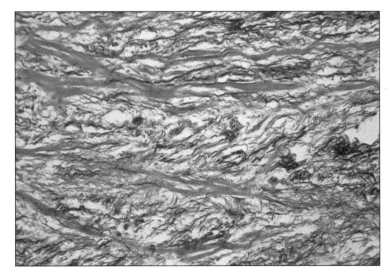

Fig. 16.15 Histological section of cardiac fibroma showing an area in which collagen fibres intermingle with smooth muscle cells (brownish). E-VG stain.

Primary malignant tumours

Angiosarcoma, rhabdomyosarcoma and mesothelioma are the most frequent primary malignancies, rhabdomyosarcomas also occurring in children and infants. A rhabdomyosarcoma is composed of malignant cells exhibiting features of striated muscle. Non-specific symptoms prevail, and cardiomegaly is the common denominator. The tumour shows no preferential sites and multiplicity is common. Intracavitary extension at multiple sites, often with destruction of valves, is a frequent finding. The diagnosis depends on the identification of rhabdomyoblasts.

Angiosarcoma is a highly malignant tumour with a distinct preference for the right side of the heart, right heart failure being the most frequent clinical finding. Histologically, these tumours are no different from angiosarcoma originating elsewhere in the body, and the same range of architectural arrangements may occur.

Mesotheliomas may primarily originate from the pericardium (Fig. 16.16, upper), and show a wide range of histological appearances, similar to that reported for primary pleural mesothelioma. The tumour grows by superficial spread and usually does not significantly invade the myocardium, although deep infiltration into the endocardium occurs occasionally (Fig. 16.16, lower). The clinical findings are often dominated by signs of pericardial effusion. Eventually, the tumour may spread circumferentially, encapsulating a major part of the heart and leading to constrictive pericardial disease. Primary pericardial mesothelioma should be distinguished from primary pleural mesothelioma extending into the pericardium (and vice versa).

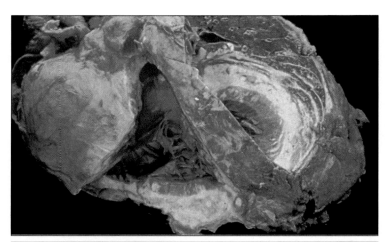

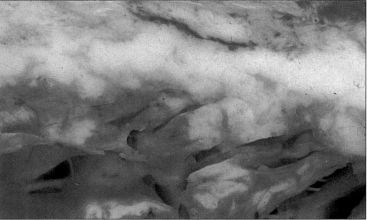

Fig. 16.16 Primary pericardial mesothelioma: (upper) extensive ingrowth into the myocardium of both ventricles. Note adhesion to lung; (lower) myocardial ingrowth near endocardial surface.

METASTATIC TUMOURS

Almost all malignant tumours may metastasize to the heart and pericardium. Direct extension may occur from primary bronchial carcinoma, oesophageal carcinoma and pleural mesothelioma. Metastatic heart disease occurs as a common complication of carcinoma of the lung, carcinoma of the breast and malignant lymphoma. With tumours as the point of departure, malignant melanomas rank high (Fig. 16.17).

Tumour deposits may vary considerably. In some instances, the epi- and pericardium are only slightly thickened, whereas in other instances distinct nodules develop in the myocardium (Fig. 16.18).

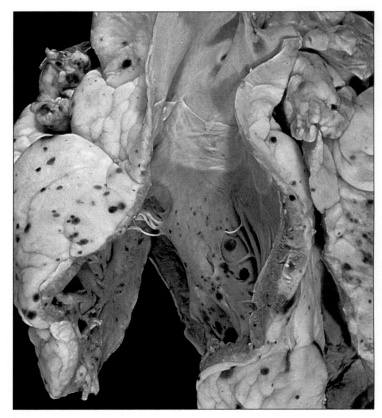

Fig. 16.17 Multiple metastases of malignant melanoma: deposits on epicardial surface, endocardially and in myocardium.

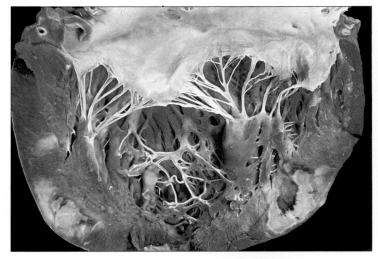

Fig. 16.18 Intramyocardial metastasis from bronchial carcinoma.

Diagnosis of metastatic tumours can be difficult since the most frequent clinical features are dyspnoea on exertion and pleural effusion. Nevertheless, the occurrence of cardiomegaly, pericardial effusion (Fig. 16.19), heart failure and cardiac arrhythmias, particularly in the setting of a malignant disease, should always raise the possibility of metastatic heart disease. It is important to note that the effusion in malignant disease is often haemorrhagic. In time, signs of constriction may develop because of extensive tumour spread which can then encapsulate the heart (Fig. 16.20).

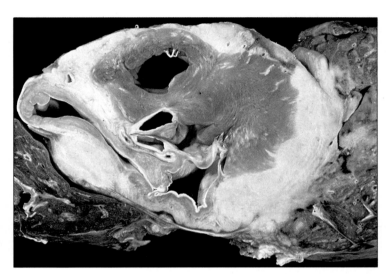

Fig. 16.20 An extensive tumour which has encapsulated the heart.

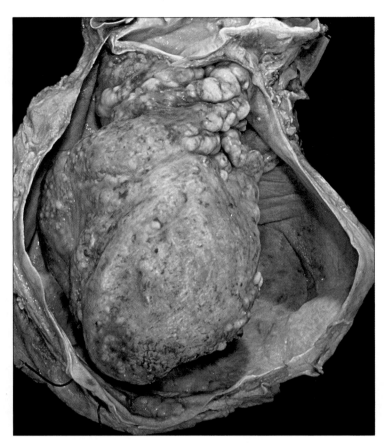

Fig. 16.19 Extensive pericardial metastasis leading to massive fluid accumulation in pericardial cavity and cardiac tamponade.

Jessica M. Mann

The first attempts at heart transplantation were carried out by Carrel and Guthrie in 1905, and the first heterotopic heart transplant was performed in a dog in 1953. The first successful human heart transplantation was performed by Dr Christian Barnard in South Africa in 1967 and, since then, more than 16,000 transplants have been performed, and heart transplantation has become an accepted treatment for end-stage cardiac failure. Data from the Registry of the International Society for Heart Transplantation show that at least 240 centres all over the world are now involved in heart and heart–lung transplantation, and that the vast majority (85%) of all transplants have been carried out since 1985. The number of children receiving new hearts has also increased from 14 procedures prior to 1980 to 900 in the period from 1985 to 1990. Over half of the recipients are younger than 5 years of age, whilst 39% are below 1 year of age.

Pooled data from the Registry of the International Society show that the commonest reason for transplantation is idiopathic cardiomyopathy, closely followed by ischaemic heart disease in adults and congenital heart disease in children. Other indications include end-stage heart failure due to valvar heart disease, refractory arrhythmias, amyloidosis, Chagas' disease and cardiac tumours.

Operative mortality for transplantation has remained stable at 10% in recent years for the adult population, although it is higher in children. Retransplantation also carries a much higher operative mortality (29%), particularly if performed within the first month after transplantation (63%). Retransplantation performed more than 6 months after the initial procedure, however, carries a much lower mortality rate (13%). Early mortality is mainly due to cardiovascular problems, including complications of surgery such as inadequate preservation of the donor heart and/or haemorrhage, and right-sided cardiac failure as seen in the setting of a very high pulmonary vascular resistance. Other causes of mortality and morbidity are failure of the kidneys and liver, pulmonary embolization and cerebrovascular accidents. Infection and rejection account for about 37% of early deaths, and for more than 70% of late deaths.

An important complement to heart transplantation is immunosuppressive therapy which, prior to 1980, was provided by azathioprine and steroids. Since the introduction of cyclosporin A in the early eighties, it has been adopted worldwide in conjunction with azathioprine, leading to a significant reduction in the dosage of steroids. This has produced a significant improvement in both short and long-term survival in those patients treated with cyclosporin, as well as bringing a decrease in the frequency of lymphoreticular neoplasms. Virtually all cardiac transplants performed at present are orthotopic (replacement of the recipient organ by the donor organ). Heterotopic transplantation of the heart (insertion of an additional heart) is a future trend which will not be included in this edition.

THE EXPLANTED HEART

The heart which is removed at transplantation will usually show dilated cardiomyopathy. There will be severe biventricular

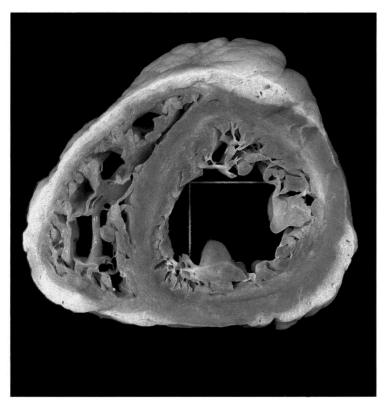

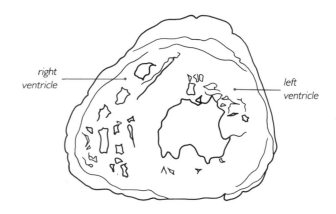

Fig. 17.1 Transverse cut of both ventricles in a patient with dilated cardiomyopathy. Biventricular dilatation is present. The thickness of the left ventricular wall is within normal limits (10mm). The coronary arteries are normal.

dilatation, with normal or minimally diseased coronary arteries, and no macroscopic evidence of acute or old myocardial infarction (Fig. 17.1). Small patchy scars, probably due to microinfarcts, can sometimes be seen in the left ventricular wall. The thickness of the ventricular wall is usually within the normal range (up to 12mm), or else only slightly increased. The apex of the left ventricle may contain old or fresh thrombus. The orifice of both mitral and tricuspid valves may be dilated, leading to valvar regurgitation, but the valves themselves are normal. Histological examination of the myocardium reveals increased interstitial fibrosis with focal myocytic hypertrophy (Figs 17.2, 17.3) and confirms the normal appearance of the coronary arteries. In most of the cases, the diagnosis of dilated cardiomyopathy will have beeñ made on clinical grounds. Care must be taken in order to avoid missing entities such as amyloidosis. Although this is still considered a relative contraindication for heart transplantation, it can be discovered in the recipient organ (Fig. 17.4). In these circumstances, amyloid can recur in the donor heart as soon as four months after transplantation.

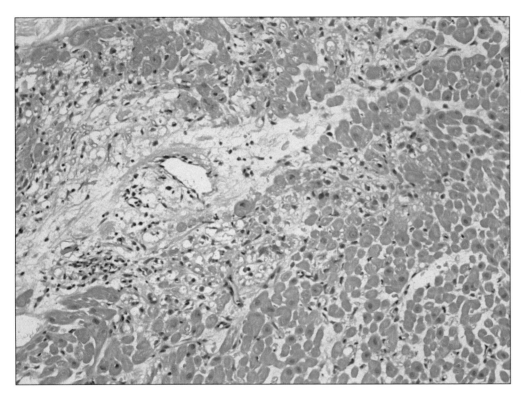

Fig. 17.2 Histological section of the left ventricular myocardium in a patient with dilated cardiomyopathy. The myocytes are vacuolated, and the interstitial fibrosis is increased.

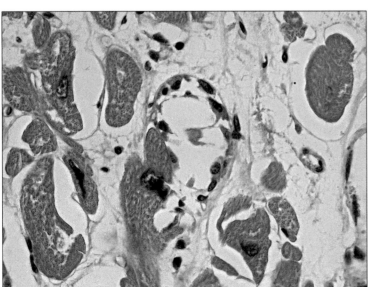

Fig. 17.3 Histological section of the myocardium (higher magnification) in a patient with dilated cardiomyopathy. Myocytic vacuolation is obvious.

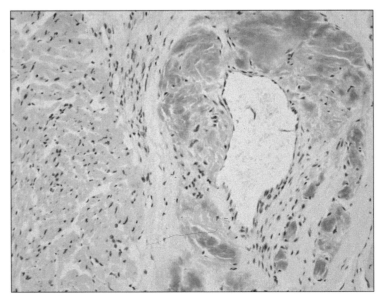

Fig. 17.4 Myocardial section from an explanted heart staining positive for amyloid with Congo red. The patient has been alive and well for 9 months after cardiac transplantation. Amyloid stains have consistently been negative on his endomyocardial biopsies.

The second largest subgroup of patients undergoing heart transplantation do so because of end-stage ischaemic heart disease. The heart, usually from a middle-aged man, may show evidence of previous coronary artery bypass surgery or other procedures such as left ventricular aneurysmectomy (Fig. 17.5). The left ventricular cavity is generally dilated (unless there has

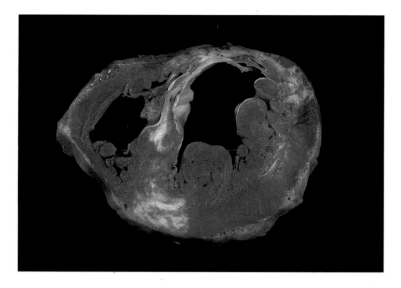

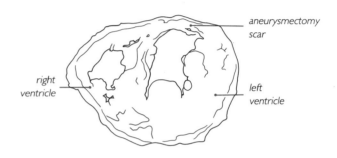

Fig. 17.5 Transverse cut of both ventricles in a patient with ischaemic heart disease. An aneurysmectomy has been performed. The anterior left ventricular wall is thin, and the endocarcium over this wall is thickened. The old anterior myocardial infarction extends into the ventricular septum. Another scar (old infarct) is present on the posteroseptal wall. The remaining myocardium is hypertrophied.

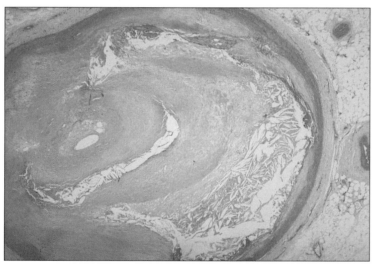

Fig. 17.6 Transverse section of the left anterior descending coronary artery in the patient from Fig. 17.5. The lumen is nearly virtual. A crescent-shaped lipid pool is seen, surrounded by fibrous tissue.

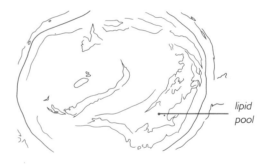

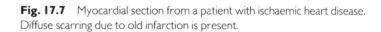

Fig. 17.7 Myocardial section from a patient with ischaemic heart disease. Diffuse scarring due to old infarction is present.

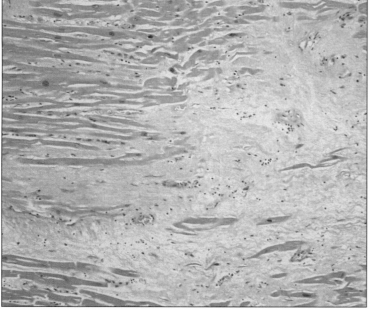

been a previous aneurysmectomy). There is usually extensive scarring due to old myocardial infarction, with thinning of the left ventricular wall and thickening of the endocardium. Thrombi may be present at the apex of the left ventricle. The coronary arteries show extensive involvement by atherosclerotic plaque (Fig. 17.6). Histological examination of the left ventricular myocardium confirms the extensive scarring (Fig. 17.7), as does the endocardial thickening, which is most striking over the papillary muscles, and the absence of acute ischaemic damage. Acute arterial occlusions due to thrombi are rarely, if ever, found.

A small percentage of patients will undergo heart transplantation because of hypertrophic cardiomyopathy. The removed hearts in these cases, instead of showing the classical picture of hypertrophic cardiomyopathy, with a significant increase in the thickness of the left ventricular wall and a small left ventricular cavity, will demonstrate a dilated left ventricular cavity, due to chronic progressive mitral regurgitation and a progressive decrease in left ventricular ejection fraction (Fig. 17.8). Endocardial thickening in the left ventricular outflow tract can be found, as well as focal fibrous thickening of the aortic leaflet of the mitral valve when it had undergone systolic anterior motion. Histological examination of the myocardium, nonetheless, will show the characteristic myocardial disarray (Fig. 17.9), together with extensive interstitial fibrosis (Fig. 17.10). The degree of coronary arterial disease in such cases will be related to the age and sex of the patient.

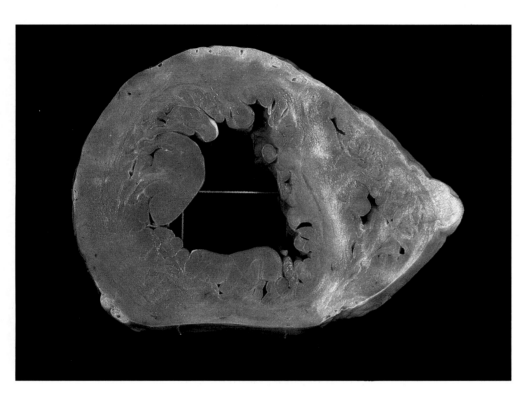

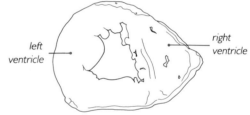

Fig. 17.8 Transverse cut of both ventricles in a patient with hypertrophic cardiomyopathy. Both ventricles are hypertrophied. The left ventricular cavity is dilated. The increase in interstitial fibrosis is evident on the ventricular septum.

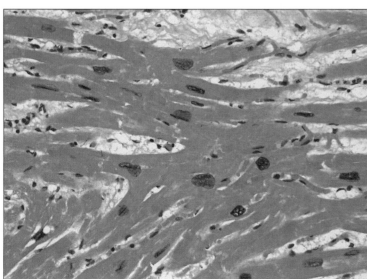

Fig. 17.9 Myocardial section from the heart shown in Fig. 17.9 showing myocardial disarray and myocytic hypertrophy.

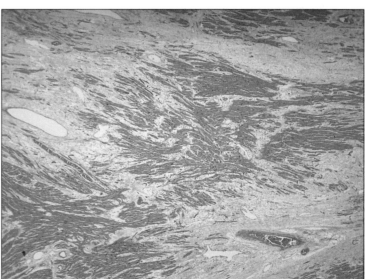

Fig. 17.10 Myocardial section showing myocardial disarray and extensive interstitial fibrosis.

ACUTE REJECTION – THE ENDOMYOCARDIAL BIOPSY

Endomyocardial biopsy is the recognized follow-up technique for patients with heart transplantation. The frequency at which endomyocardial biopsies are obtained after heart transplantation varies but, generally, they are obtained at weekly intervals during the first month after operation, and then every two weeks until discharge from hospital. Subsequently, they are performed at 3, 4 and 6 months after transplantation, and then annually, unless there is suspicion of rejection or infection. Endomyocardial biopsies have become the 'gold standard' for diagnosis and monitoring of immunosuppressive treatment in transplanted patients. They provide information about the response to an increase or change in therapy. Before the introduction of cyclosporin, it was clinical signs of left ventricular dysfunction which were used to monitor rejection. Endomyocardial biopsies were then performed to confirm the presence of acute rejection before starting treatment. Rejection in patients treated with cyclosporin, however, is characteristically a clinically silent event. Endomyocardial biopsies, therefore, must be performed routinely and graded histologically.

Since the introduction of the Caves bioptome in 1973, it has been possible to obtain right ventricular biopsies repeatedly with a minimal risk. Three to five pieces of myocardium are obtained from the right ventricle. This number of pieces is needed in order to obtain a representative amount of myocardium and to perform accurate grading of the biopsy. The sampling error is no more than 2% with such an approach. It is particularly important to take multiple biopsies in patients in whom transplantation occurred more than one year previously because of the possibility of sampling sites of previous biopsies (Figs 17.11, 17.12). The biopsies are fixed in formaldehyde, routinely processed through paraffin, and stained with haematoxylin and eosin along with Masson's trichrome in order to assess the degree of interstitial fibrosis. Additional stains, such as methyl-green pyronine, are sometimes used to demonstrate active lymphocytes. Electron microscopy is not performed routinely, since the processing of the biopsy takes too long to be useful in demonstrating acute rejection. When acute rejection is observed, it can be graded from mild to severe. The clinical decision to increase or change the immunosuppressive treatment will depend upon the histological grading, although the physician will be aware that an increased immunosuppression carries an increased risk of infection. Apart from the evaluation of rejection, the endomyocardial biopsy is also examined for the presence of infectious agents, such as toxoplasma (Fig. 17.13), cytomegalovirus and fungi.

The system of grading

The morphological features of rejection are usually graded following the system developed by Billingham at Stanford University. This system included the grades of mild, moderate and severe, together with resolving or resolved rejection. In clinical terms, the first two are easily reversible events, whereas severe rejection has been found to be much more difficult to reverse.

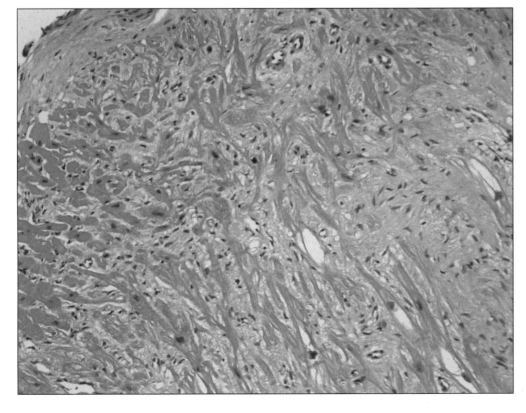

Fig. 17.11 Endomyocardial biopsy taken at the site of an old biopsy. The interstitial fibrous tissue is increased, leading to 'disorganization' of the remaining myocytes.

Mild rejection consists of a perivascular infiltrate of lympho-blasts with prominent nucleoli and pyroninophilic cytoplasm (Fig. 17.14). The endothelial cells of the small vessels in the biopsy also show increased pyroninophilia. Oedema is usually present, although this feature can easily be confused with fixation artifacts or with trauma to the tissue produced during the biopsy. The diagnosis of mild rejection, therefore, has to be made on the basis of the mononuclear infiltrate.

Moderate rejection is heralded by an increase in the peri-vascular infiltrate, which now also infiltrates between the myocardial cells (Fig. 17.15). Focal myocytic damage, evidenced by necrosis of individual myocytes, is also evident, although this is sometimes difficult to recognize, as it tends to be very localized.

Severe rejection is characterized by a marked increase in the inflammatory infiltrate, which consists of mononuclear cells

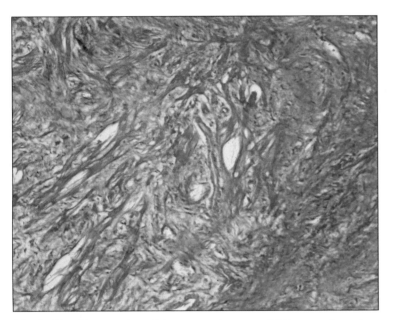

Fig. 17.12 Close-up view of the same endomyocardial biopsy as shown in Fig. 17.11, stained with Masson's trichrome to demonstrate the increase in fibrous tissue, which stains blue.

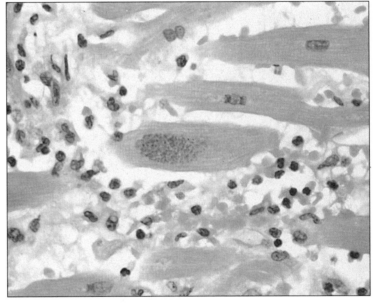

Fig. 17.13 Section of the myocardium in a transplanted patient dying with Toxoplasma infection two months after transplant. The central myocyte contains a cyst of Toxoplasma gondii.

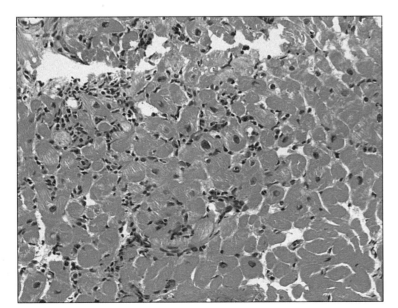

Fig. 17.14 Endomyocardial biopsy from a patient with mild rejection. A scanty perivascular infiltrate is seen in the centre of the picture. No myocytic damage is present.

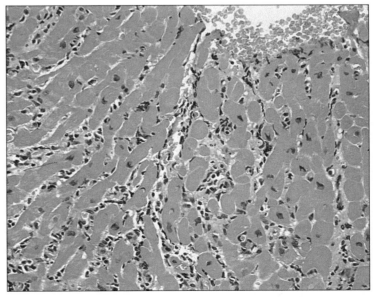

Fig. 17.15 Endomyocardial biopsy from a patient with moderate rejection. The inflammatory infiltrate now extends amongst the myocytes.

mixed with eosinophils, and neutrophils. Myocytic damage is obvious, mainly within the zones of heavy inflammatory infiltrate (Fig. 17.16). Interstitial haemorrhage can also be present.

Resolving or resolved rejection appears characteristically after 2 to 3 days of aggressive immunosuppression in those patients being treated with azathioprine. In patients treated with cyclosporin, however, damage to the myocytes takes longer to disappear. The biopsy shows a decrease in the inflammatory infiltrate when compared to the previous biopsy. Scarring can also be apparent.

The so-called Quilty effect is an accumulation of mononuclear cells (B lymphocytes) in the endocardium, with or without extension into the underlying myocardium, but in the absence of damage to the myocytes (Figs 17.17 and 17.18). It was named after the first patient in whom this pattern was recognized. The effect is not always correlated with rejection. Interestingly, it has frequently been observed in patients with high levels of cyclosporin in the blood. Its importance in relation to vascular disease

has not yet been established. Another 'cyclosporin-dependent' effect, not seen in patients treated with azathioprine, is the presence of fine and diffuse perimyocytic fibrosis.

Ischaemic changes can also be seen in biopsies soon after transplantation. They consist of focal myocytic necrosis or vacuolation, with a minimal inflammatory infiltrate surrounding the necrotic myocytes. The remaining myocardial cells are normal, and there is no perivascular or interstitial infiltrate.

Although most centres use the system developed at Stanford University, other centres dealing with large numbers of transplants have developed their own grading systems. These range from grades 0 to 10 as used at the Texas Heart Institute, to 4 grades at Pittsburgh University. It becomes difficult to compare data from different centres when there is such a disparity in grading systems. Thus, in 1990, in an attempt to establish a simple and reproducible grading system, the International Society for Heart Transplantation standardized the nomenclature for heart rejection in a system using five grades. In *Grade 0* there

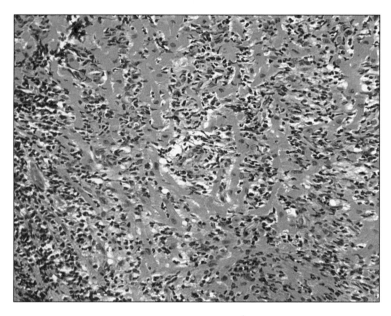

Fig. 17.16 Endomyocardial biopsy from a patient with severe rejection. The inflammatory infiltrate is extending aggressively amongst the myocytes and myocytic necrosis (loss) is obvious even at low power.

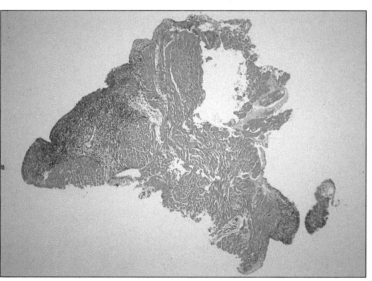

Fig. 17.17 Low power view of an endomyocardial biopsy with Quilty effect. The inflammatory infiltrate is limited to the endocardium, and does not penetrate the underlying myocardium.

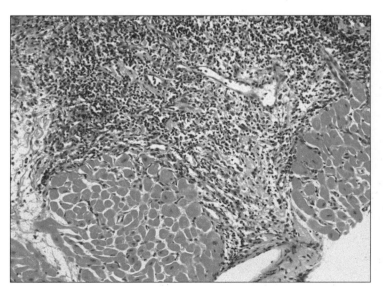

Fig. 17.18 Close-up view of the endomyocardial biopsy shown in Fig. 17.17, showing a well-defined border between the endocardial accumulation of inflammatory cells and the myocardium, which is free of inflammatory infiltrate.

is no rejection. *Grade 1* represents a perivascular or interstitial lymphocytic infiltrate which can be focal (1A) or diffuse (1B), but there is no myocytic necrosis present. *Grade 2* needs a single focus of inflammatory infiltrate, with or without myocytic necrosis limited to the area where the inflammatory infiltrate is present. *Grade 3* consists of a multifocal (3A) or diffuse (3B) inflammatory infiltrate, with or without eosinophils, but with myocytic necrosis. *Grade 4* shows an aggressive inflammatory infiltrate made up of lymphocytes, neutrophils and eosinophils. Myocytic necrosis is always seen, as well as oedema, haemorrhage and vasculitis. In this system the term 'resolving rejection' is replaced by a lesser grade than that on the previous biopsy. In a similar way, 'resolved rejection' should be replaced by grade 0 (no rejection) (Fig. 17.19).

THE POST-TRANSPLANTATION HEART

Hyperacute rejection

Episodes of rejection are considered to be due to cellular immunologic mechanisms and, whilst they can appear at any time after transplantation, 90% of all acute rejections occur within the first six months, becoming quite rare after one year in the absence of any significant alteration in the immunosuppressive regimen. There is one instance, however, in which the mechanism of rejection is mediated by antibodies, or 'vascular'. This is the 'hyperacute' rejection seen in the operating room at the time of transplantation. The graft requires huge amounts of inotropic support and lacks spontaneous electrical activity. Indeed, it is extremely difficult to induce activity, even with a pacemaker. After a while, the heart becomes cyanosed and tetanic (stone heart). Total artificial cardiac support, or emergency retransplantation, are the only two treatments available in this situation. The basic mechanism for this hyperacute rejection is uncertain, but the interaction of preformed HLA class I antibodies from the recipient with antigens on the endothelial cells of the donor heart is thought to play a role. These antibodies can be detected through a preoperative screen for lymphocytotoxic antibodies. Although it was first described in the setting of the surgical procedure, such vascular rejection has also been reported in endomyocardial biopsies.

In patients dying from hyperacute rejection 48 to 72 hours after transplantation, the donor heart shows severe biventricular dilatation (Fig. 17.20). The myocardium is flabby and shows

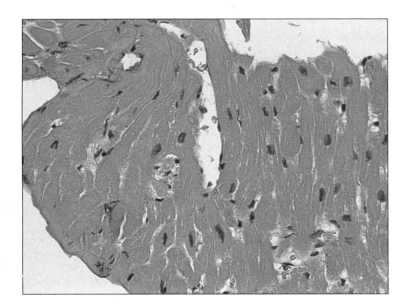

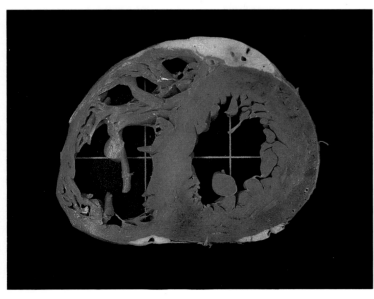

Fig. 17.19 Endomyocardial biopsy showing no rejection. There is no inflammatory infiltrate, the myocytic morphology is within normal limits.

Fig. 17.20 Transverse cut of both ventricles from a patient dying of acute rejection 48 hours after cardiac transplant. Both ventricular cavities, especially the right one, are dilated. The posteroseptal area shows some darker mottling, corresponding to interstitial haemorrhage.

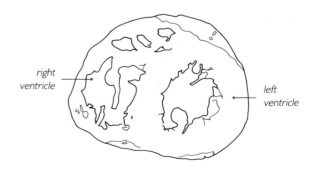

right ventricle

left ventricle

petechial haemorrhages throughout, but maximally within the subendocardium. Histological examination reveals myocardial necrosis and interstitial haemorrhage (Figs 17.21, 17.22).

The post-surgical heart

Examination of donor hearts which have been implanted for more than one year shows consistent findings. The heart weight is increased, and left ventricular hypertrophy is present (Fig. 17.23). Both the right and left ventricular cavities may be dilated, with concomitant dilatation of the tricuspid and mitral orifices leading to variable degrees of valvar regurgitation. Macroscopic scarring due to old myocardial infarction may be seen. The endocardium is generally thickened, and thrombi can be present in the left ventricular apex. The pericardium is thickened and adherent to the epicardium. If enough time from the surgical procedure has elapsed, the suture lines between the donor and recipient atria will no longer be visible (Figs 17.24, 17.25). The coronary arteries show a variable degree of vascular graft disease. This tends to be widespread throughout the epicardial arteries, and there may be fresh thrombotic occlusions which have led to acute myocardial infarction or sudden cardiac death.

Histologic examination of the myocardium reveals either well-limited areas of scarring, corresponding to old myocardial infarction, or small patchy areas of fibrosis throughout the left ventricle, probably due to old episodes of rejection or micro-infarcts (Fig. 17.26). Increased interstitial fibrosis and myocytic hypertrophy are observed in all long-term survivors, and they are not related to the number of previous episodes of rejection. Three years after transplantation, morphometric studies of myocytes demonstrate a significant increase in myocytic width, as well as in nuclear area, irrespective of the immunosuppressive regimen used.

Coronary arterial disease (vascular graft disease)

Vascular graft disease of the transplanted heart has become a major cause of death or retransplantation in those patients who survive more than 3 years. The reported incidence as diagnosed by coronary angiography is between 40 and 50% at 5 years, both for children and adults. The disease has typical angiographic features. There is a diffuse decrease in the diameter of the lumen of the epicardial coronary arteries, with lack of collateral circulation and pruning of small branches. A small percentage

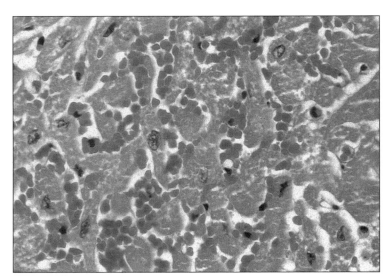

Fig. 17.21 Histologic section of the myocardium from the heart seen in Fig. 17.20 showing extensive interstitial haemorrhage.

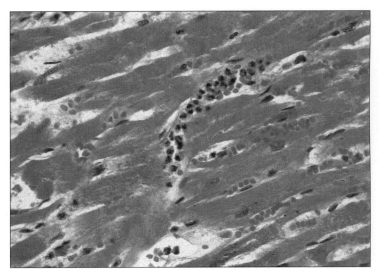

Fig. 17.22 Histologic section of the myocardium from Fig. 17.20, showing extensive myocytic necrosis and interstitial haemorrhage.

Fig. 17.23 Transverse cut of a donor heart implanted for 36 months. Both ventricles are hypertrophied and both ventricular cavities are dilated. The pericardium is thickened. No grossly visible scars are present.

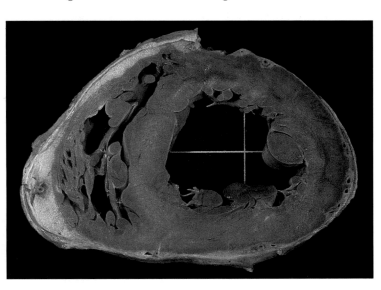

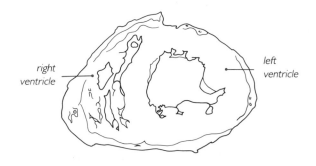

right ventricle

left ventricle

of transplanted patients, however, have angiographic images similar to those seen in non-transplanted patients with native coronary arterial disease.

The involvement of the coronary arteries is generally diffuse in all patients. Small changes in caliber, preferably measured with quantitative angiography, are important for the assessment of the development and progression of the disease. In order to be able to detect early changes, yearly coronary angiograms are performed in most recipients. Several efforts at detecting vascular graft disease with noninvasive methods in this subset of patients have not been successful. The use of cyclosporin in the immunosuppressive regimen has not changed the frequency of vascular graft disease in long-term survivors.

Many attempts have been made to find clinical predictors of vascular graft disease. Thus, a higher incidence of vascular graft disease has been discovered in those recipients with a high fasting level of plasma triglycerides, as well as in those who had been transplanted with older donor hearts. Others, however, failed to discover any correlation between the frequency of vascular graft disease and the level of triglyceride and/or cholesterol in blood, systemic hypertension, diabetes mellitus or HLA typing. Interestingly, an association has been demonstrated between the presence of cytomegalovirus infection and the occurrence of vascular graft disease.

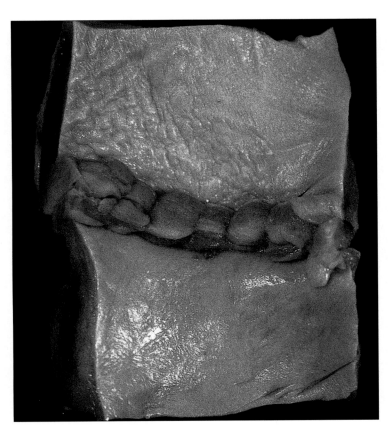

Fig. 17.24 Section through the left atrial structure in a patient dying 45 days after transplant. The surgical suture line is obvious.

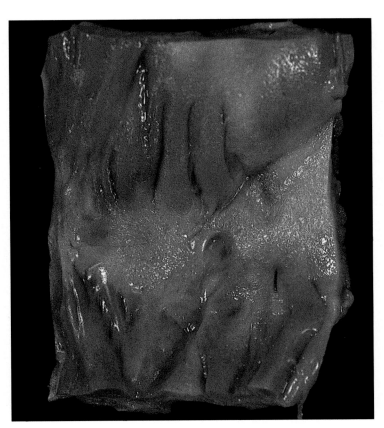

Fig. 17.25 Section through the right atrial suture in the patient dying 36 months after transplantation (Fig. 17.23). The surgical sutures are covered by white fibrous tissue, and are no longer visible on the atrial endocardial surface.

Fig. 17.26 Histological section of the myocardium shown in Fig. 17.23. Extensive patchy fibrosis is present.

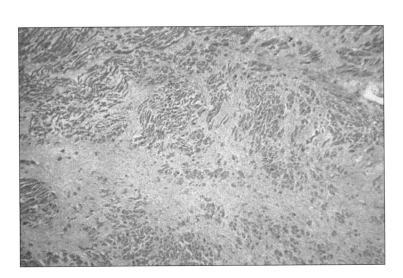

The typical histological finding of graft disease consists of concentric intimal proliferation occurring within an intact internal elastic lamina. This intimal proliferation can be seen in epicardial coronary arteries, but it also involves the smaller intra-myocardial branches. Immunohistochemistry techniques have demonstrated that the main components of the intimal proliferation are collagen, smooth muscle cells and macrophages. Foam cells are rare, and there is no lipid core as in native coronary arterial disease. The medial wall is generally spared. Calcification is rarely seen (Figs 17.27, 17.28, 17.29). If there is concomitant myocardial rejection, the intima and the adventitia may show infiltration by lymphocytes. The mechanism for intimal proliferation is not clear: some experimental studies have shown endothelial lesions as early as 20 days after transplantation. The endothelium, however, often appears intact over the diseased arterial segments. The accepted hypothesis is that of cellular or humoral immunologic injury to the endothelium early in the course of transplantation. Denervation of the heart and certain methods of cardiac preservation can also induce endothelial damage leading to later intimal proliferation. In recipients who survive for longer, the coronary arterial lesions may resemble those seen in typical coronary arterial disease, with disruption of the internal elastic lamina, involvement of the media, and frequent calcific deposits. The consequences of vascular graft disease in patients after transplantation are the same as for ordinary coronary arterial disease. These patients experience acute myocardial infarctions and sudden death. Since the vast majority of transplanted patients will have a denervated heart, however, they will not experience angina pectoris. Thus, the usual presentation is that of congestive heart failure, due to

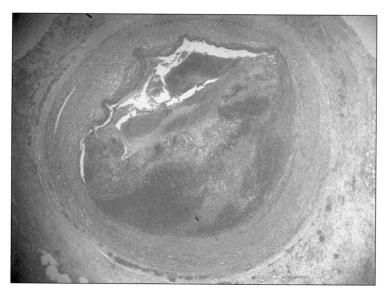

Fig. 17.27 Transverse section of the left anterior descending coronary artery from heart illustrated in Fig. 17.23. Intimal proliferation is present, with a superimposed thrombus. The lumen of the artery is significantly reduced in size. No lipid pool or calcification are seen.

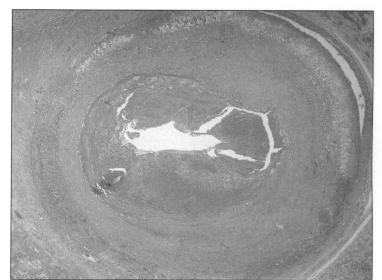

Fig. 17.28 Transverse section of the left circumflex coronary artery from the heart shown in Fig. 17.23. The intimal proliferation is concentric, and there is superimposed thrombus. Clusters of foam cells are present away from the lumen, but no lipid pool is seen as in non-transplant coronary arterial disease.

Fig. 17.29 Close-up view of the artery seen in Fig. 17.28, showing a thrombus overlying the intimal proliferation. Between the thrombus and the intima, a layer of fibrin is present. The intimal proliferation consists of collagen and smooth muscle cells. Some foam cells are present in the right lower quadrant.

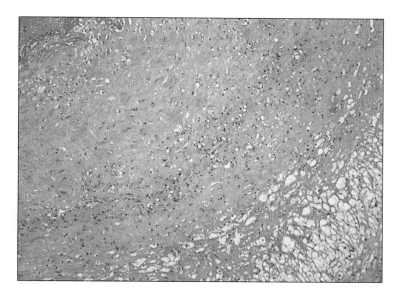

previous myocardial infarctions which have gone unnoticed. Since the coronary arterial involvement is diffuse, bypass surgery is of no help. Some isolated reports regarding percutaneous balloon angioplasty on the most severe lesions have appeared. This technique, however, has not been particularly successful, since the lesions have reappeared shortly following the procedure. Thus, the only available treatment for patients with vascular graft disease and severe myocardial involvement is retransplantation. Retransplantation itself then poses a problem due to a worldwide shortage of donors, leading to the ethical dilemma of who should receive the heart? In this respect, it should be remembered that survival after the retransplantation is much lower than after the initial transplant, and that up to half of the retransplanted patients develop vascular graft disease in their second graft.

Infections

Infections, together with rejection, are the main cause of death during the first postoperative year. In the early postoperative period (within 30 days of transplantation), infections are mainly nosocomial (Gram negative organisms and staphylococci),

whereas, in late postoperative period, opportunistic infections (such as cytomegalovirus, pneumocystis and fungi) predominate. The lungs are most frequently involved. The frequency of fatal infections has decreased since the introduction of cyclosporin as an immunosuppressive agent, as well as the total number of opportunistic infections. This is probably due, at least partly, to the reduction in steroid dosages which are possible with the use of cyclosporin.

Infection with cytomegalovirus requires a fourfold increase in serologic titers to be diagnosed. It is generally seen after the second month, and when episodes of rejection have been aggressively immunosuppressed. Infection has been reported to be more frequent when there is a mismatch between donor and recipient. Apart from being a leading cause of morbidity when it involves the lungs, cytomegalovirus has recently been found to be associated with an increased frequency of vascular graft disease. The infection is characterized by the presence of large cells, containing inclusion bodies, in both the cytoplasm and the nucleus. Both bronchiolar and alveolar epithelial cells in the lungs become enlarged and show the typical intranuclear inclusions (Figs 17.30, 17.31) which cause the nucleus to resemble

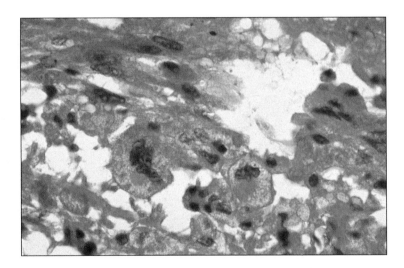

Fig. 17.30 Histologic section of the lung in a transplanted patient dying of cytomegalovirus pneumonitis. Large cells with eosinophilic cytoplasmic inclusions can be seen within the alveoli.

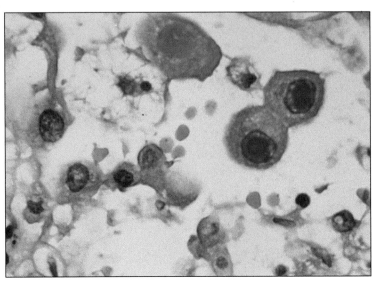

Fig. 17.31 Close-up view of the section shown in Fig. 17.30, showing the infected cells with the characteristic viral inclusions.

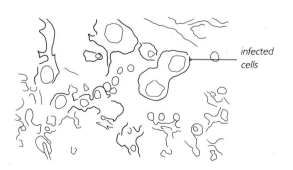

infected cells

a 'bird's eye'. Cytoplasmic inclusion bodies can reach 4 microns in diameter, and have condensed cytoplasm around them. They stain with periodic acid Schiff (PAS), whereas intranuclear inclusions stain with Masson's trichrome. In the heart, viral inclusions can be seen within the myocytes.

Infection with *Pneumocystis carinii* has a variable incidence, occurring in up to 10% of patients. It is also associated with aggressive treatment of rejection, and it generally appears 30 to 60 days after transplantation. Involvement of the lungs by pneumocystis may coincide with cytomegalovirus infection. Macroscopically, the so-called diffuse form is commonest, in which both lungs are firm and have greyish consolidated areas intercalated with normal-looking areas. Histological examination reveals a chronic interstitial pneumonia. The alveoli are distended and filled with a foamy exudate that generally has a few macrophages. This foamy exudate shows a honeycomb pattern of thin-walled cystic spaces containing the bodies of the parasite (Fig. 17.32). Cysts measuring up to 4 microns in diameter can be demonstrated with Grocott's stain (Fig. 17.33).

Neoplasms

Immunosuppression is known to cause new malignant neoplasms. Such malignancies were responsible for 11% of late deaths in patients treated with azathioprine. The figure for patients treated with cyclosporin is generally around 5%. The tumours most commonly associated with azathioprine are cutaneous malignancies, with a predominance of squamous cell carcinomas. In patients treated with cyclosporin, the most frequent neoplasm is the B cell lymphoma, which may be monoclonal or polyclonal. These lymphomas tend to appear within the first year after transplantation, rarely involving the central nervous system, but showing a special predilection for the small bowel. Clonal analysis has predictive importance, since only the polyclonal types respond to a decrease in immunosuppression. Ebstein–Barr virus has been demonstrated in the B cells.

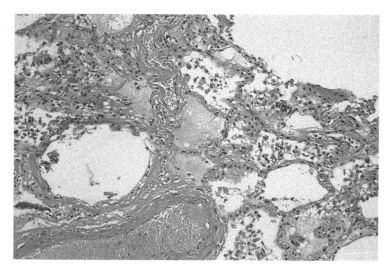

Fig. 17.32 Histological section of the lung in a transplanted patient with infection by Pneumocystis carinii. The alveoli are filled with a pale eosinophilic foamy substance.

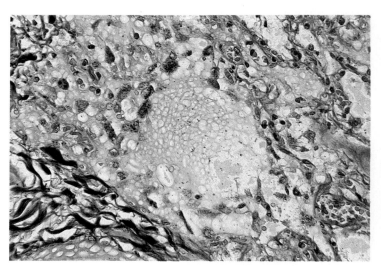

Fig. 17.33 Close-up view of the section shown in Fig. 17.32, showing an alveolus filled with Pneumocystis cysts. Grocott stain.

Index